Biomaterials

PRINCIPLES
and APPLICATIONS

Edited by

JOON B. PARK
JOSEPH D. BRONZINO

CRC PRESS

Boca Raton   London   New York   Washington, D.C.

Library of Congress Cataloging-in-Publication Data

Biomaterials : principles and applications / edited by Joon B. Park and Joseph D. Bronzino.
    p. cm.
    Includes bibliographical references and index.
    ISBN 0-8493-1491-7 (alk. paper)
    1. Biomedical materials. I. Park, Joon Bu. II. Bronzino, Joseph D., 1937–

R857.M3 P375 2002
610′.284—dc21

2002073352
CIP

Visit the CRC Press Web site at www.crcpress.com

Preface

A BIOMATERIAL IS USED to make devices to replace a part or a function of the body in a safe, reliable, economic, and physiologically acceptable manner [Hench and Erthridge, 1982]. A variety of devices and materials presently used in the treatment of disease or injury include such commonplace items as sutures, needles, catheters, plates, tooth fillings, etc. Over the years, various definitions of the term biomaterials have been proposed. For example, a *biomaterial* can be simply defined as a synthetic material used to replace part of a living system or to function in intimate contact with living tissue. The Clemson University Advisory Board for Biomaterials has formally defined a biomaterial to be "a systemically and pharmacologically inert substance designed for implantation within or incorporation with living systems." Black defined biomaterials as "a nonviable material used in a medical device, intended to interact with biological systems" [Black, 1992]. Other definitions have included "materials of synthetic as well as of natural origin in contact with tissue, blood, and biological fluids, and intended for use for prosthetic, diagnostic, therapeutic, and storage applications without adversely affecting the living organism and its components" [Bruck, 1980] and "any substance (other than drugs) or combination of substances, synthetic or natural in origin, which can be used for any period of time, as a whole or as a part of a system which treats, augments, or replaces any tissue, organ, or function of the body" [Williams, 1987]. By contrast, a *biological material* is a material such as skin or artery, produced by a biological system. Artificial materials that simply are in contact with the skin, such as hearing aids and wearable artificial limbs, are not included in our definition of biomaterials since the skin acts as a barrier with the external world.

According to these definitions one must possess knowledge in a number of different disciplines or collaborate with individuals from a wide variety of different specialties in order to properly develop and use biomaterials in medicine and dentistry (see Table 1). Table 2 provides some examples of the uses of biomaterials, which include replacement of a body part that has lost function due to disease or trauma, to assist in healing, to improve performance, and to correct abnormalities. The role of biomaterials has been influenced considerably by advances in many areas of biotechnology and science. For example, with the advent of antibiotics, infectious disease is less of a threat than in former times, so that degenerative diseases assume a greater importance. Moreover, advances in surgical technique and instruments have permitted materials to be used in ways that were not possible previously. This book is intended to familiarize the reader with the uses of materials in medicine and dentistry and provide an explanation of the scientific basis for these applications.

The performance of materials in the body can be classified in many ways. First, biomaterials may be considered from the point of view of the problem area that is to be solved, as in Table 2. Second, we may consider the body on a tissue level, an organ level (Table 3), or a system level (Table 4). Third, we may consider the classification of materials as polymers, metals, ceramics, and composites as is done in Table 5. In that vein, the role of biomaterials is governed by the interaction between the material and

TABLE 1 Fields of Knowledge to Develop Biomaterials

Discipline	Examples
Science and engineering	Materials sciences: structure–property relationship of synthetic and biological materials including metals, ceramics, polymers, composites, tissues (blood and connective tissues), etc.
Biology and physiology	Cell and molecular biology, anatomy, animal and human physiology, histopathology, experimental surgery, immunology, etc.
Clinical sciences	All the clinical specialties: dentistry, maxillofacial, neurosurgery, obstetrics and gynecology, ophthalmology, orthopedics, otolaryngology, plastic and reconstructive surgery, thoracic and cardiovascular surgery, veterinary medicine, and surgery, etc.

Source: Modified from von Recum [1994].

TABLE 2 Uses of Biomaterials

Problem Area	Examples
Replacement of diseased or damaged part	Artificial hip joint, kidney dialysis machine
Assist in healing	Sutures, bone plates, and screws
Improve function	Cardiac pacemaker, intraocular lens
Correct functional abnormality	Cardiac pacemaker
Correct cosmetic problem	Augmentation mammoplasty, chin augmentation
Aid to diagnosis	Probes and catheters
Aid to treatment	Catheters, drains

TABLE 3 Biomaterials in Organs

Organ	Examples
Heart	Cardiac pacemaker, artificial heart valve, total artificial heart
Lung	Oxygenator machine
Eye	Contact lens, intraocular lens
Ear	Artificial stapes, cochlea implant
Bone	Bone plate, intramedullary rod
Kidney	Kidney dialysis machine
Bladder	Catheter and stent

TABLE 4 Biomaterials in Body Systems

System	Examples
Skeletal	Bone plate, total joint replacements
Muscular	Sutures, muscle stimulator
Circulatory	Artificial heart valves, blood vessels
Respiratory	Oxygenator machine
Integumentary	Sutures, burn dressings, artificial skin
Urinary	Catheters, stent, kidney dialysis machine
Nervous	Hydrocephalus drain, cardiac pacemaker, nerve stimulator
Endocrine	Microencapsulated pancreatic islet cells
Reproductive	Augmentation mammoplasty, other cosmetic replacements

TABLE 5 Materials for Use in the Body

Materials	Advantages	Disadvantages	Examples
Polymers (nylon, silicone rubber, polyester, polytetrafuoroethylene, etc.)	Resilient, Easy to fabricate	Not strong, Deforms with time, may degrade	Sutures, blood vessels, hip socket, ear, nose, other soft tissues, sutures
Metals (Ti and its alloys, Co-Cr alloys, stainless steels, Au, Ag, Pt, etc.)	Strong, tough, ductile	May corrode, dense, difficult to make	Joint replacements, bone plates and screws, dental root implants, pacer and suture wires
Ceramics (aluminum oxide, calcium phosphates including hydroxyapatite, carbon)	Very biocompatible, inert, strong in compression	Brittle, not resilient, difficult to make	Dental; femoral head of hip replacement, coating of dental and orthopedic implants
Composites (carbon-carbon, wire or fiber reinforced bone cement)	Strong, tailor-made	Difficult to make	Joint implants, heart valves

the body, specifically, the effect of the body environment on the material and the effect of the material on the body [Black, 1992; Bruck, 1980; Greco, 1994; Hench and Erthridge, 1982; Park and Lakes, 1992; von Recum, 1986; Williams and Roaf, 1973].

It should be evident from any of these perspectives that most current applications of biomaterials involve structural functions even in those organs and systems which are not primarily structural in their

TABLE 6 Notable Developments Relating to Implants

Year	Investigators	Development
Late 18th–19th century		Various metal devices to fix bone fractures; wires and pins from Fe, Au, Ag, and Pt
1860–1870	J. Lister	Aseptic surgical techniques
1886	H. Hansmann	Ni-plated steel bone fracture plate
1893–1912	W.A. Lane	Steel screws and plates (Lane fracture plate)
1912	W.D. Sherman	Vanadium steel plates, first developed for medical use; lesser stress concentration and corrosion (Sherman plate)
1924	A.A. Zierold	Introduced Stellites® (CoCrMo alloy)
1926	M.Z. Lange	Introduced 18-8sMo stainless steel, better than 18-8 stainless steel
1926	E.W. Hey-Groves	Used carpenter's screw for femoral neck fracture
1931	M.N. Smith-Petersen	First femoral neck fracture fixation device made of stainless steel
1936	C.S. Venable, W.G. Stuck	Introduced Vitallium® (19-9 stainless steel), later changed the material to CoCr alloys
1938	P. Wiles	First total hip replacement prosthesis
1939	J.C. Burch, H.M. Carney	Introduced tantalum (Ta)
1946	J. and R. Judet	First biomechanically designed femoral head replacement prosthesis; first plastics (PMMA) used in joint replacements
1940s	M.J. Dorzee, A. Franceschetti	First used acrylics (PMMA) for corneal replacement
1947	J. Cotton	Introduced Ti and its alloys
1952	A.B. Voorhees, A. Jaretzta, A.B. Blackmore	First successful blood vessel replacement made of cloth for tissue ingrowth
1958	S. Furman, G. Robinson	First successful direct heart stimulation
1958	J. Charnley	First use of acrylic bone cement in total hip replacement on the advice of Dr. D. Smith
1960	A. Starr, M.L. Edwards	First commercial heart valves
1970s	W.J. Kolff	Total heart replacement

Source: Park [1984].

nature, or very simple chemical or electrical functions. Complex chemical functions such as those of the liver and complex electrical or electrochemical functions such as those of the brain and sense organs cannot be carried out by biomaterials at this time.

Historical Background

The use of biomaterials did not become practical until the advent of an aseptic surgical technique developed by Dr. J. Lister in the 1860s. Earlier surgical procedures, whether they involved biomaterials or not, were generally unsuccessful as a result of infection. Problems of infection tend to be exacerbated in the presence of biomaterials, since the implant can provide a region inaccessible to the body's immunologically competent cells. The earliest successful implants, as well as a large fraction of modern ones, were in the skeletal system. Bone plates were introduced in the early 1900s to aid in the fixation of long bone fractures. Many of these early plates broke as a result of unsophisticated mechanical design; they were too thin and had stress concentrating corners. Also, materials such as vanadium steel, which was chosen for its good mechanical properties, corroded rapidly in the body and caused adverse effects on the healing processes. Better designs and materials soon followed. Following the introduction of stainless steels and cobalt chromium alloys in the 1930s, greater success was achieved in fracture fixation, and the first joint replacement surgeries were performed. As for polymers, it was found that warplane pilots in World War II who were injured by fragments of plastic (polymethyl methacrylate) aircraft canopy did not suffer adverse chronic reactions from the presence of the fragments in the body. Polymethyl methacrylate (PMMA) became widely used after that time for corneal replacement and for replacements of sections of damaged skull bones. Following further advances in materials and in surgical technique, blood vessel replacements were tried in the 1950s and heart valve replacements and cemented joint replacements in the 1960s. Table 6 lists notable developments relating to implants. Recent years have seen many further advances.

Performance of Biomaterials

The success of biomaterials in the body depends on factors such as the material properties, design, and *biocompatibility* of the material used, as well as other factors not under the control of the engineer, including the technique used by the surgeon, the health and condition of the patient, and the activities of the patient. If we can assign a numerical value f to the probability of failure of an implant, then the *reliability* can be expressed as

$$r = 1 - f \tag{1}$$

If, as is usually the case, there are multiple modes of failure, the total reliability r_t is given by the product of the individual reliabilities $r_1 = (1 - f_1)$, etc.

$$r_t = r_1 \cdot r_2 \cdots r_n \tag{2}$$

Consequently, even if one failure mode such as implant fracture is perfectly controlled so that the corresponding reliability is unity, other failure modes such as infection could severely limit the utility represented by the total reliability of the implant. One mode of failure which can occur in a biomaterial, but not in engineering materials used in other contexts, is an attack by the body's immune system on the implant. Another such failure mode is an unwanted effect of the implant upon the body; for example, toxicity, inducing allergic reactions, or causing cancer. Consequently, biocompatibility is included as a material requirement in addition to those requirements associated directly with the function of the implant.

Biocompatibility involves the acceptance of an artificial implant by the surrounding tissues and by the body as a whole. Biocompatible materials do not irritate the surrounding structures, do not provoke an abnormal inflammatory response, do not incite allergic or immunologic reactions, and do not cause cancer. Other compatibility characteristics which may be important in the function of an implant device made of biomaterials include (1) adequate mechanical properties such as strength, stiffness, and fatigue properties; (2) appropriate optical properties if the material is to be used in the eye, skin, or tooth; and (3) appropriate density. Sterilizability, manufacturability, long-term storage, and appropriate engineering design are also to be considered.

The failure modes may differ in importance as time passes following the implant surgery. For example, consider the case of a total joint replacement in which infection is most likely soon after surgery, while loosening and implant fracture become progressively more important as time goes on. Failure modes also depend on the type of implant and its location and function in the body. For example, an artificial blood vessel is more likely to cause problems by inducing a clot or becoming clogged with thrombus than by breaking or tearing mechanically.

With these basic concepts in mind, the chapters in this book focus on biomaterials consisting of different materials such as metallic, ceramic, polymeric, and composite. Special attention is given to biologic materials in Chapters 6 through 9, while Chapter 10 addresses the hip joint prosthesis that has become one of the most common biomaterials in use today.

Defining Terms

Biomaterial: A synthetic material used to make devices to replace part of a living system or to function in intimate contact with living tissue.

Biological material: A material produced by a biological system.

Biocompatibility: Acceptance of an artificial implant by the surrounding tissues and by the body as a whole.

References

Black, J. (1992) *Biological Performance of Materials*, 2nd ed. (New York: Marcel Dekker).

Bruck, S.D. (1980) *Properties of Biomaterials in the Physiological Environment* (Boca Raton, FL: CRC Press).

Greco, R.S. (1994) *Implantation Biology* (Boca Raton, FL: CRC Press).

Hench, L.L. and Erthridge, E.C. (1982) *Biomaterials — An Interfacial Approach,* Vol. 4, A. Noordergraaf, Ed. (New York: Academic Press).

Park, J.B. (1984) *Biomaterials Science and Engineering* (New York: Plenum Press).

Park, J.B. and Lakes, R.S. (1992) *Biomaterials: An Introduction,* 2nd ed. (New York: Plenum Press).

von Recum, A. F. (1994) *Biomaterials: Educational Goals.* In: *Annual Biomaterials Society Meeting* (Boston, MA: Biomaterials Society).

von Recum, A.F. (1986) *Handbook of Biomaterials Evaluation* (New York: Macmillan Publishing Co.), pp. 97–158 and 293–502.

Williams, D.F. (1987) *Definition in Biomaterials.* In: *Progress in Biomedical Engineering* (Amsterdam: Elsevier), p. 67.

Williams, D.F. and Roaf, R. (1973) *Implants in Surgery* (London: W.B. Saunders).

Further Information

[Most important publications relating to the biomaterials area are given for further reference.]

Allgower, M., Matter, P., Perren, S. M., and Ruedi, T. 1973. *The Dynamic Compression Plate, DCP,* Springer-Verlag, New York.

Bechtol, C. O., Ferguson, A. B., and Laing, P. G. 1959. *Metals and Engineering in Bone and Joint Surgery,* Balliere, Tindall and Cox, London.

Black, J. 1992. *Biological Performance of Materials,* 2nd ed., Marcel Dekker, New York.

Bloch, B. and Hastings, G. W. 1972. *Plastic Materials in Surgery,* 2nd ed., Charles C Thomas, Springfield, IL.

Bokros, J.C., Arkins, R.J., Shim, H.S., Haubold, A.D., and Agarwal, N.K. 1976. Carbon in prosthestic devices, In: *Petroleum Derived Carbons,* M.L. Deviney and T.M. O'Grady, Eds., Am. Chem. Soc. Symp., Series No. 21, American Chemical Society, Washington, D.C.

Boretos, J.W. 1973. *Concise Guide to Biomedical Polymers,* Charles C Thomas, Springfield, IL.

Boretos, J.W. and Eden, M. (Eds.) 1984. *Contemporary Biomaterials,* Noyes, Park Ridge, NJ.

Brown, P.W. and Constantz, B. 1994. *Hydroxyapatite and Related Materials,* CRC Press, Boca Raton, FL.

Bruck, S.D. 1974. *Blood Compatible Synthetic Polymers: An Introduction,* Charles C Thomas, Springfield, IL.

Bruck, S.D. 1980. *Properties of Biomaterials in the Physiological Environment,* CRC Press, Boca Raton, FL.

Chandran, K.B. 1992. *Cardiovascular Biomechanics,* New York University Press, New York.

Charnley, J. 1970. *Acrylic Cement in Orthopedic Surgery,* Livingstone, London.

Cooney, D.O. 1976. *Biomedical Engineering Principles,* Marcel Dekker, New York.

Cranin, A.N. (Ed.) 1970. *Oral Implantology,* Charles C Thomas, Springfield, IL.

Dardik, H. (Ed.) 1978. *Graft Materials in Vascular Surgery,* Year Book Medical Publishing, Chicago.

de Groot, K., Ed. 1983. *Bioceramics of Calcium Phosphate,* CRC Press, Boca Raton, FL.

Ducheyne, P., Van der Perre, G., and Aubert, A.E., Ed. 1984. *Biomaterials and Biomechanics,* Elsevier Science, Amsterdam.

Dumbleton, J.H. and Black, J. 1975. *An Introduction to Orthopedic Materials,* Charles C Thomas, Springfield, IL.

Edwards, W.S. 1965. *Plastic Arterial Grafts,* Charles C Thomas, Springfield, IL.

Eftekhar, N.S. 1978. *Principles of Total Hip Arthroplasty,* C.V. Mosby, St. Louis, MO.

Frost, H.M. 1973. *Orthopedic Biomechanics,* Charles C Thomas, Springfield, IL.

Fung, Y.C. 1993. *Biomechanics: Mechanical Properties of Living Tissues,* 2nd ed., Springer-Verlag, New York.

Ghista, D.N. and Roaf, R. (Eds.) 1978. *Orthopedic Mechanics: Procedures and Devices,* Academic Press, London.

Greco, R.S. (Ed.) 1994. *Implantation Biology*, CRC Press, Boca Raton, FL.

Guidelines for Blood-Material Interactions, Revised 1985. Report of the National Heart, Lung, and Blood Institute Working Group, Devices and Technology Branch, NHLBI, NIH Publication No. 80-2185.

Gyers, G.H. and Parsonet, V. 1969. *Engineering in the Heart and Blood Vessels*, John Wiley & Sons, New York.

Hastings, G.W. and Williams, D.F. (Eds.) 1980. *Mechanical Properties of Biomaterials*, John Wiley & Sons, New York.

Hench, L. L. and Ethridge, E. C. 1982. *Biomaterials: An Interfacial Approach*, Academic Press, New York.

Hench, L.L. and Wilson, J. (Eds.) 1993. *An Introduction to Bioceramics*, World Scientific, Singapore.

Heppenstall, R.B. (Ed.) 1980. *Fracture Treatment and Healing*, W.B. Saunders, Philadelphia, PA.

Homsy, C.A. and Armeniades, C.D. (Eds.) 1972. Biomaterials for skeletal and cardiovascular applications, *J. Biomed. Mater. Symp.*, No. 3, John Wiley & Sons, New York.

Hulbert, S.F., Young, F.A., and Moyle, D.D. (Eds.) 1972. *J. Biomed. Mater. Res. Symp.*, No. 2.

Kawahara, H. (Ed.) 1989. *Oral Implantology and Biomaterials*, Elsevier Science, Armsterdam.

Kronenthal, R.L. and Oser, Z. (Eds.) 1975. *Polymers in Medicine and Surgery*, Plenum Press, New York.

Kuntscher, G. 1947. *The Practice of Intramedullary Nailing*, Charles C Thomas, Springfield, IL.

Lee, H. and Neville, K. 1971. *Handbook of Biomedical Plastics*, Pasadena Technology Press, Pasadena, CA.

Lee, S.M. (Ed.) 1987. *Advances in Biomaterials*, Technomic, Lancaster, PA.

Leinninger, R.I. 1972. Polymers as surgical implants, *CRC Crit. Rev. Bioeng.*, 2:333–360.

Levine, S.N. (Ed.) 1968. Materials in Biomedical Engineering, *Ann. N.Y. Acad. Sci.*, 146.

Lynch, W. 1982. *Implants: Reconstructing Human Body*, Van Nostrand Reinhold, New York.

Martz, E.O., Goel, V.K., Pope, M.H., and Park, J.B., Materials and design of spinal implants — a review. *J. Biomed. Mat. Res. (Appl. Biomater.)*, 38:267–288, 1997.

Mears, D.C. 1979. *Materials and Orthopedic Surgery*, Williams & Wilkins, Baltimore, MD.

Oonishi, H. Aoki, H. and Sawai, K. (Eds.) 1989. *Bioceramics*, Ishiyaku EuroAmerica, Tokyo.

Park, J.B. 1979. *Biomaterials: An Introduction*, Plenum Press, New York.

Park, J.B. 1984. *Biomaterials Science and Engineering*, Plenum Press, New York.

Park, J.B. and Lakes, R.S. 1992. *Biomaterials: An Introduction*, 2nd ed., Plenum Press, New York.

Park, K., Shalaby, W.S.W., and Park, H. 1993. *Biodegradable Hydrogels for Drug Delivery*, Technomic, Lancaster, PA.

Rubin, L.R. (Ed.) 1983. *Biomaterials in Reconstructive Surgery*, C.V. Mosby, St. Louis, MO.

Savastano, A.A. (Ed.) 1980. *Total Knee Replacement*, Appleton-Century-Crofts, New York.

Sawyer, P.N. and Kaplitt, M.H. 1978. *Vascular Grafts*, Appleton-Century-Crofts, New York.

Schaldach, M. and Hohmann, D. (Eds.) 1976. *Advances in Artificial Hip and Knee Joint Technology*, Springer-Verlag, Berlin.

Schnitman, P.A. and Schulman, L.B. (Eds.) 1980. *Dental Implants: Benefits and Risk*, A NIH-Harvard Consensus Development Conference, NIH Pub. No. 81-1531, U.S. Dept. Health and Human Services, Bethesda, MD.

Sharma, C.P. and Szycher, M. (Ed.) 1991. *Blood Compatible Materials and Devices*, Technomic, Lancaster, PA.

Stanley, J.C., Burkel, W.E., Lindenauer, S.M., Bartlett, R.H., and Turcotte, J.G. (Eds.) 1972. *Biologic and Synthetic Vascular Prostheses*, Grune & Stratton, New York.

Stark, L. and Agarwal, G. (Eds.) 1969. *Biomaterials*, Plenum, New York.

Swanson, S.A.V. and Freeman, M.A.R. (Eds.) 1977. *The Scientific Basis of Joint Replacement*, John Wiley & Sons, New York.

Syrett, B.C. and Acharya, A. (Eds.) 1979. *Corrosion and Degradation of Implant Materials*, ASTM STP 684, American Society for Testing and Materials, Philadelphia, PA.

Szycher, M. (Ed.) 1991. *High Performance Biomaterials*, Technomic, Lancaster, PA.

Szycher, M. and Robinson, W.J. (Ed.) 1980. *Synthetic Biomedical Polymers, Concepts and Applications*, Technomic, Lancaster, PA.

Taylor, A.R. 1970. *Endosseous Dental Implants*, Butterworths, London.

Uhthoff, H.K. (Ed.) 1980. *Current Concepts of Internal Fixation of Fractures*, Springer-Verlag, Berlin.

Venable, C.S. and Stuck, W.C. 1947 *The Internal Fixation of Fractures*, Charles C Thomas, Springfield, IL.

Webster, J. G. (Ed.) 1988. *Encyclopedia of Medical Devices and Instrumentation*, John Wiley & Sons, New York.

Williams, D.F. and Roaf, R. 1973. *Implants in Surgery*, W.B. Saunders, London.

Williams, D.F. (Ed.) 1976. *Compatibility of Implant Materials*, Sector Pub. Ltd., London, 1976.

Williams, D.F. (Ed.) 1981. *Fundamental Aspects of Biocompatibility*, Vols. I and II, CRC Press, Boca Raton, FL.

Williams, D.F. (Ed.) 1981. *Systemic Aspects of Blood Compatibility*, CRC Press, Boca Raton, FL.

Williams, D.F. (Ed.) 1982. *Biocompatibility in Clinical Practice*, Vols. I and II, CRC Press, Boca Raton, FL.

Wright, V. (Ed.) 1969. *Lubrication and Wear in Joints*, J.B. Lippincott, Philadelphia, PA.

Yamamuro, T., Hench, L.L., and Wilson J. (Ed.) 1990. *CRC Handbook of Bioactive Ceramics*, Vols. I and II, CRC Press, Boca Raton, FL.

Journals of Interest

Acta Orthopaedica Scandinavica

American Association of Artificial Internal Organs: Transactions

Annals of Biomedical Engineering

Biomaterials

Biomedical Materials and Engineering

Clinical Orthopaedics and Related Research

CRC Critical Review in Bioengineering

International Orthopaedics

Journal of Applied Biomaterials

Journal of Arthoplasty

Journal of Biomechanics

Journal of Biomedical Engineering

Journal of Biomedical Materials Research

Journal of Bone and Joint Surgery

Journal of Medical Engineering and Technology

Journal of Orthopaedic Research

Medical Engineering and Physics

Transactions of the American Society of Artificial Internal Organs (held annually in spring): *Extended Abstracts*

Transactions of the Orthopaedic Research Society Meeting (held annually during February): *Abstracts*

Transactions of the Society for Biomaterials (held annually during April and May): *Abstracts*

Society for Biomaterials: **http://www.biomaterials.org/index.html**

Contributors

Editors

Joon B. Park
University of Iowa
Iowa City, Iowa

Joseph D. Bronzino
Trinity College
Hartford, Connecticut

W. G. Billotte
University of Dayton
Dayton, Ohio

John C. Keller
University of Iowa
Iowa City, Iowa

Shu-Tung Li
Collagen Matrix, Inc.
Franklin Lakes, New Jersey

Karen J. L. Burg
Carolinas Medical Center
Charlotte, North Carolina

Gilson Khang
Chonbuk National University
Chonju, Korea

Adolfo Llinás
Pontificia Universidad Javeriana
Bogota, Columbia

K. B. Chandran
University of Iowa
Iowa City, Iowa

Young Kon Kim
Inje University
Kyungnam, Korea

Sang-Hyun Park
University of California
Los Angeles, California

Chih-Chang Chu
Cornell University
Ithaca, New York

Roderic S. Lakes
University of Wisconsin-
  Madison
Madison, Wisconsin

S. W. Shalaby
Poly-Med, Inc.
Anderson, South Carolina

Robin Coger
Massachusetts General Hospital
Harvard University Medical
  School and the Shriners Burn
  Institutes
Cambridge, Massachusetts

Hai Bang Lee
Korea Research Institute of
  Chemical Technology
Chungnam, Korea

Mehmet Toner
Massachusetts General Hospital
Harvard University Medical
  School and the Shriners Burn
  Institutes
Cambridge, Massachusetts

Vijay K. Goel
University of Toledo
Toledo, Ohio

Jin Ho Lee
Hannam University
Taejon, Korea

Contents

1

Metallic Biomaterials

Joon B. Park
University of Iowa

Young Kon Kim
Inje University

1.1 Introduction

Metals are used as biomaterials due to their excellent electrical and thermal conductivity and mechanical properties. Since some electrons are independent in metals, they can quickly transfer an electric charge and thermal energy. The mobile free electrons act as the binding force to hold the positive metal ions together. This attraction is strong, as evidenced by the closely packed atomic arrangement resulting in high specific gravity and high melting points of most metals. Since the metallic bond is essentially nondirectional, the position of the metal ions can be altered without destroying the crystal structure resulting in a plastically deformable solid.

Some metals are used as passive substitutes for hard tissue replacement such as total hip and knee joints, for fracture healing aids as bone plates and screws, spinal fixation devices, and dental implants because of their excellent mechanical properties and corrosion resistance. Some metallic alloys are used for more active roles in devices such as vascular stents, catheter guide wires, orthodontic archwires, and cochlea implants.

The first metal alloy developed specifically for human use was the "vanadium steel" which was used to manufacture bone fracture plates (Sherman plates) and screws. Most metals such as iron (Fe), chromium (Cr), cobalt (Co), nickel (Ni), titanium (Ti), tantalum (Ta), niobium (Nb), molybdenum (Mo), and tungsten (W) that were used to make alloys for manufacturing implants can only be tolerated by the body in minute amounts. Sometimes those metallic elements, in naturally occurring forms, are essential in red blood cell functions (Fe) or synthesis of a vitamin B_{12} (Co), but cannot be tolerated in large amounts in the body [Black, 1992]. The biocompatibility of the metallic implant is of considerable concern because these implants can corrode in an *in vivo* environment [Williams, 1982]. The consequences of corrosion are the disintegration of the implant material per se, which will weaken the implant, and the harmful effect of corrosion products on the surrounding tissues and organs.

1.2   Stainless Steels

The first stainless steel utilized for implant fabrication was the 18-8 (type 302 in modern classification), which is stronger and more resistant to corrosion than the vanadium steel. Vanadium steel is no longer used in implants since its corrosion resistance is inadequate *in vivo*. Later 18-8sMo stainless steel was introduced which contains a small percentage of molybdenum to improve the corrosion resistance in chloride solution (salt water). This alloy became known as *type 316 stainless steel*. In the 1950s the carbon content of 316 stainless steel was reduced from 0.08 to a maximum amount of 0.03% (all are weight percent unless specified) for better corrosion resistance to chloride solution and to minimize the sensitization, and hence became known as type *316L stainless steel*. The minimum effective concentration of chromium is 11% to impart corrosion resistance in stainless steels. The chromium is a reactive element, but it and its alloys can be *passivated* by 30% nitric acid to give excellent corrosion resistance.

The *austenitic stainless steels*, especially types 316 and 316L, are most widely used for implant fabrication. These cannot be hardened by heat treatment but can be hardened by cold-working. This group of stainless steels is nonmagnetic and possesses better corrosion resistance than any others. The inclusion of molybdenum enhances resistance to *pitting corrosion* in salt water. The American Society for Testing and Materials (ASTM) recommends type 316L rather than 316 for implant fabrication. The specifications for 316L stainless steel are given in Table 1.1. The only difference in composition between the 316L and 316 stainless steel is the maximum content of carbon, i.e., 0.03% and 0.08%, respectively, as noted earlier.

The nickel stabilizes the austenitic phase [γ, face centered cubic crystal (fcc) structure] at room temperature

TABLE 1.1   Compositions of 316L Stainless Steel [American Society for Testing and Materials, F139–86, p.61, 1992]

Element	Composition (%)
Carbon	0.03 max
Manganese	2.00 max
Phosphorus	0.03 max
Sulfur	0.03 max
Silicon	0.75 max
Chromium	17.00–20.00
Nickel	12.00–14.00
Molybdenum	2.00–4.00

and enhances corrosion resistance. The austenitic phase formation can be influenced by both the Ni and Cr contents as shown in Fig. 1.1 for 0.10% carbon stainless steels. The minimum amount of Ni for maintaining austenitic phase is approximately 10%.

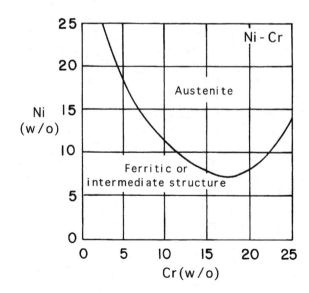

FIGURE 1.1   The effect of Ni and Cr contents on the austenitic phase of stainless steels containing 0.1% C [Keating, 1956].

TABLE 1.2 Mechanical Properties of 316L Stainless Steel for Implants [American Society for Testing and Materials, F139–86, p.61, 1992]

Condition	Ultimate Tensile Strength, min. (MPa)	Yield Strength (0.2% offset), min. (MPa)	Elongation 2 in. (50.8mm), min. (%)	Rockwell Hardness
Annealed	485	172	40	95 HRB
Cold-worked	860	690	12	—

Table 1.2 gives the mechanical properties of 316L stainless steel. A wide range of properties exists depending on the heat treatment (annealing to obtain softer materials) or cold working (for greater strength and hardness). Figure 1.2 shows the effect of cold working on the yield and ultimate tensile strength of 18-8 stainless steels. The engineer must consequently be careful when selecting materials of this type. Even the 316L stainless steels may corrode inside the body under certain circumstances in a highly stressed and oxygen depleted region, such as the contacts under the screws of the bone fracture plate. Thus, these stainless steels are suitable for use only in *temporary* implant devices such as fracture plates, screws, and hip nails. Surface modification methods such as anodization, passivation, and glow-discharge nitrogen implantation are widely used in order to improve corrosion resistance, wear resistance, and fatigue strength of 316L stainless steel [Bordiji et al., 1996].

FIGURE 1.2 Effect of cold-work on the yield and ultimate tensile strength of 18-8 stainless steel [ASTM, 1980].

1.3 CoCr Alloys

There are basically two types of cobalt-chromium alloys: (1) the castable CoCrMo alloy and (2) the CoNiCrMo alloy which is usually *wrought* by (hot) *forging*. The castable CoCrMo alloy has been used for many decades in dentistry and, relatively recently, in making artificial joints. The wrought CoNiCrMo alloy is relatively new, now used for making the stems of prostheses for heavily loaded joints such as the knee and hip.

The ASTM lists four types of CoCr alloys which are recommended for surgical implant applications: (1) cast CoCrMo alloy (F75), (2) wrought CoCrWNi alloy (F90), (3) wrought CoNiCrMo alloy (F562), and (4) wrought CoNiCrMoWFe alloy (F563). The chemical compositions of each are summarized in Table 1.3. At the present time only two of the four alloys are used extensively in implant fabrications, the castable CoCrMo and the wrought CoNiCrMo alloy. As Table 1.3 shows, the compositions are quite different from each other.

The two basic elements of the CoCr alloys form a solid solution of up to 65% Co. The molybdenum is added to produce finer grains which results in higher strengths after casting or forging. The chromium enhances corrosion resistance as well as solid solution strengthening of the alloy.

TABLE 1.3   Chemical Compositions of CoCr Alloys [American Society for Testing and Materials, F75–87, p.42; F90–87, p.47; F562–84, p.150, 1992]

Element	CoCrMo (F75) Min.	Max.	CoCrWNi (F90) Min.	Max.	CoNiCrMo (F562) Min.	Max.	CoNiCrMoWFe (F563) Min.	Max.
Cr	27.0	30.0	19.0	21.0	19.0	21.0	18.00	22.00
Mo	5.0	7.0	—	—	9.0	10.5	3.00	4.00
Ni	—	2.5	9.0	11.0	33.0	37.0	15.00	25.00
Fe	—	0.75	—	3.0	—	1.0	4.00	6.00
C	—	0.35	0.05	0.15	—	0.025	—	0.05
Si	—	1.00	—	1.00	—	0.15	—	0.50
Mn	—	1.00	—	2.00	—	0.15	—	1.00
W	—	—	14.0	16.0	—	—	3.00	4.00
P	—	—	—	—	—	0.015	—	—
S	—	—	—	—	—	0.010	—	0.010
Ti	—	—	—	—	—	1.0	0.50	3.50
Co		Balance						

FIGURE 1.3   Relationship between ultimate tensile strength and the amount of cold-work for CoNiCrMo alloy [Devine and Wulff, 1975].

The CoNiCrMo alloy originally called MP35N (Standard Pressed Steel Co.) contains approximately 35% Co and Ni each. The alloy is highly corrosion resistant to seawater (containing chloride ions) under stress. Cold working can increase the strength of the alloy considerably as shown in Fig. 1.3. However, there is a considerable difficulty of cold working on this alloy, especially when making large devices such as hip joint stems. Only hot-forging can be used to fabricate a large implant with the alloy.

The abrasive wear properties of the wrought CoNiCrMo alloy are similar to the cast CoCrMo alloy (about 0.14 mm/yr in joint simulation tests with ultra high molecular weight polyethylene acetabular cup); however, the former is not recommended for the bearing surfaces of joint prostheses because of its poor frictional properties with itself or other materials. The superior fatigue and ultimate tensile strength of the wrought CoNiCrMo alloy make it suitable for the applications which require long service life without fracture or stress fatigue. Such is the case for the stems of the hip joint prostheses. This advantage is better appreciated when the implant has to be replaced, since it is quite difficult to remove the failed piece of implant embedded deep in the femoral medullary canal. Furthermore, the revision arthroplasty is usually inferior to the primary surgery in terms of its function due to poorer fixation of the implant.

The mechanical properties required for CoCr alloys are given in Table 1.4. As with the other alloys, the increased strength is accompanied by decreased ductility. Both the cast and wrought alloys have excellent corrosion resistance.

TABLE 1.4 Mechanical Property Requirements of CoCr Alloys (ASTM F76, F90, F562) [American Society for Testing and Materials, F75–87, p.42; F90–87, p.47; F562–84, p.150, 1992]

Property	Cast CoCrMo (F75)	Wrought CoCrWNi (F90)	Wrought CoNiCrMo (F562)	
			Solution Annealed	Cold-Worked and Aged
Tensile strength (MPa)	655	860	793–1000	1793 min.
Yield strength (0.2% offset) (MPa)	450	310	240–655	1585
Elongation (%)	8	10	50.0	8.0
Reduction of area (%)	8	—	65.0	35.0
Fatigue strength (MPa)[a]	310	—	—	—

[a] From Semlitsch [1980].

Experimental determination of the rate of nickel release from the CoNiCrMo alloy and 316L stainless steel in 37°C Ringer's solution showed an interesting result. Although the cobalt alloy has more initial release of nickel ions into the solution, the *rate* of release was about the same (3×10^{-10} g/cm^2/day) for both alloys [Richards Mfg. Company, 1980]. This is rather surprising since the nickel content of the CoNiCrMo alloy is about three times that of 316L stainless steel.

The metallic products released from the prosthesis because of wear, corrosion, and fretting may impair organs and local tissues. *In vitro* studies have indicated that particulate Co is toxic to human osteoblast-like cell lines and inhibits synthesis of type-I collagen, osteocalcin, and alkaline phosphatase in the culture medium. However, particulate Cr and CoCr alloys are well tolerated by cell lines with no significant toxicity. The toxicity of metal extracts *in vitro* have indicated that Co and Ni extracts at 50% concentration appear to be highly toxic since all viability parameters were altered after 24 h. However, Cr extract seems to be less toxic than Ni and Co [Granchi et al., 1996].

The modulus of elasticity for the CoCr alloys does not change with the changes in their ultimate tensile strength. The values range from 220 to 234 GPa, which are higher than other materials such as stainless steels. This may have some implications of different load transfer modes to the bone in artificial joint replacements, although the effect of the increased modulus on the fixation and longevity of implants is not clear. Low wear (average linear wear on the MeKee-Farrar component was 4.2 μm/yr) has been recognized as an advantage of metal-on-metal hip articulations because of its hardness and toughness [Schmalzried et al., 1996].

1.4 Ti Alloys

Pure Ti and Ti6Al4V

Attempts to use titanium for implant fabrication dates to the late 1930s. It was found that titanium was tolerated in cat femurs, as was stainless steel and Vitallium® (CoCrMo alloy). Titanium's lightness (4.5 g/cm^3; see Table 1.5) and good mechanochemical properties are salient features for implant application.

There are four grades of unalloyed commercially pure (cp) titanium for surgical implant applications as given in Table 1.6. The impurity contents separate them; oxygen, iron, and nitrogen should be controlled carefully. Oxygen in particular has a great influence on the ductility and strength.

One titanium alloy (Ti6Al4V) is widely used to manufacture implants and its chemical requirements are given in Table 1.7. The main alloying elements of the alloy are aluminum (5.5~6.5%) and vanadium (3.5~4.5%). The Ti6Al4V alloy has approximately the same fatigue strength (550 MPa) of CoCr alloy

TABLE 1.5 Specific Gravities of Some Metallic Implant Alloys

Alloys	Density (g/cm^3)
Ti and its alloys	4.5
316 Stainless steel	7.9
CoCrMo	8.3
CoNiCrMo	9.2
NiTi	6.7

TABLE 1.6 Chemical Compositions of Ti and Its Alloy [American Society for Testing and Materials, F67–89, p.39; F136–84, p.55, 1992]

Element	Grade 1	Grade 2	Grade 3	Grade 4	Ti6Al4V[a]
Nitrogen	0.03	0.03	0.05	0.05	0.05
Carbon	0.10	0.10	0.10	0.10	0.08
Hydrogen	0.015	0.015	0.015	0.015	0.0125
Iron	0.20	0.30	0.30	0.50	0.25
Oxygen	0.18	0.25	0.35	0.40	0.13
Titanium			Balance		

[a] Aluminum 6.00% (5.50~6.50), vanadium 4.00% (3.50~4.50), and other elements 0.1% maximum or 0.4% total. All are maximum allowable weight percent.

TABLE 1.7 Mechanical Properties of Ti and Its Alloys (ASTM F136) [American Society for Testing and Materials, F67–89, p.39; F136–84, p.55, 1992 and Davidson et al., 1994]

Property	Grade 1	Grade 2	Grade 3	Grade 4	Ti6Al4V	Ti13Nb13Zr
Tensile strength (MPa)	240	345	450	550	860	1030
Yield strength (0.2% offset) (MPa)	170	275	380	485	795	900
Elongation (%)	24	20	18	15	10	15
Reduction of area (%)	30	30	30	25	25	45

after rotary bending fatigue tests [Imam et al., 1983]. Titanium is an allotropic material, which exists as a hexagonal close packed structure (hcp, α-Ti) up to 882°C and body-centered cubic structure (bcc, β-Ti) above that temperature. Titanium alloys can be strengthened and mechanical properties varied by controlled composition and thermomechanical processing techniques. The addition of alloying elements to titanium enables it to have a wide range of properties: (1) Aluminum tends to stabilize the α-phase, that is increase the transformation temperature from α- to β-phase (Fig. 1.4); (2) vanadium stabilizes the β-phase by lowering the temperature of the transformation from α to β.

The α-alloy has a single-phase microstructure (Fig. 1.5a) which promotes good weldability. The stabilizing effect of the high aluminum content of these groups of alloys makes excellent strength characteristics and oxidation resistance at high temperature (300~600°C). These alloys cannot be heat-treated for precipitation hardening since they are single-phased.

The addition of controlled amounts of β-stabilizers causes the higher strength β-phase to persist below the transformation temperature which results in the two-phase system. The precipitates of β-phase will appear by heat treatment in the solid solution temperature and subsequent quenching, followed by aging at a somewhat lower temperature. The aging cycle causes the coherent precipitation of some fine α particles from the metastable β; imparting α structure may produce local strain field capable of absorbing deformation energy. Cracks are stopped or deterred at the α particles, so that the hardness is higher than for the solid solution (Fig. 1.5b).

The higher percentage of β-stabilizing elements (13%V in Ti13V11Cr3Al alloy) results in a microstructure that is substantially β which can be strengthened by heat treatment (Fig. 1.5c). Another Ti alloy (Ti13Nb13Zr) with 13% Nb and 13% Zr showed *martensite* structure after being water quenched and aged, which showed high corrosion resistance with low modulus ($E = 79$ MPa) [Davidson et al., 1994]. Formation of plates of martensite induces considerable elastic distortion in the parent crystal structure and increases strength (Fig. 1.5d).

The mechanical properties of the commercially pure titanium and its alloys are given in Table 1.7. The modulus of elasticity of these materials is about 110 GPa except for the 13Nb13Zr alloy. From Table 1.7 one can see that the higher impurity content of the cp-Ti leads to higher strength and reduced ductility. The strength of the material varies from a value much lower than that of 316 stainless steel or

FIGURE 1.4 Part of phase diagram of Ti-Al-V at 4 w/o V [Smith and Hughes, 1966].

FIGURE 1.5 Microstructure of Ti alloys (all are 500×) [Hille, 1966]. (a) Annealed α-alloy. (b) Ti6Al4V, α–β alloy, annealed. (c) β-alloy, annealed. (d) Ti6Al4V, heat-treated at 1650°C and quenched [Imam et al., 1983].

the CoCr alloys to a value about equal to that of annealed 316 stainless steel of the cast CoCrMo alloy. However, when compared by the specific strength (strength per density) the titanium alloys exceed any other implant materials as shown in Fig. 1.6. Titanium, nevertheless, has poor shear strength, making it less desirable for bone screws, plates, and similar applications. It also tends to gall or seize when in sliding contact with itself or another metal.

Titanium derives its resistance to corrosion by the formation of a solid oxide layer to a depth of 10 nm. Under *in vivo* conditions the oxide (TiO_2) is the only stable reaction product. However, micromotion at the cement–prosthesis and cement–bone are inevitable; consequently, titanium oxide and titanium alloy particles are released in cemented joint prostheses. Sometimes this wear debris accumulates as periprosthetic fluid collects and triggers giant cell response around the implants. This cystic collection continues

FIGURE 1.6 Yield strength to density ratio of some implant materials [Hille, 1966].

to enlarge and aspiration reveals "dark" heavily stained fluid containing titanium wear particles and histiocytic cells. Histological examination of the stained soft tissue showed "fibrin necrotic debris" and collagenous, fibrous tissue containing a histiocytic and foreign body giant cell infiltrate. The metallosis, black staining of the periprosthetic tissues, has been implicated in knee implants [Breen and Stoker, 1993].

The titanium implant surface consists of a thin oxide layer and the biological fluid of water molecules, dissolved ions, and biomolecules (proteins with surrounding water shell) as shown in Fig. 1.7. The microarchitecture (microgeometry, roughness, etc.) of the surface and its chemical compositions are important due to the following reasons:

1. Physical nature of the surface either at the atomic, molecular, or higher level relative to the dimensions of the biological units may cause different contact areas with biomolecules, cells, etc. The different contact areas, in turn, may produce different perturbations and types of bonding of the biological units, which may influence their conformation and function.
2. Chemical composition of the surface may produce different types of bonding to the biomolecules, which may then also affect their properties and function. Metals undergo chemical reactions at the surface depending on the environment which cause the difficulties of understanding the exact nature of the interactions.

The surface–tissue interaction is dynamic rather than static, i.e., it will develop into new stages as time passes, especially during the initial period after implantation. During the initial few seconds after implantation, there will be only water, dissolved ions, and free biomolecules in the closest proximity of the surface but no cells. The composition of biofluid will then change continuously as inflammatory and healing processes proceed, which in turn also probably causes changes in the composition of the adsorbed layer of biomolecules on the implant surface until quasiequilibrium sets in. Eventually, cells and tissues will approach the surface and, depending on the nature of the adsorbed layer, they will respond in specific ways that may further modify the adsorbed biomolecules. The type of cells closest to the surface and their activities will change with time. For example, depending on the type of initial interaction, the final

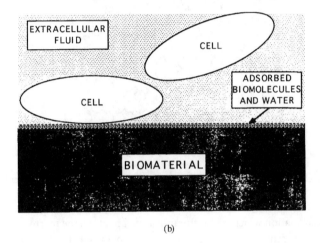

FIGURE 1.7 (a) Interface between a titanium implant and bioliquid and (b) the cell surface interaction [Kasemo and Lausma, 1988].

results may be fibrous capsule formation or tissue integration [Hazan et al., 1993; Kasemo and Lausma, 1988; Takatsuka et al., 1995; Takeshita et al., 1997; Yan et al., 1997].

Osseointegration is defined as direct contact without intervening soft tissue between viable remodeled bone and an implant. Surface roughness of titanium alloys have a significant effect on the bone apposition to the implant and on the bone implant interfacial pull out strength. The average roughness increased from 0.5 to 5.9 μm and the interfacial shear strength increased from 0.48 to 3.5 MPa [Feighan et al., 1995]. Highest levels of osteoblast cell attachment are obtained with rough sand blast surfaces where cells differentiated more than those on the smooth surfaces [Keller et al., 1994]. Chemical changes of the titanium surface following heat treatment are thought to form a TiO_2 hydrogel layer on top of the TiO_2 layer, as shown in Fig. 1.8. The TiO_2 hydrogel layer may induce the apatite crystal formation [Kim et al., 1996].

In general, on the rougher surfaces there are lower cell numbers, decreased rate of cellular proliferation, and increased matrix production compared to smooth surfaces. Bone formation appears to be strongly related to the presence of transforming growth factor β_1 in the bone matrix [Kieswetter et al., 1996].

TiNi Alloys

The *titanium–nickel* alloys show unusual properties i.e., after it is deformed the material can snap back to its previous shape following heating of the material. This phenomenon is called *shape memory effect* (SME). The SME of TiNi alloy was first observed by Buehler and Wiley at the U.S. Naval Ordnance Laboratory [Buehler et al., 1963]. The equiatomic TiNi or NiTi alloy (Nitinol) exhibits an exceptional SME near room temperature: if it is plastically deformed below the transformation temperature, it reverts

FIGURE 1.8   Chemical change of titanium implant surface of alkali following heat treatment [Kim et al., 1996].

back to its original shape as the temperature is raised. The SME can be generally related to a diffusionless martensitic phase transformation which is also thermoelastic in nature, the thermoelasticity being attributed to the ordering in the parent and martensitic phases [Wayman and Shimizu, 1972]. Another unusual property is the superelasticity, which is shown schematically in Fig. 1.9. As can be seen, the stress does not increase with increased strain after the initial elastic stress region and upon release of the stress or strain the metal springs back to its original shape in contrast to other metals such as stainless steel. The superlastic property is utilized in orthodontic archwires since the conventional stainless steel wires are too stiff and harsh for the tooth. In addition, the shape memory effect can also be utilized.

Some possible applications of shape memory alloys are orthodontic dental archwire, intracranial aneurysm clip, *vena cava* filter, contractile artificial muscles for an artificial heart, vascular stent, catheter guide wire, and orthopedic staple [Duerig et al., 1990].

In order to develop such devices, it is necessary to understand fully the mechanical and thermal behavior associated with the martensitic phase transformation. A widely known NiTi alloy is 55-Nitinol (55 weight % or 50 atomic % Ni), which has a single phase and the mechanical memory plus other properties, for example, high acoustic damping, direct conversion of heat energy into mechanical energy, good fatigue properties, and low temperature ductility. Deviation from the 55-Nitinol (near stoichiometric NiTi) in the Ni-rich direction yields a second group of alloys which are also completely nonmagnetic but differ from 55-Nitinol in their ability to be thermally hardened to higher hardness levels. Shape recovery capability decreases and heat treatability increases rapidly as the Ni content approaches 60%. Both 55- and 60-Nitinols have a relatively low modulus of elasticity and can be tougher and more resilient than stainless steel, NiCr, or CoCr alloys.

Efficiency of 55-Nitinol shape recovery can be controlled by changing the final annealing temperatures during preparation of the alloy device [Lee et al., 1988]. For the most efficient recovery, the shape is fixed by constraining the specimen in a desired configuration and heating to 482~510°C. If the annealed wire is deformed at a temperature below the shape recovery temperature, shape recovery will occur upon heating, provided the deformation has not exceeded crystallographic strain limits (~8% strain in tension). The NiTi alloys also exhibit good biocompatibility and corrosion resistance *in vivo*.

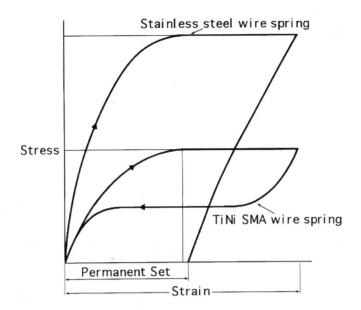

FIGURE 1.9 Schematic illustration of the stainless steel wire and TiNi SMA wire springs for orthodontic archwire behavior (modified from [Wayman and Duerig, 1990]).

There is no significant difference between titanium and NiTi in the inhibition of mitosis in human fibroblasts. NiTi showed lower percentage bone and bone contact area than titanium and the Ti6Al4V alloy [Takeshita et al., 1997].

The mechanical properties of NiTi alloys are especially sensitive to the stoichiometry of composition (typical composition is given in Table 1.8) and the individual thermal and mechanical history. Although much is known about the processing, mechanical behavior, and properties relating to the shape memory effect, considerably less is known about the thermomechanical and physical metallurgy of the alloy.

TABLE 1.8 Chemical Composition of NiTi Alloy Wire

Element	Composition(%)
Ni	54.01
Co	0.64
Cr	0.76
Mn	0.64
Fe	0.66
Ti	Balance

1.5 Dental Metals

Dental *amalgam* is an alloy made of liquid mercury and other solid metal particulate alloys made of silver, tin, copper, etc. The solid alloy is mixed with (liquid) mercury in a mechanical vibrating mixer and the resulting material is packed into the prepared cavity. One of the solid alloys is composed of at least 65% silver and not more than 29% tin, 6% copper, 2% zinc, and 3% mercury. The reaction during setting is thought to be

$$\gamma + Hg \to \gamma + \gamma_1 + \gamma_2 \tag{1.1}$$

in which the γ phase is Ag_3Sn, the γ_1 phase is Ag_2Hg_3, and the γ_2 phase is Sn_7Hg. The phase diagram for the Ag-Sn-Hg system shows that over a wide compositional range all three phases are present. The final composition of dental amalgams typically contain 45 to 55% mercury, 35 to 45% silver, and about 15% tin after fully set in about one day.

Gold and gold alloys are useful metals in dentistry as a result of their durability, stability, and corrosion resistance [Nielsen, 1986]. Gold fillings are introduced by two methods: casting and malleting. *Cast* restorations are made by taking a wax impression of the prepared cavity, making a mold from this impression in a material such as gypsum silica, which tolerates high temperature, and casting molten gold in the mold. The patient is given a temporary filling for the intervening time. Gold *alloys* are used for cast restorations, since they have mechanical properties which are superior to those of pure gold. Corrosion resistance is retained in these alloys provided they contain 75% or more of gold and other noble metals. Copper alloyed with gold significantly increases its strength. Platinum also improves the strength, but no more than about 4% can be added, or the melting point of the alloy is elevated excessively. Silver compensates for the color of copper. A small amount of zinc may be added to lower the melting point and to scavenge oxides formed during melting. Gold alloys of different composition are available. Softer alloys containing more than 83% gold are used for inlays which are not subjected to much stress. Harder alloys containing less gold are chosen for crowns and cusps which are more heavily stressed.

Malleted restorations are built up in the cavity from layers of *pure* gold foil. The foils are welded together by pressure at ambient temperature. In this type of welding, the metal layers are joined by thermal diffusion of atoms from one layer to the other. Since intimate contact is required in this procedure, it is particularly important to avoid contamination. The pure gold is relatively soft, so this type of restoration is limited to areas not subjected to much stress.

1.6   Other Metals

Several other metals have been used for a variety of specialized implant applications. *Tantalum* has been subjected to animal implant studies and has been shown very biocompatible. Due to its poor mechanical properties (Table 1.9) and its high density (16.6 g/cm^3) it is restricted to few applications such as wire sutures for plastic and neurosurgery and as a radioisotope for bladder tumors.

Platinum group metals (PGM) such as Pt, Pd, Rh, Ir, Ru, and Os are extremely corrosion resistant but have poor mechanical properties [Wynblatt, 1986]. They are mainly used as alloys for electrodes such as pacemaker tips because of their high resistance to corrosion and low threshold potentials for electrical conductivity.

Thermoseeds made of 70% Ni and 30% Cu have been produced which possess Curie points in the therapeutic hyperthermia range, approximately 40 to 50°C [Ferguson et al., 1992]. Upon the application of an alternating magnetic field, eddy currents are induced, which will provide a continuous heat source through resistive heating of the material. As the temperature of a ferromagnetic substance nears its Curie point, however, there is a loss of ferromagnetic properties and a resulting loss of heat output. Thus, self-regulation of temperature is achieved and can be used to deliver a constant hyperthermic temperature extracorporeally at any time and duration.

Surface modifications of metal alloys such as coatings by plasma spray, physical or chemical vapor deposition, ion implantaion, and fluidized bed deposition have been used in industry [Smith, 1993]. Coating implants with tissue compatible materials such as hydroxyapatite, oxide ceramics, Bioglass®, and pyrolytic carbon are typical applications in implants. Such efforts have been largely ineffective if the implants are permanent and particularly if the implants are subjected to a large loading. The main problem is the delamination of the coating or eventual wear of the coating. The added cost of coating or ion implanting hinders the use of such techniques unless the technique shows unequivocal superiority compared to the non-treated implants.

TABLE 1.9   Mechanical Properties of Tantalum [American Society for Testing and Materials, F560–86, p.143, 1992]

Property	Annealed	Cold-Worked
Tensile strength (MPa)	207	517
Yield strength (0.2% offset) (MPa)	138	345
Elongation (%)	20–30	2
Young's modulus (GPa)	—	190

1.7 Corrosion of Metallic Implants

Corrosion is the unwanted chemical reaction of a metal with its environment, resulting in its continued degradation to oxides, hydroxides, or other compounds. Tissue fluid in the human body contains water, dissolved oxygen, proteins, and various ions such as chloride and hydroxide. As a result, the human body presents a very aggressive environment for metals used for implantation. Corrosion resistance of a metallic implant material is consequently an important aspect of its biocompatibility.

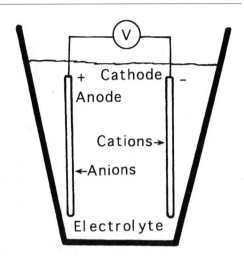

FIGURE 1.10   Electrochemical cell.

Electrochemical Aspects

The lowest free energy state of many metals in an oxygenated and hydrated environment is that of the *oxide*. Corrosion occurs when metal atoms become ionized and go into solution, or combine with oxygen or other species in solution to form a compound which flakes off or dissolves. The body environment is very aggressive in terms of corrosion since it is not only aqueous but also contains chloride ions and proteins. A variety of chemical reactions occur when a metal is exposed to an aqueous environment, as shown in Fig. 1.10. The electrolyte, which contains ions in solution, serves to complete the electric circuit. In the human body, the required ions are plentiful in the body fluids. Anions are negative ions which migrate toward the anode, and cations are positive ions which migrate toward the cathode. At the anode, or positive electrode, the metal oxidizes by losing valence electrons as in the following:

$$M \rightarrow M^{+n} + ne^- \tag{1.2}$$

At the cathode, or negative electrode, the following reduction reactions are important:

$$M^{+n} + ne^- \rightarrow M \tag{1.3}$$

$$M^{++} + OH^- + 2e^- \rightarrow MOH \tag{1.4}$$

$$2H_3O^+ + 2e^- \rightarrow H_2\uparrow + 2H_2O \tag{1.5}$$

$$1/2O_2 + H_2O + 2e^- \rightarrow 2OH^- \tag{1.6}$$

The tendency of metals to corrode is expressed most simply in the standard electrochemical series of Nernst potentials, shown in Table 1.10. These potentials are obtained in electrochemical measurements in which one electrode is a standard hydrogen electrode formed by bubbling hydrogen through a layer of finely divided platinum black. The potential of this reference electrode is defined to be zero. Noble metals are those which have a potential higher than that of a standard hydrogen electrode; base metals have lower potentials.

If two dissimilar metals are present in the same environment, the one which is most negative in the galvanic series will become the anode, and bimetallic (or galvanic) corrosion will occur. Galvanic corrosion can be much more rapid than the corrosion of a single metal. Consequently, implantation of dissimilar metals (mixed metals) is to be avoided. Galvanic action can also result in corrosion within a single metal, if there is inhomogeneity in the metal or in its environment, as shown in Fig. 1.11.

TABLE 1.10   Standard Electrochemical Series

Reaction	ΔE_o (V)
Li$\leftrightarrow$Li$^+$	−3.05
Na$\leftrightarrow$Na$^+$	−2.71
Al$\leftrightarrow$Al^{+++}	−1.66
Ti$\leftrightarrow$Ti^{+++}	−1.63
Cr$\leftrightarrow$Cr^{++}	−0.56
Fe$\leftrightarrow$Fe^{++}	−0.44
Cu$\leftrightarrow$Cu^{++}	−0.34
Co$\leftrightarrow$Co^{++}	−0.28
Ni$\leftrightarrow$Ni^{++}	−0.23
H$_2$$\leftrightarrow$2H$^+$	0.00
Ag$\leftrightarrow$Ag$^+$	+0.80
Au$\leftrightarrow$Au$^+$	+1.68

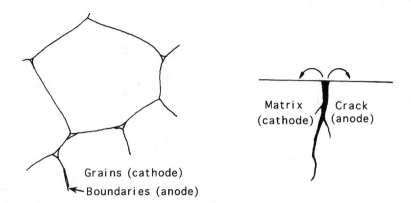

FIGURE 1.11   Micro-corrosion cells. (Left) Grain boundaries are anodic with respect to the grain interior. (Right) Crevice corrosion due to oxygen-deficient zone in metal's environment.

The potential difference, E, actually observed depends on the concentration of the metal ions in solution according to the Nernst equation,

$$E = E_o + \left(RT/nF\right)\ln\left[M^{+n}\right] \tag{1.7}$$

in which R is the gas constant, E_o is the standard electrochemical potential, T is the absolute temperature, F is Faraday's constant (96,487 C/mole), and n is the number of moles of ions.

The order of nobility observed in actual practice may differ from that predicted thermodynamically. The reasons are that some metals become covered with a *passivating* film of reaction products which protects the metal from further attack. The dissolution reaction may be strongly irreversible so that a potential barrier must be overcome. In this case, corrosion may be inhibited even though it remains energetically favorable. The kinetics of corrosion reactions are not determined by the thermodynamics alone.

Pourbaix Diagrams in Corrosion

The Pourbaix diagram is a plot of regions of *corrosion, passivity,* and *immunity* as they depend on electrode potential and pH [Pourbaix, 1974]. The Pourbaix diagrams are derived from the Nernst equation and from the solubility of the degradation products and the equilibrium constants of the reaction. For the sake of definition, the *corrosion region* is set arbitrarily at a concentration of greater than 10^{-6} gram atom/L (molar) or more of metal in the solution at equilibrium. This corresponds to about 0.06 mg/L for metals such as iron and copper, and 0.03 mg/L for aluminum. *Immunity* is defined as equilibrium between metal and its ions at less than 10^{-6} molar. In the region of immunity, the corrosion is energetically impossible. Immunity is also referred to as cathodic protection. In the passivation domain, the stable solid constituent is an oxide, hydroxide, hydride, or a salt of the metal. *Passivity* is defined as equilibrium between a metal and its reaction products (oxides, hydroxides, etc.) at a concentration of 10^{-6} molar or less. This situation is useful if reaction products are adherent. In the biomaterials setting, passivity may or may not be adequate; disruption of a passive layer may cause an increase in corrosion. The equilibrium state may not occur if reaction products are removed by the tissue fluid. Materials differ in their propensity to re-establish a passive layer which has been damaged. This layer of material may protect the underlying metal if it is firmly adherent and nonporous; in that case further corrosion is prevented. Passivation can also result from a concentration polarization due to a buildup of ions near the electrodes. This is not likely to occur in the body since the ions are continually replenished. Cathodic depolarization reactions can aid in the passivation of a metal by virtue of an energy barrier which hinders the kinetics. Equations (1.5) and (1.6) are examples.

FIGURE 1.12 Pourbaix diagram for chromium, showing regions associated with various body fluids (modified from [Black, 1992]).

There are two diagonal lines in the diagrams shown in Fig. 1.12. The top oxygen line represents the upper limit of the stability of water and is associated with oxygen-rich solutions or electrolytes near oxidizing materials. In the region above this line, oxygen is evolved according to $2H_2O \rightarrow O_2\uparrow + 4H^+ + 4e^-$. In the human body, saliva, intracellular fluid, and interstitial fluid occupy regions near the oxygen line, since they are saturated with oxygen. The lower hydrogen diagonal line represents the lower limit of the stability of water. Hydrogen gas is evolved according to Eq. (1.5). Aqueous corrosion occurs in the region between these diagonal lines on the Pourbaix diagram. In the human body, urine, bile, the lower gastrointestinal tract, and secretions of ductless glands occupy a region somewhat above the hydrogen line.

The significance of the Pourbaix diagram is as follows. Different parts of the body have different pH values and oxygen concentrations. Consequently, a metal that performs well (is immune or passive) in one part of the body may suffer an unacceptable amount of corrosion in another part. Moreover, pH can change dramatically in tissue that has been injured or infected. In particular, normal tissue fluid has a pH of about 7.4, but in a wound it can be as low as 3.5, and in an infected wound the pH can increase to 9.0.

Pourbaix diagrams are useful, but do not tell the whole story; there are some limitations. Diagrams are made considering equilibrium among metal, water, and reaction products. The presence of other ions, e.g., chloride, may result in very much different behavior and large molecules in the body may also change the situation. Prediction of passivity may in some cases be optimistic, since reaction rates are not considered.

Rate of Corrosion and Polarization Curves

The regions in the Pourbaix diagram specify whether corrosion will take place, but they do not determine the rate. The rate, expressed as an electric current density [current per unit area], depends upon electrode potential as shown in the polarization curves shown in Fig. 1.13. From such curves, it is possible to calculate the number of ions per unit time liberated into the tissue, as well as the depth of metal removed by corrosion in a given time. An alternative experiment is one in which the weight loss of a specimen of metal due to corrosion is measured as a function of time.

The rate of corrosion also depends on the presence of synergistic factors, such as those of mechanical origin (uneven distribution of mechanical stress). The stressed alloy failures occur due to the propagation of cracks in corrosive environments. For example, in corrosion fatigue (stress corrosion cracking), repetitive deformation of a metal in a corrosive environment results in acceleration of both the corrosion and the fatigue microdamage. Since the body environment involves both repeated mechanical loading and a chemically aggressive environment, fatigue testing of implant materials should always be performed

FIGURE 1.13   Potential-current density curves for some biomaterials [Greener et al., 1972].

under physiological environmental conditions, under Ringer's solution at body temperature. In *fretting corrosion*, rubbing of one part on another disrupts the passivation layer, resulting in accelerated corrosion. In *pitting*, the corrosion rate is accelerated in a local region. Stainless steel is vulnerable to pitting. Localized corrosion can occur if there is inhomogeneity in the metal or in the environment. *Grain boundaries* in the metal may be susceptible to the initiation of corrosion, as a result of their higher energy level. *Crevices* are also vulnerable to corrosion, since the chemical environment in the crevice may differ from that in the surrounding medium. The area of contact between a screw and a bone plate, for example, can suffer crevice corrosion.

Corrosion of Available Metals

Choosing a metal for implantation should take into account the corrosion properties discussed above. Metals which are in current use as biomaterials include gold, cobalt chromium alloys, type 316 stainless steel, cp-titanium, titanium alloys, nickel–titanium alloys, and silver–tin–mercury amalgam.

The noble metals are immune to corrosion and would be ideal materials if corrosion resistance were the only concern. Gold is widely used in dental restorations and in that setting it offers superior performance and longevity. Gold is not, however, used in orthopedic applications as a result of its high density, insufficient strength, and high cost.

Titanium is a base metal in the context of the electrochemical series; however, it forms a robust passivating layer and remains passive under physiological conditions. Corrosion currents in normal saline are very low: 10^{-8} A/cm^2. Titanium implants remain virtually unchanged in appearance. Ti offers superior corrosion resistance but is not as stiff or strong as steel or CoCr alloys.

Cobalt–chromium alloys, like titanium, are passive in the human body. They are widely used in orthopedic applications. They do not exhibit pitting corrosion.

Stainless steels contain enough chromium to confer corrosion resistance by passivity. The passive layer is not as robust as in the case of titanium or the cobalt chrome alloys. Only the most corrosion resistant of the stainless steels are suitable for implants. These are the austenitic types—316, 316L, and 317—which contain molybdenum. Even these types of stainless steel are vulnerable to pitting and to crevice corrosion around screws.

The phases of dental amalgam are passive at neutral pH, and the transpassive potential for the γ_2 phase is easily exceeded, due to interphase galvanic couples or potentials due to differential aeration under dental plaque. Amalgam, therefore, often corrodes and is the most active (corrosion prone) material used in dentistry.

Corrosion of an implant in the clinical setting can result in symptoms such as local pain and swelling in the region of the implant, with no evidence of infection; cracking or flaking of the implant as seen on x-ray films; and excretion of excess metal ions. At surgery, gray or black discoloration of the surrounding tissue may be seen and flakes of metal may be found in the tissue. Corrosion also plays a role in the mechanical failures of orthopedic implants. Most of these failures are due to fatigue, and the presence of a saline environment certainly exacerbates fatigue. The extent to which corrosion influences fatigue in the body is not precisely known.

Stress Corrosion Cracking

When an implant is subjected to stress, the corrosion process could be accelerated due to the mechanical energy. If the mechanical stress is repeated then fatigue stress corrosion takes place such as in the femoral stem of the hip joint and hip nails made of stainless steels [Dobbs and Scales, 1979; Sloter and Piehler, 1979]. However, other mechanisms of corrosion such as fretting may also be involved at point of contact such as in the counter-sink of the hip nail or bone fracture plate for the screws.

1.8   Manufacturing of Implants

Stainless Steels

The austenitic stainless steels work-harden very rapidly as shown in Fig. 1.2 and therefore cannot be cold-worked without intermediate heat treatments. The heat treatments should not induce, however, the formation of chromium carbide (CCr_4) in the grain boundaries; this may cause corrosion. For the same reason, the austenitic stainless steel implants are not usually welded.

The distortion of components by the heat treatments can occur but this problem can be solved by controlling the uniformity of heating. Another undesirable effect of the heat treatment is the formation of surface oxide scales which have to be removed either chemically (acid) or mechanically (sand-blasting). After the scales are removed the surface of the component is polished to a mirror or mat finish. The surface is then cleaned, degreased, and passivated in nitric acid (ASTM Standard F86). The component is washed and cleaned again before packaging and sterilizing.

CoCr Alloys

The CoCrMo alloy is particularly susceptible to work-hardening so that the normal fabrication procedure used with other metals cannot be employed. Instead, the alloy is cast by a lost wax (or investment casting) method which involves making a wax pattern of the desired component. The pattern is coated with a refractory material, first by a thin coating with a slurry (suspension of silica in ethyl silicate solution) followed by complete investing after drying: (1) the wax is then melted out in a furnace (100~150°C), (2) the mold is heated to a high temperature burning out any traces of wax or gas-forming materials, (3) molten alloy is poured with gravitational or centrifugal force, and (4) the mold is broken after cooled. The mold temperature is about 800~1000°C and the alloy is at 1350~1400°C.

Controlling the mold temperature will have an effect on the grain size of the final cast; coarse ones formed at higher temperatures will decrease the strength. However, a high processing temperature will result in larger carbide precipitates with greater distances between them, resulting in a less brittle material. Again there is a complementary (trade-off) relationship between strength and toughness.

Ti and Its Alloys

Titanium is very reactive at high temperature and burns readily in the presence of oxygen. Therefore, it requires an inert atmosphere for high temperature processing or is processed by vacuum melting. Oxygen diffuses readily in titanium and the dissolved oxygen embrittles the metal. As a result, any hot-working or forging operation should be carried out below 925°C. Machining at room temperature is not the solution to all the problems since the material also tends to gall or seize the cutting tools. Very sharp tools with slow speeds and large feeds are used to minimize this effect. Electrochemical machining is an attractive means.

Defining Terms

Amalgam: An alloy obtained by mixing silver tin alloy with mercury.

Anode: Positive electrode in an electrochemical cell.

Cathode: Negative electrode in an electrochemical cell.

Corrosion: Unwanted reaction of metal with environment. In a Pourbaix diagram, it is the region in which the metal ions are present at a concentration of more than 10^{-6} molar.

Crevice corrosion: A form of localized corrosion in which concentration gradients around pre-existing crevices in the material drive corrosion processes.

Curie temperature: Transition temperature of a material from ferromagnetic to paramagnetic.

Galvanic corrosion: Dissolution of metal driven by macroscopic differences in electrochemical potential, usually as a result of dissimilar metals in proximity.

Galvanic series: Table of electrochemical potentials (voltage) associated with the ionization of metal atoms. These are called Nernst potentials.

Hyperthermia: Application of high enough thermal energy (heat) to suppress the cancerous cell activities. Above 41.5°C (but below 60°C) is needed to have any effect.

Immunity: Resistance to corrosion by an energetic barrier. In a Pourbaix diagram, it is the region in which the metal is in equilibrium with its ions at a concentration of less than 10^{-6} molar. Noble metals resist corrosion by immunity.

Martensite: A metastable structure formed by quenching of the austenite (g) structure in alloys such as steel and Ti alloys. They are brittle and hard and therefore are further treated with heat to make them tougher.

Nernst potential: Standard electrochemical potential measured with respect to a standard hydrogen electrode.

Noble: Type of metal with a positive standard electrochemical potential.

Passivation: Production of corrosion resistance by a surface layer of reaction products (normally an oxide layer that is impervious to gas and water).

Passivity: Resistance to corrosion by a surface layer of reaction products. In a Pourbaix diagram, it is the region in which the metal is in equilibrium with its reaction products at a concentration of less than 10^{-6} molar.

Pitting: A form of localized corrosion in which pits form on the metal surface.

Pourbaix diagram: Plot of electrical potential vs. pH for a material in which the regions of corrosion, passivity, and immunity are identified.

Shape memory effect (SME): Thermoelastic behavior of some alloys which can revert back to their original shape when the temperature is greater than the phase transformation temperature of the alloy.

Superelasticity: Minimal stress increase beyond the initial strain region resulting in very low modulus in the region for some shape memory alloys.

References

ASTM. (1980). *Annual Book of ASTM Standards* (Philadelphia, PA: American Society for Testing and Materials).

Black, J. (1992). *Biological Performance of Materials*, 2nd ed. (New York: Marcel Dekker).

Bordiji, K., Jouzeau, J., Mainard, D., Payan, E., Delagoutte, J., and Netter, P. (1996). Evaluation of the effect of three surface treatments on the biocompatibility of 316L stainless steel using human differentiated cells. *Biomaterials* 17, 491–500.

Breen, D. J. and Stoker, D. J. (1993). Titanium lines: a manifestation of metallosis and tissue response to titanium alloy megaprostheses at the knee. *Clin. Radiol.* 43, 274–277.

Buehler, W. J., Gilfrich, J. V., and Wiley, R. C. (1963). Effect of low-temperature phase changes on the mechanical properties of alloys near composition Ti–Ni. *J. Appl. Phys.* 34, 1475–1477.

Davidson, J. A., Mishra, A. K., Kovacs, P., and Poggie, R. A. (1994). New surface hardened, low-modulus, corrosion-resistant Ti–13Nb–13Zr alloy for total hip arthroplasty. *Biomed. Mater. Eng.* 4, 231–243.

Devine, T. M. and Wulff, J. (1975). Cast vs. wrought cobalt-chromium surgical implant alloys. *J. Biomed. Mater. Res.* 9, 151–167.

Dobbs, H. S. and Scales, J. T. (1979). Fracture and corrosion in stainless steel hip replacement stems. In: *Corrosion and Degradation of Implant Materials,* B. C. Syrett and A. Acharya, Eds. (Philadelphia, PA: American Society for Testing and Materials), pp. 245–258.

Duerig, T. W., Melton, K. N., Stockel, D., and Wayman, C. M. (1990). *Engineering Aspects of Shape Memory Alloys* (London: Butterworth-Heinemann).

Feighan, J. E., Goldberg, V. M., Davy, D., Parr, J. A., and Stevenson, S. (1995). The influence of surface-blasting on the incorporation of titanium-alloy implants in a rabbit intramedullary model. *J. Bone Joint Surg.* 77A, 1380–1395.

Ferguson, S. D., Paulus, J. A., Tucker, R. D., Loening, S. A., and Park, J. B. (1992). Effect of thermal treatment on heating characteristics of Ni–Cu alloy for hyperthermia: preliminary studies. *J. Appl. Biomater.* 4, 55–60.

Granchi, D., Ciapetti, G., Savarino, L., Cavedagna, D., Donati, M. E., and Pizzoferrato, A. (1996). Assessment of metal extract toxicity on human lymphocytes cultured *in vitro. J. Biomed. Mater. Res.* 31, 183–191.

Greener, E. H., Harcourt, J. K., and Lautenschlager, E. P. (1972). *Materials Science in Dentistry* (Baltimore, MD: Williams & Wilkins).

Hazan, R., Brener, R., and Oron, U. (1993). Bone growth to metal implants is regulated by their surface chemical properties. *Biomaterials* 14, 570–574.

Hille, G. H. (1966). Titanium for surgical implants. *J. Mater.* 1, 373–383.

Imam, M. A., Fraker, A. C., Harris, J. S., and Gilmore, C. M. (1983). Influence of heat treatment on the fatigue lives of Ti–6Al–4V and Ti–4.5Al–5Mo–1.5CR. In: *Titanium Alloys in Surgical Implants,* H. A. Luckey and F. E. Kubli, Eds. (Philadelphia, PA: ASTM Special Technical Publication 796), pp. 105–119.

Kasemo, B. and Lausma, J. (1988). Biomaterial and implant surface: a surface science approach. *Int. J. Oral Maxillofac Impl.* 3, 247–259.

Keating, F. H. (1956). *Chromium-Nickel Austenitic Steels* (London: Butterworth).

Keller, J. C., Stanford, C. M., Wightman, J. P., Draughn, R. A., and Zaharias, R. (1994). Characterizations of titanium implant surfaces. III. *J. Biomed. Mater. Res.* 28, 939–946.

Kieswetter, K., Schwartz, Z., Hummert, T. W., Cochran, D. L., Simpson, J., and Boyan, B. D. (1996). Surface roughness modulates the local production of growth factors and cytokines by osteoblast-like MG-63 cells. *J. Biomed. Mater. Res.* 32, 55–63.

Kim, H., Miyaji, F., Kokubo, T., and Nakamura, T. (1996). Preparation of bioactive Ti and its alloys via simple chemical surface treatment. *J. Biomed. Mater. Res.* 32, 409–417.

Lee, J. H., Park, J. B., Andreasen, G. F., and Lakes, R. S. (1988). Thermomechanical study of Ni–Ti alloys. *J. Biomed. Mater. Res.* 22, 573–588.

Nielsen, J. P. (1986). *Dental Noble-Metal Casting Alloys: Composition and Properties.* In: *Encyclopedia of Materials Science and Engineering,* M. B. Bever, Ed. (Oxford, Cambridge: Pergamon Press), pp. 1093–1095.

Pourbaix, M. (1974). *Atlas of Electrochemical Equilibria in Aqueous Solutions,* 2nd ed. (Houston/CEBEL-COR, Brussels: NACE).

Richards Mfg. Company. (1980). Biophase Implant Material, technical information publication 3846 (Memphis, TN).

Schmalzried, T. P., Peters, P. C., Maurer, B. T., Bragdon, C. R., and Harris, W. H. (1996). Long-duration metal-on-metal total hip arthroplasties with low wear of the articulating surfaces. *J. Arthroplasty* 11, 322–331.

Semlitch, M. (1980). Properties of wrought CoNiCrMo alloy Protasul-10, a highly corrosion and fatigue resistant implant material for joint endoprotheses. *Eng. Med.* 9, 201–207.

Sloter, L. E. and Piehler, H. R. (1979). Corrosion-fatigue performance of stainless steel hip nails—Jewett type. In: *Corrosion and Degradation of Implant Materials*, B. C. Syrett and A. Acharya, Eds. (Philadelphia, PA: American Society for Testing and Materials), pp. 173–195.

Smith, C. J. E. and Hughes, A. N. (1966). The corrosion-fatigue behavior of a titanium–6w/o aluminum–4w/o vanadium alloy. *Eng. Med.* 7, 158–171.

Smith, W. F. (1993). *Structure and Properties of Engineering Alloys*, 2nd ed. (New York: McGraw-Hill).

Takatsuka, K., Yamamuro, T., Nakamura, T., and Kokubo, T. (1995). Bone-bonding behavior of titanium alloy evaluated mechanically with detaching failure load. *J. Biomed. Mater. Res.* 29, 157–163.

Takeshita, F., Ayukawa, Y., Iyama, S., Murai, K., and Suetsugu, T. (1997). Long-term evaluation of bone–titanium interface in rat tibiae using light microscopy, transmission electron microscopy, and image processing. *J. Biomed. Mater. Res.* 37, 235–242.

Wayman, C. M. and Duerig, T. W. (1990). An introduction of martensite and shape memory. In: *Engineering Aspects of Shape Memory Alloys*, T. W. Duerig, K. N. Melton, D. Stockel, and C. M. Wayman, Eds. (London: Butterworth-Heinemann), pp. 3–20.

Wayman, C. M. and Shimizu, K. (1972). The shape memory ('Marmem') effect in alloys. *Metal Sci. J.* 6, 175–183.

Williams, D. F. (1982). *Biocompatibliity in Clinical Practice* (Boca Raton, FL: CRC Press).

Wynblatt, P. (1986). *Platinum Group Metals and Alloys*. In: *Encyclopedia of Materials Science and Engineering*, M. B. Bever, Ed. (Oxford, Cambridge: Pergamon Press), pp. 3576–3579.

Yan, W., Nakamura, T., Kobayashi, M., Kim, H., Miyaji, F., and Kokubo, T. (1997). Bonding of chemically treated titanium implants to bone. *J. Biomed. Mater. Res.* 37, 267–275.

Further Reading

American Society for Testing and Materials. 1992. *Annual Book of ASTM Standards*, Vol. 13, *Medical Devices and Services*, American Society for Testing and Materials, Philadelphia, PA .

Bardos, D. I. 1977. Stainless steels in medical devices, in *Handbook of Stainless Steels*. Peckner, D. and Bernstein, I. M., Eds. pp. 1–10, McGraw-Hill, New York.

Bechtol, C. O., Ferguson, Jr., A. B., and Laing, P. G. 1959. *Metals and Engineering in Bone and Joint Surgery*, Williams & Wilkins, Baltimore, MD.

Comte, T. W. 1984. Metallurgical observations of biomaterials, in *Contemporary Biomaterials*, Boretos, J. W. and Eden, M., Eds., pp. 66–91, Noyes, Park Ridge, NJ.

Duerig, T. W., Melton, K. N., Stockel, D., and Wayman, C. M., Eds. 1990. *Engineering Aspects of Shape Memory Alloys*, Butterworth-Heinemann, London.

Dumbleton, J. H. and Black, J. 1975. *An Introduction to Orthopaedic Materials*, Charles C Thomas, Springfield, IL.

Fontana, M. G. and Greene, N. O. 1967. *Corrosion Engineering*, pp. 163–168, McGraw-Hill, New York.

Greener, E. H., Harcourt, J. K., and Lautenschlager, E. P. 1972. *Materials Science in Dentistry*, Williams & Wilkins, Baltimore, MD.

Hildebrand, H. F. and Champy, M., Eds. 1988. *Biocompatibility of Co–Cr–Ni Alloys*. Plenum Press, New York.

Levine, S. N., Ed. 1968. *Materials in Biomedical Engineering*, Annals of New York Academy of Science, Vol. 146. New York.

Luckey, H. A., Ed. 1983. *Titanium Alloys in Surgical Implants*, ASTM Special Technical Publication 796, Philadelphia, PA.

Mears, D. C. 1979. *Materials and Orthopaedic Surgery*, Williams & Wilkins, Baltimore, MD.

Park, J. B. 1984. *Biomaterials Science and Engineering*, Plenum Press, New York.

Perkins, J., Ed. 1975. *Shape Memory Effects in Alloys*, Plenum Press, New York.

Puckering, F. B., Ed. 1979. *The Metallurgical Evolution of Stainless Steels*, 1–42, American Society for Metals and the Metals Society, Metals Park, OH.

Smith, W. F. 1993. *Structure and Properties of Engineering Alloys*, 2nd ed., McGraw-Hill, New York.

Weinstein, A., Horowitz, E., and Ruff, A. W., Eds. 1977. *Retrieval and Analysis of Orthopaedic Implants*, NBS, U.S. Department of Commerce, Washington, D.C.

Williams, D. F. and Roaf, R. 1973. *Implants in Surgery*, W.B. Saunders, London.

2

Ceramic Biomaterials

W. G. Billotte
University of Dayton

2.1 Introduction

Ceramics are defined as the art and science of making and using solid articles that have as their essential component inorganic nonmetallic materials [Kingery et al., 1976]. Ceramics are refractory, polycrystalline compounds, usually inorganic, including silicates, metallic oxides, carbides and various refractory hydrides, sulfides, and selenides. Oxides such as Al_2O_3, MgO, SiO_2, and ZrO_2 contain metallic and nonmetallic elements and ionic salts, such as $NaCl$, $CsCl$, and ZnS [Park and Lakes, 1992]. Exceptions to the preceding include covalently bonded ceramics such as diamond and carbonaceous structures such as graphite and pyrolized carbons [Park and Lakes, 1992].

Ceramics in the form of pottery have been used by humans for thousands of years. Until recently, their use was somewhat limited because of their inherent brittleness, susceptibility to notches or microcracks, low tensile strength, and low impact strength. However, within the last 100 years, innovative techniques for fabricating ceramics have led to their use as "high tech" materials. In recent years, humans have realized that ceramics and their composites can also be used to augment or replace various parts of the body, particularly bone. Thus, the ceramics used for the latter purposes are classified as *bioceramics*. Their relative inertness to the body fluids, high compressive strength, and aesthetically pleasing appearance led to the use of ceramics in dentistry as dental crowns. Some carbons have found use as implants especially for blood interfacing applications such as heart valves. Due to their high specific strength as fibers and their biocompatibility, ceramics are also being used as reinforcing components of composite implant materials and for tensile loading applications such as artificial tendons and ligaments [Park and Lakes, 1992].

Unlike metals and polymers, ceramics are difficult to shear plastically due to the (ionic) nature of the bonding and minimum number of slip systems. These characteristics make the ceramics nonductile and are responsible for almost zero creep at room temperature [Park and Lakes, 1992]. Consequently, ceramics

TABLE 2.1   Desired Properties of Implantable Bioceramics

1. Should be nontoxic
2. Should be noncarcinogenic
3. Should be nonallergic
4. Should be noninflammatory
5. Should be biocompatible
6. Should be biofunctional for its lifetime in the host

are very susceptible to notches or microcracks because instead of undergoing plastic deformation (or yield) they will fracture elastically on initiation of a crack. At the crack tip the stress could be many times higher than the stress in the material away from the tip, resulting in a *stress concentration* which weakens the material considerably. The latter makes it difficult to predict the tensile strength of the material (ceramic). This is also the reason ceramics have low tensile strength compared to compressive strength. If a ceramic is flawless, it is very strong even when subjected to tension. Flawless glass fibers have twice the tensile strengths of high strength steel (~7 GPa) [Park and Lakes, 1992].

Ceramics are generally hard; in fact, the measurement of hardness is calibrated against ceramic materials. Diamond is the hardest, with a hardness index of 10 on Mohs scale, and talc ($Mg_3Si_3O_{10}COH$) is the softest ceramic (Mohs hardness 1), while ceramics such as alumina (Al_2O_3; hardness 9), quartz (SiO_2; hardness 8), and apatite ($Ca_5P_3O_{12}F$; hardness 5) are in the middle range. Other characteristics of ceramic materials are (1) their high melting temperatures and (2) low conductivity of electricity and heat. These characteristics are due to the chemical bonding within ceramics.

In order to be classified as a bioceramic, the ceramic material must meet or exceed the properties listed in Table 2.1. The number of specific ceramics currently in use or under investigation cannot be accounted for in the space available for bioceramics in this book. Thus, this chapter will focus on a general overview of the relatively bioinert, bioactive or surface reactive ceramics, and biodegradable or resorbable bioceramics.

Ceramics used in fabricating implants can be classified as nonabsorbable (relatively inert), bioactive or surface reactive (semi-inert) [Hench, 1991, 1993], and biodegradable or resorbable (non-inert) [Hentrich et al., 1971; Graves et al., 1972]. Alumina, zirconia, silicone nitrides, and carbons are inert bioceramics. Certain glass ceramics and dense hydroxyapatites are semi-inert (bioreactive), and calcium phosphates and calcium aluminates are resorbable ceramics [Park and Lakes, 1992].

2.2   Nonabsorbable or Relatively Bioinert Bioceramics

Relatively Bioinert Ceramics

Relatively bioinert ceramics maintain their physical and mechanical properties while in the host. They resist corrosion and wear and have all the properties listed for bioceramics in Table 2.1. Examples of relatively bioinert ceramics are dense and porous aluminum oxides, zirconia ceramics, and single-phase calcium aluminates (Table 2.2). Relatively bioinert ceramics are typically used as structural-support implants. Some of these are bone plates, bone screws, and femoral heads (Table 2.3). Examples of nonstructural support uses are ventilation tubes, sterilization devices [Feenstra and de Groot, 1983] and drug delivery devices (see Table 2.3).

Alumina (Al_2O_3)

The main source of high purity alumina (aluminum oxide, Al_2O_3) is bauxite and native corundum. The commonly available alumina (alpha, α) can be prepared by calcining alumina trihydrate. The chemical composition and density of commercially available "pure" calcined alumina are given in Table 2.4. The American Society for Testing and Materials (ASTM) specifies that alumina for implant use should contain 99.5% pure alumina and less than 0.1% combined SiO_2 and alkali oxides (mostly Na_2O) [F603-78].

TABLE 2.2 Examples of Relatively Bioinert Bioceramics

Type	Ref.
1. Pyrolitic carbon-coated devices	Adams and Williams, 1978
	Bokros et al., 1972
	Bokros, 1972
	Chandy and Sharma, 1991
	Dellsperger and Chandran, 1991
	Kaae, 1971
	More and Silver, 1990
	Shimm and Haubold, 1980
	Shobert, 1964
2. Dense and nonporous aluminum oxides	Hench, 1991
	Hentrich et al., 1971
	Krainess and Knapp, 1978
	Park, 1991
	Ritter et al., 1979
	Shackelford, 1988
3. Porous aluminum oxides	Hench, 1991
	Hentrich et al., 1971
	Park, 1991
	Ritter et al., 1979
	Shackelford, 1988
4. Zirconia ceramics	Barinov and Baschenko, 1992
	Drennan and Steele, 1991
	Hench, 1991
	Kumar et al., 1989
5. Dense hydroxyapatites	Bajpai, 1990
	Cotell et al., 1992
	Fulmer et al., 1992
	Huaxia et al., 1992
	Kijima and Tsutsumi, 1979
	Knowles et al., 1993
	Meenan et al., 1992
	Niwa et al., 1980
	Posner et al., 1958
	Schwartz et al., 1993
	Valiathan et al., 1993
	Whitehead et al., 1993
6. Calcium aluminates	Hammer et al., 1972
	Hentrich et al., 1971
	Hulbert and Klawitter, 1971

Alpha alumina has a rhombohedral crystal structure ($a = 4.758$ Å and $c = 12.991$ Å). Natural alumina is known as sapphire or ruby, depending on the types of impurities which give rise to color. The single-crystal form of alumina has been used successfully to make implants [Kawahara, 1989; Park 1991]. Single-crystal alumina can be made by feeding fine alumina powders onto the surface of a seed crystal which is slowly withdrawn from an electric arc or oxy-hydrogen flame as the fused powder builds up. Single crystals of alumina up to 10 cm in diameter have been grown by this method [Park and Lakes, 1992].

The strength of polycrystalline alumina depends on its grain size and porosity. Generally, the smaller the grains, the lower the porosity and the higher the strength [Park and Lakes, 1992]. The ASTM standard (F603-78) requires a flexural strength greater than 400 MPa and elastic modulus of 380 GPa (Table 2.5).

Aluminum oxide has been used in the area of orthopedics for more than 25 years [Hench, 1991]. Single-crystal alumina has been used in orthopedics and dental surgery for almost 20 years. Alumina is usually a quite hard material; its hardness varies from 20 to 30 GPa. This high hardness permits its use as an abrasive (emery) and as bearings for watch movements [Park and Lakes, 1992]. Both polycrystalline

TABLE 2.3 Uses of Bioinert Bioceramics

Use	Ref.
1. In reconstruction of acetabular cavities	Boutin, 1981
	Dorlot et al., 1986
2. As bone plates and screws	Zimmermann et al., 1991
3. In the form of ceramic-ceramic composites	Boutin, 1981
	Chignier et al., 1987
	Sedel et al.,1991
	Terry et al., 1989
4. In the form of ceramic-polymer composites	Hulbert, 1992
5. As drug delivery devices	Buykx et al., 1992
6. As femoral heads	Boutin, 1981
	Dörre, 1991
	Ohashi et al., 1988
	Oonishi, 1992
7. As middle ear ossicles	Grote, 1987
8. In the reconstruction of orbital rims	Heimke, 1992
9. As components of total and partial hips	Feenstra and de Groot, 1983
10. In the form of sterilization tubes	Feenstra and de Groot, 1983
11. As ventilation tubes	Feenstra and de Groot, 1983
12. In the repair of the cardiovascular area	Chignier et al., 1987
	Ely and Haubold, 1993

TABLE 2.4 Chemical Composition of Calcined Alumina

Chemical	Composition (Weight %)
Al_2O_3	99.6
SiO_2	0.12
Fe_2O_3	0.03
Na_2O	0.04

Source: Park, J. B., and Lakes, R. S. 1992. Ceramic implant materials. In: *Biomaterials — An Introduction*, 2nd ed., J. B. Park and R. S. Lakes, Eds., p. 121, Plenum Press, New York.

TABLE 2.5 Physical Property Requirements of Alumina and Partially Stabilized Zirconia

Property	Alumina	Zirconia
Elastic modulus (GPa)	380	190
Flexural strength (GPa)	>0.4	1.0
Hardness, Mohs	9	6.5
Density (g/cm³)	3.8–3.9	5.95
Grain size (µm)	4.0	0.6

Note: Both ceramics contain 3 mole% Y_2O_3.
Source: J.B. Park, personal communication, 1993.

and single-crystal alumina have been used clinically. The high hardness is accompanied by low friction and wear and inertness to the *in vivo* environment. These properties make alumina an ideal material for use in joint replacements [Park and Lakes, 1992]. Aluminum oxide implants in bones of rhesus monkeys have shown no signs of rejection or toxicity for 350 days (Graves et al., 1972; Hentrich et al., 1971). One of the most popular uses for aluminum oxide is in total hip prostheses. Aluminum oxide hip prostheses with an ultra-high-molecular-weight polyethylene (UHMWPE) socket have been claimed to be a better device than a metal prosthesis with a UHMWPE socket [Oonishi, 1992]. However, the key for success of any implant, besides the correct surgical implantation, is the highest possible quality control during fabrication of the material and the production of the implant [Hench, 1991].

Zirconia (ZrO_2)

Pure zirconia can be obtained from chemical conversion of zircon ($ZrSiO_4$), which is an abundant mineral deposit [Park and Lakes, 1992]. Zirconia has a high melting temperature ($T_m = 2953$ K) and chemical stability with $a = 5.145$ Å, $b = 0.521$ Å, $c = 5.311$ Å, and $\beta = 99°14$ in [Park and Lakes, 1992]. It undergoes a large volume change during phase changes at high temperature in pure form; therefore, a dopant oxide such as Y_2O_3 is used to stabilize the high temperature (cubic) phase. We have used 6 mole% Y_2O_3 as dopant to make zirconia for implantation in bone [Hentrich et al., 1971]. Zirconia produced in this manner is referred to as *partially stabilized* zirconia [Drennan and Steele, 1991]. However, the physical properties of zirconia are somewhat inferior to that of alumina (Table 2.5).

High-density zirconia oxide showed excellent compatibility with autogenous rhesus monkey bone and was completely nonreactive to the body environment for the duration of the 350-day study [Hentrich et al., 1971]. Zirconia has shown excellent biocompatibility and good wear and friction when combined with ultra-high-molecular-weight polyethylene [Kumar et al., 1989; Murakami and Ohtsuki, 1989].

Carbons

Carbons can be made in many allotropic forms: crystalline diamond, graphite, noncrystalline glassy carbon, and quasicrystalline pyrolitic carbon. Among these, only pyrolitic carbon is widely utilized for implant fabrication; it is normally used as a surface coating. It is also possible to coat surfaces with diamond. Although the techniques of coating with diamond have the potential to revolutionize medical device manufacturing, they are not yet commercially available [Park and Lakes, 1992].

FIGURE 2.1   Crystal structure of graphite. (*Source:* Shobert E.I. 1964. *Carbon and Graphite.* New York, Academic Press.)

The crystalline structure of carbon, as used in implants, is similar to the graphite structure shown in Fig. 2.1. The planar hexagonal arrays are formed by strong covalent bonds in which one of the valence electrons or atoms is free to move, resulting in high but anisotropic electric conductivity. Since the bonding between the layers is stronger than the van der Waals force, it has been suggested that the layers are *cross-linked*. However, the remarkable lubricating property of graphite cannot be attained unless the cross-links are eliminated [Park and Lakes, 1992].

The poorly crystalline carbons are thought to contain unassociated or unoriented carbon atoms. The hexagonal layers are not perfectly arranged, as shown in Fig. 2.2. Properties of individual crystallites seem to be highly anisotropic. However, if the crystallites are randomly dispersed, the aggregate becomes isotropic [Park and Lakes, 1992].

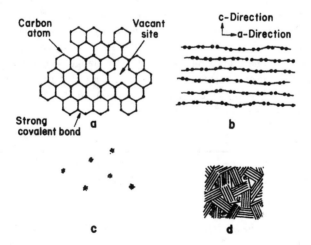

FIGURE 2.2   Schematic presentation of poorly crystalline carbon. (a) Single-layer plane. (b) Parallel layers in a crystallite. (c) Unassociated carbon. (d) An aggregate of crystallites, single layers, and unassociated carbon. (*Source:* Bokros J. C. 1972. Deposition structure and properties of pyrolitic carbon. In: *Chemistry and Physics of Carbon*, Vol. 5, pp. 70–81, Marcel Dekker, New York.)

FIGURE 2.3 Fracture stress vs. density for unalloyed LTI pyrolite carbons. (*Source:* Kaae, J. L. 1971. Structure and mechanical properties of isotropic pyrolitic carbon deposited below 1600°C. *J. Nucl. Mater.* 38:42–50.)

FIGURE 2.4 Elastic modulus vs. density for unalloyed LTI pyrolite carbons. (*Source:* Kaae, J. L. 1971. Structure and mechanical properties of isotropic pyrolitic carbon deposited below 1600°C. *J. Nucl. Mater.* 38:42–50.)

The mechanical properties of carbon, especially pyrolitic carbon, are largely dependent on its density, as shown in Figs. 2.3 and 2.4. The increased mechanical properties are directly related to increased density, which indicates that the properties of pyrolitic carbon depend mainly on the aggregate structure of the material [Park and Lakes, 1992].

Graphite and glassy carbon have a much lower mechanical strength than pyrolitic carbon (Table 2.6). However, the average modulus of elasticity is almost the same for all carbons. The strength of pyrolitic carbon is quite high compared to graphite and glassy carbon. Again, this is due to the fewer number of flaws and unassociated carbons in the aggregate.

Table 2.6 Properties of Various Types of Carbon

Property	Type of Carbon		
	Graphite	Glassy	Pyrolitic[a]
Density (g/cm$_3$)	1.5–1.9	1.5	1.5–2.0
Elastic modulus (GPa)	24	24	28
Compressive strength (MPa)	138	172	517 (575[a])
Toughness (Mn/cm^3)[b]	6.3	0.6	4.8

[a] 1.0 w/o Si-alloyed pyrolitic carbon, Pyrolite™ (Carbomedics, Austin, TX).
[b] 1 m-N/cm^3 = 1.45 × 10^{-3} in-lb/in^3.
Source: Park, J. B. and Lakes, R. S. 1992. Ceramic implant materials. In: *Biomaterials — An Introduction*, 2nd ed., J. B. Park and R. S. Laker, Eds., p. 133, Plenum Press, New York.

TABLE 2.7 Mechanical Properties of Carbon Fiber-Reinforced Carbon

Property	Fiber Lay-Up	
	Unidirectional	0-90° Crossply
Flexural modulus (GPa)		
Longitudinal	140	60
Transverse	7	60
Flexural strength (MPa)		
Longitudinal	1200	500
Transverse	15	500
Interlaminar shear strength (MPa)	18	18

Source: Adams, D. and Williams, D. F. 1978. Carbon fiber-reinforced carbon as a potential implant material. *J. Biomed. Mater. Res.* 12:38.

A composite carbon which is reinforced with carbon fiber has been considered for making implants. However, the carbon–carbon composite is highly anisotropic, and its density is in the range of 1.4 to 1.45 g/cm³ with a porosity of 35 to 38% (Table 2.7).

Carbons exhibit excellent compatibility with tissue. Compatibility of pyrolitic carbon-coated devices with blood have resulted in extensive use of these devices for repairing diseased heart valves and blood vessels (Park and Lakes, 1992).

Pyrolitic carbons can be deposited onto finished implants from hydrocarbon gas in a *fluidized bed* at a controlled temperature and pressure. The anisotropy, density, crystallite size, and structure of the deposited carbon can be controlled by temperature, composition of the fluidized gas, the bed geometry, and the residence time (velocity) of the gas molecules in the bed. The microstructure of deposited carbon should be highly controlled, since the formation of growth features associated with uneven crystallization can result in a weaker material (Fig. 2.5). It is also possible to introduce various elements into the fluidized gas and co-deposit them with carbon. Usually silicon (10 to 20 w/o) is co-deposited (or alloyed) to increase hardness for applications requiring resistance to abrasion, such as heart valve discs.

Recently, success was achieved in depositing pyrolitic carbon onto the surfaces of blood vessel implants made of polymers. This type of carbon is called ultra-low-temperature isotropic (ULTI) carbon instead of low-temperature isotropic (LTI) carbon. The deposited carbon has excellent compatibility with blood and is thin enough not to interfere with the flexibility of the grafts [Park and Lakes, 1992].

The vitreous or glassy carbon is made by controlled pyrolysis of polymers such as phenolformaldehyde, Rayon (cellulose), and polyacrylnitrite at a high temperature in a controlled environment. This process is particularly useful for making carbon fibers and textiles which can be used alone or as components of composites.

2.3   Biodegradable or Resorbable Ceramics

Although plaster of Paris was used in 1892 as a bone substitute [Peltier, 1961], the concept of using synthetic resorbable ceramics as bone substitutes was introduced in 1969 [Hentrich et al., 1969; Graves et al., 1972]. *Resorbable ceramics*, as the name implies, degrade upon implantation in the host. The resorbed material is replaced by endogenous tissues. The rate of degradation varies from material to material. Almost all bioresorbable ceramics except Biocoral and plaster of Paris (calcium sulfate dihydrate) are variations of calcium phosphate (Table 2.8). Examples of resorbable ceramics are aluminum calcium phosphate, coralline, plaster of Paris, hydroxyapatite, and tricalcium phosphate (Table 2.8).

Calcium Phosphate

Calcium phosphate has been used in the form of artificial bone. This material has been synthesized and used for manufacturing various forms of implants, as well as for solid or porous coatings on other implants (Table 2.9).

FIGURE 2.5 Microstructure of carbons deposited in a fluidized bed. (a) A granular carbon with distinct growth features. (b) An isotropic carbon without growth features. Both under polarized light, 240×. (*Source:* Bokros, J. C., LaGrange, L. D., and Schoen, G. J. 1972. Control of structure of carbon for use in bioengineering, *Chem. Phys. Carbon,* 9:103–171.)

Calcium phosphate can be crystallized into salts such as hydroxyapatite and β-whitlockite depending on the Ca:P ratio, presence of water, impurities, and temperature. In a wet environment and at lower temperatures (<900°C), it is more likely that hydroxyl- or hydroxyapatite will form, while in a dry atmosphere and at a higher temperature, β-whitlockite will be formed [Park and Lakes, 1992]. Both forms are very tissue compatible and are used as bone substitutes in a granular form or a solid block. The apatite form of calcium phosphate is considered to be closely related to the mineral phase of bone and teeth.

TABLE 2.8 Examples of Biodegradable/Resorbable Bioceramics

Type	Ref.
1. Aluminum–calcium–phosphorous oxides	Bajpai et al., 1985
	Mattie and Bajpai, 1988
	Wyatt et al., 1976
2. Glass fibers and their composites	Alexander et al., 1987
	Zimmermann et al., 1991
3. Corals	Bajpai, 1983
	Guillemin et al., 1989
	Khavari and Bajpai, 1993
	Sartoris et al., 1986
	Wolford et al., 1987
4. Calcium sulfates, including plaster of Paris	Bajpai, 1983
	Peltier, 1961
	Scheidler and Bajpai, 1992
5. Ferric–calcium–phosphorous oxides	Fuski et al., 1993
	Larrabee et al., 1993
	Stricker et al., 1992
6. Hydroxyapatites	Bajpai and Fuchs, 1985
	Bajpai, 1983
	Jenei et al., 1986
	Ricci et al., 1986
7. Tricalcium phosphate	Bajpai, 1983
	Bajpai et al., 1988
	Lemons et al., 1988
	Morris and Bajpai, 1989
8. Zinc–calcium–phosphorous oxides	Arar et al., 1989
	Bajpai, U.S. Patent No. 4,778,471
	Binzer and Bajpai, 1987
	Gromofsky et al., 1988
9. Zinc–sulfate–calcium–phosphorous oxides	Scheidler and Bajpai, 1992

TABLE 2.9 Uses of Biodegradable/Resorbable Bioceramics

Use	Ref.
1. As drug delivery devices	Abrams and Bajpai, 1994
	Bajpai, 1992
	Bajpai, 1994
	Benghuzzi et al., 1991
	Moldovan and Bajpai, 1994
	Nagy and Bajpai, 1994
2. For repairing bone damaged due to disease or trauma	Bajpai, 1990
	Gromofsky et al., 1988
	Khavari and Bajpai, 1993
	Morris and Bajpai, 1987
	Scheidler and Bajpai, 1992
3. For filling space vacated by bone screws, donor bone, excised tumors, and diseased bone loss	Bajpai and Fuchs, 1985
	Ricci et al., 1986
4. For repairing and fusion of spinal and lumbo-sacral vertebrae	Bajpai et al., 1984
	Yamamuro et al., 1988
5. For repairing herniated discs	Bajpai et al., 1984
6. For repairing maxillofacial and dental defects	Freeman et al., 1981
7. Hydroxyapatite ocular implants	De Potter et al., 1994
	Shields et al., 1993

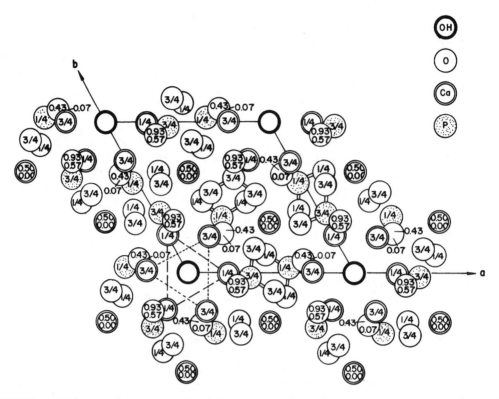

FIGURE 2.6 Hydroxyapatite structure projected down the c-axis onto the basal plane. (*Source:* Posner, A. S., Perloff, A., and Diorio, A. D. 1958. Refinement of hydroxyapatite structure, *Acta. Cryst.* 11:308–309.)

The mineral part of bone and teeth is made of a crystalline form of calcium phosphate similar to hydroxyapatite [$Ca_{10}(PO_4)_6(OH)_2$]. The apatite family of mineral [$A_{10}(BO_4)_6X_2$] crystallizes into hexagonal rhombic prisms and has unit cell dimensions $a = 9.432$ Å and $c = 6.881$ Å. The atomic structure of hydroxyapatite projected down the c-axis onto the basal plane is shown in Fig. 2.6. Note that the hydroxyl ions lie on the corners of the projected basal plane and they occur at equidistant intervals (3.44 Å) along the columns perpendicular to the basal plane and parallel to the c-axis. Six of the ten calcium ions in the unit cell are associated with the hydroxyls in these columns, resulting in strong interactions among them [Park and Lakes, 1992].

The ideal Ca:P ratio of hydroxyapatite is 10:6 and the calculated density is 3.219 g/cm³. Substitution of OH with fluoride gives the apatite greater chemical stability due to the closer coordination of fluoride (symmetric shape) as compared to the hydroxyl (asymmetric, two atoms) by the nearest calcium. This is why fluoridation of drinking water helps in resisting caries of the teeth [Park and Lakes, 1992].

The mechanical properties of synthetic calcium phosphates vary considerably (Table 2.10). The wide variations in properties of polycrystalline calcium phosphates are due to the variations in the structure and manufacturing processes. Depending on the final firing conditions, the calcium phosphate can be calcium hydroxyapatite or β-whitlockite. In many instances, both types of structures exist in the same final product [Park and Lakes, 1992].

Polycrystalline hydroxyapatite has a high elastic modulus (40 to 117 GPa). Hard tissue such as bone, dentin, and dental enamel are natural composites which contain hydroxyapatite (or a similar mineral), as well as protein, other organic materials, and water. Enamel is the stiffest hard tissue, with an elastic modulus of 74 GPa, and contains the most mineral. Dentin ($E = 21$ GPa) and compact bone ($E = 12$ to 18 GPa) contain comparatively less mineral. The Poisson's ratio for the mineral or synthetic hydroxyapatite is about 0.27, which is close to that of bone (≈ 0.3) [Park and Lakes, 1992].

Table 2.10 Physical Properties of Calcium Phosphate

Property	Value
Elastic modulus (GPa)	4.0–117
Compressive strength (MPa)	294
Bending strength (MPa)	147
Hardness (Vickers, GPa)	3.43
Poisson's ratio	0.27
Density (theoretical, g/cm^3)	3.16

Source: Park, J. B. and Lakes, R. S. 1992. Ceramic implant materials. In: *Biomaterials — An Introduction*, 2nd ed., J. B. Park and R. S. Laker, Eds., p. 125, Plenum Press, New York.

Hontsu et al. (1997) were able to deposit an amorphous HA film on Ti, α-Al$_2$O$_3$, SiO//Si(100), and SrTiO$_3$ using a pulsed ArF excimer laser. Upon heat treatment the amorphous film was converted to the crystalline form of HA. The HA film's electrical properties were measured for the first time (Table 2.14).

Among the most important properties of hydroxyapatite as a biomaterial is its excellent biocomaptibility. Hydroxyapatite appears to form a direct chemical bond with hard tissues [Piattelli and Trisi, 1994]. On implantation of hydroxyapatite particles or porous blocks in bone, new lamellar cancellous bone forms within 4 to 8 weeks [Bajpai and Fuchs, 1985]. Scanning electron micrograph (500×) of a set and hardened hydroxyapatite–cysteine composite is shown in Fig. 2.7. The composite sets and hardens on addition of water.

Many different methods have been developed to make precipitates of hydroxyapatite from an aqueous solution of Ca(NO$_3$)$_2$ and NaH$_2$PO$_4$. There has been successful use of modifications to Jarcho and colleagues' wet precipitation procedure for synthesizing hydroxyapatites for use as bone implants [Jarcho et al., 1979; Bajpai and Fuchs, 1985] and drug delivery devices [Abrams and Bajpai, 1994; Bajpai, 1992, 1994; Parker and Bajpai, 1993]. The dried, filtered precipitate is placed in a high-temperature furnace

FIGURE 2.7 Scanning electron micrograph (500×) of a set and hardened hydroxyapatite (HA)–cysteine composite. The small white cysteine particles can be seen on the larger HA particles.

and calcined at 1150°C for 1 h. The calcined powder is then ground in a ball mill, and the particles are separated by an automatic sieve shaker and sieves. The sized particles are then pressed in a die and sintered at 1200°C for 36 h for making drug delivery devices [Abrams and Bajpai, 1994; Bajpai, 1989, 1992]. Above 1250°C, hydroxyapatite shows a second precipitation phase along the grain boundaries [Park and Lakes, 1992].

Aluminum–Calcium–Phosphate (ALCAP) Ceramics

Initially we fabricated a calcium aluminate ceramic containing phosphorous pentoxide [Hentrich et al., 1969, 1971; Graves et al., 1972]. Aluminum–calcium–phosphorous oxide ceramic (ALCAP) was developed later [Bajpai and Graves, 1980]. ALCAP has insulating dielectric properties but no magnetic or piezoelectric properties [Allaire et al., 1989]. ALCAP ceramics are unique because they provide a multipurpose crystallographic system where one phase of the ceramic on implantation can be more rapidly resorbed than the others [Bajpai, 1983; Mattie and Bajpai, 1988; Wyatt et al., 1976]. ALCAP is prepared from stock powders of aluminum oxide, calcium oxide, and phosphorous pentoxide. A ratio of 50:34:16 by weight of AlO_2:CaO:P_2O_5 is used to obtain the starting mixture for calcining at 1350°C in a high-temperature furnace for 12 h. The calcined material is ground in a ball mill and sieved by an automatic siever to obtain particles of the desired size. The particulate powder is then pressed into solid blocks or hollow cylinders (green shape) and sintered at 1400°C for 36 h to increase the mechanical strength. ALCAP ceramic implants have given excellent results in terms of biocompatibility and gradual replacement of the ceramic material with endogenous bone [Bajpai, 1982; Mattie and Bajpai, 1988]. A scanning electron micrograph (1000×) of sintered porous ALCAP is shown in Fig. 2.8.

Coralline

Coral is a natural substance made by marine invertebrates. According to Holmes et al. [1984], the marine invertebrates live in the limestone exostructure, or coral. The porous structure of the coral is unique for each species of marine invertebrate [Holmes et al., 1984]. Corals for use as bone implants are selected

FIGURE 2.8   Scanning electron micrograph (1000×) of sintered porous ALCAP.

on the basis of structural similarity to bone [Holmes et al., 1984]. Coral provides an excellent structure for the ingrowth of bone, and the main component, calcium carbonate, is gradually resorbed by the body [Khavari and Bajpai, 1993]. Corals can also be converted to hydroxyapatite by a hydrothermal exchange process. Interpore 200, a coral hydroxyapatite, resembles cancellous bone [Sartoris et al., 1986]. Both pure coral (Biocoral) and coral transformed to hydroxyapatite are currently used to repair traumatized bone, replace diseased bone, and correct various bone defects.

Biocoral is composed of crystalline calcium carbonate or aragonite, the metastable form of calcium carbonate. The compressive strength of Biocoral varies from 26 (50% porous) to 395 MPa (dense) and depends on the porosity of the ceramic. Likewise, the modulus of elasticity (Young's modulus) of Biocoral varies from 8 (50% porous) to 100 GPa (dense) [Biocoral, 1989].

Tricalcium Phosphate (TCP) Ceramics

A multicrystalline porous form of β-tricalcium phosphate [β-$Ca_3(PO_4)_2$] has been used successfully to correct periodontal defects and augment bony contours [Metsger et al., 1982]. X-ray diffraction of β-tricalcium phosphate shows an average interconnected porosity of over 100 μm [Lemons et al., 1979]. Often tribasic calcium phosphate is mistaken for β-tricalcium phosphate. According to Metsger and colleagues [1982], tribasic calcium phosphate is a nonstoichiometric compound often bearing the formula of hydroxyapatite [$Ca_{10}(PO_4)_6(OH)_2$].

β-Tricalcium phosphate is prepared by a wet precipitation procedure from an aqueous solution of $Ca(NO_3)_2$ and NaH_2PO_4 [Bajpai et al., 1988]. The precipitate is calcined at 1150°C for 1 h, ground, and sieved to obtain the desired size particles for use as bone substitutes [Bajpai et al., 1988; Bajpai, 1990] and for making ceramic matrix drug delivery systems [Morris and Bajpai, 1989; Nagy and Bajpai, 1994; Moldovan and Bajpai, 1994]. These particles are used as such or pressed into cylindrical shapes and sintered at 1150 to 1200°C for 36 h to achieve the appropriate mechanical strength for use as drug delivery devices [Bajpai, 1989, 1992, 1994; Benghuzzi et al., 1991]. A scanning electron micrograph (500×) of a set and hardened TCP-cysteine composite is shown in Fig. 2.9. The composite sets and hardens on the addition of water. TCP is usually more soluble than synthetic hydroxyapatite and, on implantation, allows good bone ingrowth and eventually is replaced by endogenous bone.

Zinc–Calcium–Phosphorous Oxide (ZCAP) Ceramics

Zinc is essential for human metabolism and is a component of at least 30 metalloenzymes [Pories and Strain, 1970]. In addition, zinc may also be involved in the process of wound healing [Pories and Strain, 1970]. Thus zinc–calcium–phosphorous oxide polyphasic (ZCAP) ceramics were synthesized to repair bone defects and deliver drugs [Binzer and Bajpai, 1987; Bajpai, 1988, 1993; Arar and Bajpai, 1992]. ZCAP is prepared by a thermal mixing of zinc oxide, calcium oxide, and phosphorous pentoxide powders [Bajpai, 1988]. ZCAP, like ALCAP, has insulating dielectric properties but no magnetic or piezoelectric properties [Allaire et al., 1989]. Various ratios of these powders have been used to produce the desired material [Bajpai, 1988]. The oxide powders are mixed in a ball mill and subsequently calcined at 800°C for 24 h. The calcined ceramic is then ground and sieved to obtain the desired size particles. Scanning electron micrograph (500×) of a set and hardened ZCAP-cysteine composite is shown in Fig. 2.10. The composite sets and hardens on addition of water. To date, ZCAP ceramics have been used to repair experimentally induced defects in bone and for delivering drugs [Binzer and Bajpai, 1987; Bajpai, 1993].

Zinc–Sulfate–Calcium–Phosphate (ZSCAP) Ceramics

Zinc–sulfate–calcium–phosphate polyphasic (ZSCAP) ceramics are prepared from stock powders of zinc sulfate, zinc oxide, calcium oxide, and phosphorous pentoxide [Bajpai, 1988]. A ratio of 15:30:30:25 by weight of $ZnSO_4$:ZnO:CaO:P_2O_5 is mixed in a crucible and allowed to cool for 30 min after the exothermal reaction has subsided. The cooled mixture is calcined in a crucible at 650°C for 24 h. The calcined ceramic is ground in a ball mill and the particles of the desired size are separated by sieving in an automatic

FIGURE 2.9 Scanning electron micrograph (500×) of a set and hardened TCP–cysteine composite. The small white cysteine particles can be seen on the larger TCP particles.

FIGURE 2.10 Scanning electron micrograph (500×) of a set and hardened ZCAP–cysteine composite. The small white cysteine particles have blended with the ZCAP particles.

FIGURE 2.11 Scanning electron micrograph (2000×) of a set and hardened ZSCAP particles (45–63 μm). Sulfate is hardly visible between the cube-shaped ZCAP particles.

siever. Scanning electron micrograph (2000×) of set and hardened ZSCAP particles (45 to 63 μm) is shown in Fig. 2.11. ZSCAP sets and hardens on addition of water. ZSCAP particles, on implantation in bone, set and harden on contact with blood and have been used to repair experimentally induced defects in bone [Scheidler and Bajpai, 1992].

Ferric–Calcium–Phosphorous–Oxide (FECAP) Ceramics

Ferric–calcium–phosphorous–oxide polyphasic (FECAP) ceramic is prepared from powders of ferric (III) oxide, calcium oxide, and phosphorous pentoxide [Fuski et al., 1993; Larrabee et al., 1993; Stricker et al., 1992]. The powders are combined in various ratios by weight and mixed in a blender. Blocks of the mixture are then pressed in a die by means of a hydraulic press and calcined at 1100°C for 12 h. The calcined ceramic blocks are crushed and ground in a ball mill. The calcined ceramic is ground in a ball mill and the particles of the desired size are separated by sieving in an automatic siever. A scanning electron micrograph (1000×) of a set and hardened FECAP-α ketoglutaric acid composite is shown in Fig. 2.12. The composite sets and hardens on the addition of water. Studies conducted to date suggest complete resorption of FECAP particles implanted in bone within 60 days [Larrabee et al., 1993]. This particular ceramic could be used in patients suffering from anemia and similar diseases [Fuski et al., 1993].

2.4 Bioactive or Surface-Reactive Ceramics

Upon implantation in the host, surface-reactive ceramics form strong bonds with adjacent tissue. Examples of surface-reactive ceramics are dense nonporous glasses, Bioglass and Ceravital, and hydroxyapatites (Table 2.11). One of their many uses is the coating of metal prostheses. This coating provides a stronger bonding to the adjacent tissues, which is very important for prostheses. A list of the uses of surface-reactive ceramics is shown in Table 2.12.

FIGURE 2.12   Scanning electron micrograph (1000×) of a set and hardened FECAP–α-ketoglutaric acid composite. Plate-shaped FECAP particles have been aggregated by the acid.

Table 2.11   Examples of Surface-Reactive Bioceramics

Type	Ref.
1. Bioglass and Ceravital™	Ducheyne, 1985
	Gheyson et al., 1983
	Hench, 1991
	Hench, 1993
	Ogino et al., 1980
	Ritter et al., 1979
2. Dense and nonporous glasses	Andersson et al., 1992
	Blencke et al., 1978
	Li et al., 1991
	Ohtsuki et al., 1992
	Ohura et al., 1992
	Schepers et al., 1993
	Takatsuko et al., 1993
3. Hydroxyapatite	Bagambisa et al., 1993
	Bajpai, 1990
	Fredette et al., 1989
	Huaxia et al., 1992
	Knowles and Bonfield, 1993
	Niwa et al., 1980
	Park and Lakes, 1992
	Posner et al., 1958
	Schwartz et al., 1993
	Whitehead et al., 1993

TABLE 2.12   Uses of Surface-Reactive Bioceramics

Use	Ref.
1. For coating of metal prostheses	Cotell et al., 1992
	Huaxia et al., 1992
	Ritter et al., 1979
	Takatsuko et al., 1993
	Whitehead et al., 1993
2. In reconstruction of dental defects	Hulbert et al., 1987
	Gheysen et al., 1983
	Schepers et al., 1988
	Schepers et al., 1989
3. For filling space vacated by bone screws, donor bone, excised tumors, and diseased bone loss	Hulbert et al., 1987
	Schepers et al., 1993
	Terry et al., 1989
4. As bone plates and screws	Doyle, 1990
	Ducheyne and McGuckin, 1990
	Yamamuro et al., 1988
5. As replacements of middle ear ossicles	Feenstra and de Groot, 1983
	Grote, 1987
	Hench, 1991
	Hench, 1993
	Reck et al., 1988
6. For lengthening of rami	Feenstra and de Groot, 1983
7. For correcting periodontal defects	Feenstra and de Groot, 1983
	Hulbert, 1992
8. In replacing subperiosteal teeth	Hulbert, 1992

Glass Ceramics

Several variations of Bioglass and Ceravital glass ceramics have been used by various workers within the last decade. Glass ceramics used for implantation are silicon-oxide-based systems with or without phosphorous pentoxide.

Glass ceramics are polycrystalline ceramics made by controlled crystallization of glasses developed by S. D. Stookey of Corning Glass Works in the early 1960s [Park and Lakes, 1992]. Glass ceramics were first utilized in photosensitive glasses, in which small amounts of copper, silver, and gold are precipitated by ultraviolet light irradiation. These metallic precipitates help to nucleate and crystallize the glass into a fine-grained ceramic that possesses excellent mechanical and thermal properties. Both Bioglass and Ceravital glass ceramics have been used as implants [Yamamuro et al., 1990].

The formation of glass ceramics is influenced by the nucleation and growth of small (<1-μm diameter) crystals as well as the size distribution of these crystals. It is estimated that about 10^{12} to 10^{15} nuclei per cubic centimeter are required to achieve such small crystals. In addition to the metallic agents already mentioned, Pt groups, TiO_2, ZrO_2, and P_2O_5 are widely used for nucleation and crystallization. The nucleation of glass is carried out at temperatures much lower than the melting temperature. During processing the melt viscosity is kept in the range of 10^{11} and 10^{12} Poise for 1 to 2 h. In order to obtain a larger fraction of the microcrystalline phase, the material is further heated to an appropriate temperature for maximum crystal growth. Deformation of the product, phase transformation within the crystalline phases, or redissolution of some of the phases should be avoided. The crystallization is usually more than 90% complete with grain sizes 0.1 to 1 μm. These grains are much smaller than those of conventional ceramics. Figure 2.13 shows a schematic representation of the temperature–time cycle for a glass ceramic [Park and Lakes, 1992].

The glass ceramics developed for implantation are SiO_2-CaO-Na_2O-P_2O_5 and Li_2O-ZnO-SiO_2 systems. Two major groups are experimenting with the SiO_2-CaO-Na_2O-P_2O_5 glass ceramic. One group varied

FIGURE 2.13 Temperature–time cycle for a glass ceramic. (*Source:* Kingery, W. D., Bowen, H. K., and Uhlmann, D. R. 1976. *Introduction to Ceramics*, 2nd ed., p. 368. John Wiley & Sons, New York.)

TABLE 2.13 Compositions of Bioglass and Ceravital Glass Ceramics

Type	Code	SiO_2	CaO	Na_2O	P_2O_5	MgO	K_2O
Bioglass	42S5.6	42.1	29.0	26.3	2.6	—	—
	(45S5)46S5.2	46.1	26.9	24.4	2.6	—	—
	49S4.9	49.1	25.3	23.8	2.6	—	—
	52S4.6	52.1	23.8	21.5	2.6	—	—
	55S4.3	55.1	22.2	20.1	2.6	—	—
	60S3.8	60.1	19.6	17.7	2.6	—	—
Ceravital	Bioactive[a]	40–50	30–35	5–10	10–15	2.5–5	0.5–3
	Nonbioactive[b]	30–35	25–30	3.5–7.5	7.5–12	1–2.5	0.5–2

[a] The Ceravital® composition is in weight % while the Bioglass® compositions are in mol %.

[b] In addition, Al_2O_3 (5.0–15.0), TiO_2(1.0–5.0), and Ta_2O_5 (5–15) are added.

Source: Park, J. B. and Lakes, R. S. 1992. Ceramic implant materials. In: *Biomaterials — An Introduction*, 2nd ed., J. B. Park and R. S. Laker, Eds., p. 127. Plenum Press, New York.

the compositions (except for P_2O_5) in order to obtain the best glass ceramic composition for inducing direct bonding with bone (Table 2.13). The bonding to bone is related to the simultaneous formation of a calcium phosphate and SiO_2-rich film layer on the surface, as exhibited by the 46S5.2 type Bioglass. If a SiO_2-rich layer forms first and a calcium phosphate film develops later (46 to 55 mol % SiO_2 samples) or no phosphate film is formed (60 mole % SiO_2) then direct bonding with bone does not occur [Park and Lakes, 1992]. The approximate region of the SiO_2-CaO-Na_2O system for the tissue–glass–ceramic reaction is shown in Fig. 2.14. As can be seen, the best region (region A) for good tissue bonding is the composition given for 46S5.2 type Bioglass (see Table 2.13) [Park and Lakes, 1992].

Ceravital

The composition of Ceravital is similar to that of Bioglass in SiO_2 content but differs somewhat in other components (see Table 2.13). In order to control the dissolution rate, Al_2O_3, TiO_2, and Ta_2O_5 are added in Ceravital glass ceramic. The mixtures, after melting in a platinum crucible at 1500°C for 3 h, are annealed and cooled. The nucleation and crystallization temperatures are 680°C and 750°C, respectively, each for 24 h. When the size of crystallites reaches approximately 4 Å and the characteristic needle structure is not formed, the process is stopped to obtain a fine-grain-structured glass ceramic. [Park and Lakes, 1993]

Glass ceramics have several desirable properties compared to glasses and ceramics. The thermal coefficient of expansion is very low, typically 10^{-7} to 10^{-5}°C^{-1}, and in some cases it can even be made negative. Due to the controlled grain size and improved resistance to surface damage, the tensile strength of these materials can be increased by at least a factor of two, from about 100 to 200 MPa. The resistance to scratching and abrasion of glass ceramics is similar to that of sapphire [Park and Lakes, 1992].

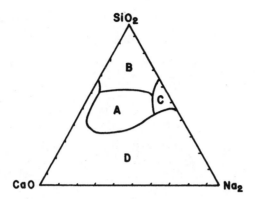

FIGURE 2.14   Approximate regions of the tissue–glass–ceramic bonding for the SiO_2-CaO-Na_2O system. (A) Bonding within 30 days. (B) Nonbonding; reactivity is too low. (C) Nonbonding; reactivity is too high. (D) Bonding does not form glass. (*Source:* Hench, L. L. and Ethridge, E. C. 1982. *Biomaterials: An Interfacial Approach.* p.147, Academic Press, New York.)

A transmission electron micrograph of Bioglass glass ceramic implanted in the femur of rats for 6 weeks showed intimate contacts between the mineralized bone and the Bioglass (Fig. 2.15). The mechanical strength of the interfacial bond between bone and Bioglass ceramic is on the same order of magnitude as the strength of the bulk glass ceramic (850 kg/cm^2 or 83.3 MPa), which is about three fourths that of the host bone strength [Park and Lakes, 1992].

A negative characteristic of the glass ceramic is its brittleness. In addition, limitations on the compositions used for producing a biocompatibile (or osteoconductive) glass ceramic hinders the production of a glass ceramic which has substantially higher mechanical strength. Thus, glass ceramics cannot be used for making major load-bearing implants such as joint implants. However, they can be used as fillers for bone cement, dental restorative composites, and coating material (see Table 2.12). A glass ceramic containing 36 wt% of magnetite in a β-wollastonite- and CaOSiO$_2$-based glassy matrix has been synthesized for treating bone tumors by hyperthermia [Kokubo et al., 1992].

2.5   Deterioration of Ceramics

It is of great interest to know whether the inert ceramics such as alumina undergo significant static or dynamic fatigue. Even for the biodegradable ceramics, the rate of degradation *in vivo* is of paramount importance. Controlled degradation of an implant with time on implantation is desirable. Above a critical stress level, the fatigue strength of alumina is reduced by the presence of water. This is due to the delayed crack growth, which is accelerated by the water molecules [Park and Lakes, 1992]. Reduction in strength occurs if water penetrates the ceramic. Decrease in strength was not observed in samples which did not show water marks on the fractured surface (Fig. 2.16). The presence of a small amount of silica in one sample lot may have contributed to the permeation of water molecules that is detrimental to the strength [Park and Lakes, 1992]. It is not clear whether the static fatigue mechanism operates in single-crystal alumina. It is reasonable to assume that static fatigue will occur if the ceramic contains flaws or impurities, because these will act as the source of crack initiation and growth under stress [Park and Lakes, 1992].

Studies of the fatigue behavior of vapor-deposited pyrolitic carbon fibers (4000 to 5000 Å thick) onto a stainless steel substrate showed that the film does not break unless the substrate undergoes plastic deformation at 1.3×10^{-2} strain and up to one million cycles of loading. Therefore, the fatigue is closely related to the substrate, as shown in Fig. 2.17. Similar substrate–carbon adherence is the basis for the pyrolitic carbon deposited polymer arterial grafts [Park and Lakes, 1992].

The fatigue life of ceramics can be predicted by assuming that the fatigue fracture is due to the slow growth of preexisting flaws. Generally, the strength distribution, σ_i, of ceramics in an inert environment can be correlated with the probability of failure F by the following equation:

FIGURE 2.15 Transmission electron micrograph of well-mineralized bone (b) juxtaposed to the glass-ceramic (c), which fractured during sectioning (51, 500×). Insert (a) is the diffraction pattern from ceramic area and (b) is from bone area. (*Source:* Beckham, C. A., Greenlee, T. K., Jr., Crebo, A. R., 1971. Bone formation at a ceramic implant interface, *Calc. Tiss. Res.* 8:165–171.)

$$\text{Ln Ln}\left(\frac{1}{1-F}\right) = m \text{ Ln}\left(\frac{s_i}{s_o}\right) \tag{2.1}$$

Both m and s_o are constants in the equation. Figure 2.18 shows a good fit for Bioglass-coated alumina [Park and Lakes, 1992].

A minimum service life (t_{min}) of a specimen can be predicted by means of a proof test wherein it is subjected to stresses that are greater than those expected in service. Proof tests also eliminate the weaker pieces. This minimum life can be predicted from the following equation:

$$t_{min} = B\,\sigma_P^{N-2}\sigma_a^{-N} \tag{2.2}$$

Here σ_p is the proof test stress, σ_a is the applied stress, and B and N are constants.

FIGURE 2.16 Flexural strength of dense alumina rods after aging under stress in Ringer's solution. Lot 1 and 2 are from different batches of production. (*Source:* Krainess, F. E. and Knapp, W. J. 1978. Strength of a dense alumina ceramic after aging *in vitro*. *J. Biomed. Mater. Res.* 12:245.)

FIGURE 2.17 Strain vs. number of cycles to failure (○ = absence of fatigue cracks in carbon film; ● = fracture of carbon film due to fatigue failure of substrates; □ = data from substrate determined in single-cycle tensile test). (*Source:* Shimm, H. S. and Haubold, A. D. 1980. The fatigue behavior of vapor deposited carbon films. *Biomater. Med. Dev. Art. Org.* 8:333–344.)

FIGURE 2.18 Plot of Ln Ln $[1/(1-F)]$ vs. Ln s for Bioglass-coated alumina in a *tris*-hydroxyaminomethane buffer and liquid nitrogen. F is the probability of failure and S is strength. (*Source:* Ritter, J. E., Jr., Greenspan, D. C., Palmer, R. A., and Hench, L. L. 1979. Use of fracture of an alumina and bioglass coated alumina, *J. Biomed. Mater. Res.* 13:260.)

FIGURE 2.19   Plot of Eq. (2.3) for alumina after proof testing. $N = 43.85$, $m = 13.21$, and $\sigma_o = 55728$ psi. (*Source:* Ritter, J. E., Jr., Greenspan, D. C., Palmer, R. A., and Hench, L. L. 1979. Use of fracture of an alumina and bioglass coated alumina, *J. Biomed. Mater. Res.* 13:261.)

Equation (2.2), after rearrangement, reads as follows:

$$t_{\min} = \sigma_a^2 = B\left(\sigma_P / \sigma_a\right)^{N-2} \tag{2.3}$$

Figure 2.19 shows a plot of Eq. (2.3) for alumina on a logarithmic scale [Park and Lakes, 1992].

2.6 Bioceramic Manufacturing Techniques

In order to fabricate bioceramics in more and more complex shapes, scientists are investigating the use of old and new manufacturing techniques. These techniques range from the adaptation of an age-old pottery technique to the latest manufacturing methods for high-temperature ceramic parts for airplane engines. No matter where the technique is perfected, the ultimate goal is the fabrication of bioceramic particles or devices in a desired shape in a consistent manner with the desired properties. The technique used to fabricate the bioceramic device will depend greatly on the ultimate application of the device, whether it is for hard-tissue replacement or the integration of the device within the surrounding tissue.

Hard-Tissue Replacement

Hard-tissue replacement implies that the bioceramic device will be used for load-bearing applications. Although it is desirable to have a device with a sufficient porosity for the surrounding tissue to infiltrate and attach to the device, the most important and immediate property is the strength of the device. In order to accomplish this, one must manufacture a bioceramic implant with a density and strength sufficient to mimic that of bone. However, if the bioceramic part is significantly stronger than the surrounding bone, one runs into the common problem seen with metals called *stress shielding*. The

TABLE 2.14 Electrical Properties of an HA Film

Dielectric constant (ε_r)	5.7 (25°C 1 MHz)
Loss tangent (tan δ)	<2%
Breakdown electric field	10^4 V cm^{-1}

Source: Hontsu et al., 1997.

density of the bioceramic greatly determines its overall strength. As the density increases so does the overall strength of the bioceramic. Some of the techniques used to manufacture dense bioceramics are injection molding, gel casting, bicontinuous microemulsion, inverse microemulsion, emulsion, and additives.

Injection molding is a common technique used to form plastic parts for many commercial applications such as automobile parts. Briefly, the process involves forcing a heated material into a die and then ejecting the formed piece from the die. Injection molding allows for making complex shapes. Cihlar and Trunec (1996) found that by calcining (1273 K, 3 h) and milling the hydroxyapatite (HA) prior to mixing with a binder, an ethylene vinyl acetate copolymer (EVA)/HA mixture of 63% HA, they achieved 98% relative density with only 16% shrinkage using injection molding. The maximum flexural strength was 60 MPa for HA products sintered at 1473 K. However, this is still not strong enough for load-bearing applications. They also observed that HA decomposed to α-TCP at temperatures greater than 1573 K [Cihlar and Trunec, 1996].

In gel casting, HA is formed using the standard chemical precipitation. The calcium phosphate precipitant (30% w/v) is then mixed with glycerol and filtered. The "gel cake" is sintered at 1200°C for 2 h. This has yielded a density of >99% and a highly uniform microstructure [Varma and Sivakumar, 1996].

Bicontinuous microemulsion, inverse microemulsion, and emulsion are all wet chemistry based methods to produce nanometer-size HA powders. All three methods yield >97% relative density upon sintering at 1200°C for 2 h. The biocontinuous and inverse microemulsion resulted in the two smallest HA particle sizes, 22 and 24 nm, respectively [Lim et al., 1997].

Another strategy to increase the density of ceramics is to use additives or impurities in small weight percents during sintering. The main disadvantages to this technique include (1) the possible decomposition of the original pure bioceramic and (2) all or portions of the bioceramic being non-biocompatible.

Suchanek et al. (1997) studied the addition of several different additives to HA in 5 wt% amounts. The additives studied were K_2CO_3, Na_2CO_3, H_3BO_3, KF, $CaCl_2$, KCl, KH_2PO_4, $(KPO_3)_n$, $Na_2Si_2O_5$, $Na_2P_2O_7$, Na_3PO_4, $(NaPO_3)_n$, $Na_5P_3O_{10}$, and β-NaCaPO$_4$. HA has a fracture toughness of 1 MPa·m$^{1/2}$, whereas human bone has a fracture toughness of 2 to 12 MPa·m$^{1/2}$. One of the ways to improve the mechanical properties is to improve the densification of HA. Suchanek et al. (1997) found that the following additives (5 wt.%) did not improve the densification of HA: H_3BO_3, $CaCl_2$, KCl, KH_2PO_4, $(KPO_3)_n$, and $Na_2Si_2O_5$. The densification of HA was improved through the addition (5 wt.%) of K_2CO_3, Na_2CO_3, KF, $Na_2P_2O_7$, Na_3PO_4, $(NaPO_3)_n$, $Na_5P_3O_{10}$, and β-NaCaPO$_4$. However, H_3BO_3, $CaCl_2$, KH_2PO_4, $(KPO_3)_n$, $Na_2Si_2O_5$, K_2CO_3, Na_2CO_3, and KF produced the formation of β-TCP or CaO. The sodium phosphates used in this study were added to HA without the formation of β-TCP or CaO. The only compound that improved densification, did not cause formation of β-TCP or CaO, and provided a weak interface for HA was β-NaCaPO$_4$.

Another additive that has been investigated to improve the performance of HA is lithium (Li). The addition of lithium can increase the microhardness and produces a fine microstructure in HA. Fanovich et al. (1998) found that the addition of 0.2 wt% of Li to HA produced the maximum microhardness (5.9 GPa). However, the addition of high amounts of Li to HA results in abnormal grain growth and large pores. Furthermore, Li addition to HA results in the formation of β-TCP upon sintering.

Zirconia has been used as an additive to HA in order to improve its mechanical strength. Kawashima et al. (1997) found that addition of partially stabilized zirconia (PSZ) to HA can be used to increase the fracture toughness to 2.8 MPa·m$^{1/2}$. Bone has a fracture toughness of 2–12 MPa·m$^{1/2}$ [Suchanek et al., 1997]. PSZ was added to HA in different percentages (17, 33, 50 wt%) and it was found that 50 wt% PSZ

Table 2.15   Bioceramic Manufacturing Techniques for Hard Tissue
Replacement or Tissue Integration

Manufacturing Technique	Ref.
Hard Tissue Replacement	
Injection molding	Cihlar and Trunec, 1996
Bicontinuous microemulsion	Lim et al., 1997
Inverse microemulsion	
Emulsion	
Additives	Fanovich et al., 1998; Kawashima et al., 1997; Suchanek et al., 1997
Tissue Integration	
Drip casting	Liu, 1996; Lyckfeldt and Ferreira, 1998
Starch consolidation	Lyckfeldt and Ferreira, 1998]
Polymeric sponge method	
Foaming method	
Organic additives	
Gel casting	
Slip casting	
Direct coagulation consolidation	
Hydrolysis-assisted solidification	
Freezing	

had the highest fracture toughness. The surface energy of the PSZ–HA was not significantly different from HA alone. This suggests that the PSZ–HA composite could be biocompatible because of the similarity of the surface with HA [Kawashima et al., 1997].

Tissue Integration

The porosity is a critical factor for growth and integration of a tissue into the bioceramic implant. In particular the open porosity, that which is connected to the outside surface, is critical to the integration of tissue into the ceramic especially if the bioceramic is inert. Several methods have been developed to form porous ceramics, two of which are starch consolidation and drip casting.

In starch consolidation (Table 2.15), starch powders of a specific size are mixed with a bioceramic slurry at a predetermined weight percent. Upon heating, the starch will uptake water from the slurry mixture and swell. Upon sintering of the starch–bioceramic mixture, the starch is burned out and the pores are left in their place. Starch consolidation has been used to form complex shapes in alumina with ultimate porosities between 23 and 70 vol%. By controlling the starch content, one can control the ultimate porosity and resulting pore sizes. Large pores formed using starch consolidation in alumina were in the size range 10 to 80 μm whereas small pores varied between 0.5 and 9.5 μm [Lyckfeldt and Ferreira, 1998].

Liu (1996) used a drip casting technique (Table 2.15) to form porous HA granules with pore sizes from 95 to 400 μm. The granules had a total porosity from 24 to 76 vol%. The HA was made into a slurry using water and poly(vinyl butyral) powders. The slurry was then dripped onto a spherical mold surface. This technique is similar to that of drip casting by dripping an HA slurry into a liquid nitrogen bath. In both instances, calcining and sintering procedures are used to produce the final product [Liu, 1996].

Acknowledgments

The author is grateful to Dr. Joon B. Park for inviting him to write this chapter and for providing the basic shell from his book to expand upon. The author thanks his wife, Zoe, for her patience and understanding and Dr. M. C. Hofmann for her support and help.

In Memoriam

In memory of Dr. P. K. Bajpai, who left us early in 1998, I would like to share our lab's recipe for hydroxyapatite. Dr. Bajpai's lab and research at the University of Dayton have ended after 30-plus years, but I felt it would be fitting to share this recipe as a way to encourage other scientists to continue exploring the possibilities of bioceramics.

Hydroxyapatite Synthesis Method

Prepare the following solutions:

Solution 1: Dissolve 157.6 g calcium nitrate tetrahydrate $[Ca(NO_3)_2 4H_2O]$ in 500 ml DI water. Bring the solution to a pH of 11 by adding ≈ 70 ml ammonium hydroxide $[NH_4OH]$. Bring the solution to 800 ml with DI water.

Solution 2: Dissolve 52.8 g ammonium phosphate dibasic $[(NH_4)_2HPO_4]$ in 500 ml DI water. Bring the solution to a pH of 11 by adding ≈ 150 ml ammonium hydroxide $[NH_4OH]$. Add DI water until the precipitate is completely dissolved, 250–350 ml.

Special note: If you use calcium nitrate $[Ca(NO_3)_{2n}H_2O]$ instead of calcium nitrate tetrahydrate you need to recalculate the amount of calcium nitrate to add to make Solution 1 on the basis of the absence of the extra four waters. If you do not, you will have to add a large amount of ammonium hydroxide to pH the solution.

1. Add one half of Solution 1 to a 2-L separatory funnel.
2. Add one half of Solution 2 to a 2-L separatory funnel.
3. Titrate both solutions into a 4-L beaker with heat and constant stirring.
4. Boil gently for 30 min.
5. Repeat steps 1–4 for the rest of Solutions 1 and 2.
6. Let cool completely, allowing precipitate to settle to bottom of beaker.
7. Pour contents of beaker into 250-ml polypropylene bottles.
8. Centrifuge bottles for 10 min at (10,000 rpm) 16,000 *g*.
9. Collect precipitate from the six bottles into two and resuspend with DI water.
10. Fill the four empty bottles with the reaction mixture and centrifuge all six as before.
11. Collect precipitant from the two bottles that were resuspended with DI water.
12. Combine remaining four bottles into two bottles and resuspend with DI water.
13. Repeat steps 10–12 as necessary.
14. Dry precipitate for 24–48 h at 70°C.
15. Calcine the precipitate for 1 h at 1140°C.
16. Grind and sieve product as desired.

Defining Terms

Alumina: Aluminum oxide (Al_2O_3), which is very hard (Mohs hardness is 9) and strong. Single crystals are called sapphire or ruby depending on color. Alumina is used to fabricate hip joint socket components or dental root implants.

Calcium phosphate: A family of calcium phosphate ceramics including aluminum calcium phosphate, ferric calcium phosphate, hydroxyapatite and tricalcium phosphate (TCP), and zinc calcium phosphate, which are used to substitute or augment bony structures and deliver drugs.

Glass-ceramics: A glass crystallized by heat treatment. Some of those have the ability to form chemical bonds with hard and soft tissues. Bioglass and Ceravital are well-known examples.

Hydroxyapatite: A calcium phosphate ceramic with a calcium to phosphorus ratio of 5/3 and nominal composition $Ca_{10}(PO_4)_6(OH)_2$. It has good mechanical properties and excellent biocompatibility. Hydroxyapatite is the mineral constituent of bone.

LTI carbon: A silicon alloyed pyrolitic carbon deposited onto a substrate at low temperature with isotropic crystal morphology. It is highly compatible with blood and used for cardiovascular implant fabrication such as artificial heart valve.

Maximum radius ratio: The ratio of atomic radii computed by assuming the largest atom or ion which can be placed in a crystal's unit cell structure without deforming the structure.

Mohs scale: A hardness scale in which 10 (diamond) is the hardest and 1 (talc) is the softest.

References

Abrams L and Bajpai PK. 1994. Hydroxyapatite ceramics for continuous delivery of heparin. *Biomed. Sci. Instrumen.* 30:169–174.

Adams D and Williams DF. 1978. Carbon fiber-reinforced carbon as a potential implant material, *J. Biomed. Mater. Res.* 12:35–42.

Alexander H, Parsons JR, Ricci JL, Bajpai PK, and Weiss AB. 1987. Calcium-based ceramics and composites in bone reconstruction. *Crit. Rev.* 4:43–47.

Allaire M, Reynolds D, and Bajpai PK. 1989. Electrical properties of biocompatible ALCAP and ZCAP ceramics. *Biomed. Sci. Instrumen.* 25:163–168.

Andersson OH, Guizhi L, Kangasniemi K, and Juhanoja J. 1992. Evaluation of the acceptance of glass in bone, *J. Mat. Sci.: Mater. Med.* 3:145–150.

Annual Book of ASTM Standards, part 46, F603-78, American Society for Testing and Materials, Philadelphia, 1980.

Arar HA and Bajpai PK. 1992. Insulin delivery by zinc calcium phosphate (ZCAP) ceramics. *Biomed. Sci. Instrumen.* 28:172–178.

Bagambisa FB, Joos U, and Schilli W. 1993. Mechanisms and structure of the bond between bone and hydroxyapatite ceramics. *J. Biomed. Mater. Res.* 27:1047–1055.

Bajpai PK, Fuchs CM, and Strnat MAP. 1985. Development of alumino-calcium phosphorous oxide (ALCAP) ceramic cements. In: *Biomedical Engineering. IV. Recent Developments.* Proceedings of the Fourth Southern Biomedical Engineering Conference, Jackson, MS, B Sauer, Ed., pp. 22–25. Pergamon Press, New York, pp. 22–25.

Bajpai PK. 1994. Ceramic drug delivery systems. In: *Biomedical Materials Research in The Far East* (I). X Zhang and Y Ikada, Eds., pp. 41–42. Kobunshi Kankokai, Kyoto, Japan.

Bajpai PK. 1993. Zinc-based ceramic cysteine composite for repairing vertebral defects. *J.I.S.* 6:346.

Bajpai PK. 1992. Ceramics: a novel device for sustained long term delivery of drugs. In: *Bioceramics*, Vol. 3, JA Hulbert and SF Hulbert, Eds., pp. 87–99. Rose-Hulman Institute of Technology, Terre Haute, IN.

Bajpai PK. 1990. Ceramic amino acid composites for repairing traumatized hard tissues. In: *Handbook of Bioactive Ceramics*, Vol. II: *Calcium Phosphate and Hydroxylapatite Ceramics*, T Yamamuro, LL Hench, and J Wilson-Hench, Eds., pp. 255–270. CRC Press, Boca Raton, FL.

Bajpai PK. 1989. Ceramic implantable drug delivery system. *Trends Biomater. Artif. Org.* 3:203–211.

Bajpai PK. 1988. ZCAP Ceramics. U.S. Patent No. 4,778,471.

Bajpai PK. 1983. Biodegradable scaffolds in orthopedic, oral, and maxillo facial surgery. In: *Biomaterials in Reconstructive Surgery*, LR Rubin, Ed., pp. 312–328. C.V. Mosby, St. Louis, MO.

Bajpai PK, Fuchs CM, and McCullum DE. 1988. Development of tricalcium phosphate ceramic cements. In: *Quantitative Characterization and Performance of Porous Implants for Hard Tissue Applications*, ASTM STP 953, JE Lemons, Ed., pp. 377–388. American Society for Testing and Materials, Philadelphia, PA.

Bajpai PK and Fuchs CM. 1985. Development of a hydroxyapatite bone grout. In: *Proceedings of the First Annual Scientific Session of the Academy of Surgical Research*, San Antonio, TX, CW Hall, Ed., pp. 50–54. Pergamon Press, New York.

Bajpai PK, Graves GA Jr, Wilcox LG, and Freeman MJ. 1984. Use of resorbable alumino–calcium–phosphorous–oxide ceramics (ALCAP) in health care. *Trans. Soc. Biomat.* 7:353.

Bajpai PK and Graves GA Jr. 1980. Porous Ceramic Carriers for Controlled Release of Proteins, Polypeptide Hormones and other Substances within Human and/or Mammalian Species. U.S. Patent No. 4,218,255.

Barinov SM and Bashenko YuV. 1992. Application of ceramic composites as implants: result and problem. In: *Bioceramics and the Human Body*, A Ravaglioli and A Krajewski, Eds., pp. 206–210. Elsevier Applied Science, London.

Beckham CA, Greenlee TK Jr, and Crebo AR. 1971. Bone formation at a ceramic implant interface. *Calc. Tiss. Res.* 8:165–171.

Benghuzzi HA, Giffin BF, Bajpai PK, and England BG. 1991. Successful antidote of multiple lethal infections with sustained delivery of difluoromethylornithine by means of tricalcium phosphate drug delivery devices. *Trans. Soc. Biomat.* 24:53.

Binzer TJ and Bajpai PK. 1987. The use of zinc–calcium–phosphorous oxide (ZCAP) ceramics in reconstructive bone surgery, *Digest of Papers, Sixth Southern Biomedical Engineering Conference*. Dallas, TX, RC Eberhart, Ed., pp. 182–185. McGregor and Werner, Washington, D.C.

Biocoral. 1989. From coral to biocoral, p. 46. *Innoteb*, Paris, France.

Blencke BA, Bromer H, Deutscher KK. 1978. Compatibility and long-term stability of glass-ceramic implants. *J. Biomed. Mater. Res.* 12:307–318.

Bokros JC. 1972. Deposition structure and properties of pyrolitic carbon. *Chem. Phys. Carbon.* 5:70–81.

Bokros JC, LaGrange LD, and Schoen GJ. 1972. Control of structure of carbon for use in bioengineering. *Chem. Phys. Carbon* 9:103–171.

Boutin P. 1981. T.H.R. using alumina–alumina sliding and a metallic stem: 1330 cases and an 11-year follow-up. In: *Orthopaedic Ceramic Implants*, Vol. 1, H Oonishi and HY Ooi Eds., Japanese Society of Orthopaedic Ceramic Implants, Tokyo.

Buykx WJ, Drabarek E, Reeve KD, Anderson N, Mathivanar R, and Skalsky M. 1992. *Development of Porous Ceramics for Drug Release and Other Applications*. In: *Bioceramics*, Vol. 3. JE Hulbert and SF Hulbert, Eds., pp. 349–354. Rose Hulman Institute of Technology, Terre Haute, IN.

Chandy T and Sharma CP. 1991. Biocomaptibility and toxicological screening of materials. In: *Blood Compatible Materials and Devices*, CP Sharma and M Szycher, Eds., pp. 153–166. Technomic, Lancaster, PA.

Chignier E, Monties JR, Butazzoni B, Dureau G, and Eloy R. 1987. Haemocompatibility and biological course of carbonaceous composites for cardiovascular devices. *Biomaterials*. 8:18–23.

Cihlar J and Trunec M. 1996. Injection moulded hydroxyapatite ceramics. *Biomaterials* 17: 1905–1911.

Cotell CM, Chrisey DB, Grabowski KS, Sprague JA, and Gossett CR. 1992. Pulsed laser deposition of hydroxyapatite thin films on Ti-6Al-4V, *J. Appl. Biomat.* 3:87–93.

de Groot K. 1983. *Bioceramics of Calcium Phosphate*. CRC Press, Boca Raton, FL.

De Potter P, Shields CL, Shields JL, and Singh AD. 1994. Use of the hydroxyapatite ocular implant in the pediatric population. *Arch. Ophthalmol.* 112:208–212.

Dellsperger KC and Chandran KB. 1991. Prosthetic heart valves. In: *Blood Compatible Materials and Devices*, CP Sharma and M Szycher, Eds., Technomic, Lancaster, PA.

Dorlot JM, Christel P, and Meunier A. 1988. Alumina hip prostheses: long term behaviors. In: *Bioceramics, Proceedings of 1st International Symposium on Ceramics in Medicine*, H Oonishi, H Aoki, and K Sawai, Eds., pp. 236–301. Ishiyaku EuroAmerica, Inc., Tokyo.

Dörre E. 1991. Problems concerning the industrial production of alumina ceramic components for hip prosthesis. In: *Bioceramics and the Human Body*, A Ravaglioli and A Krajewski, Eds., pp. 454–460. Elsevier Applied Science, London.

Doyle C. 1990. Composite bioactive ceramic-metal materials. In: *Handbook of Bioactive Ceramics*. T Yamamuro, LL Hench, and J Wilson, Eds., pp. 195–208. CRC Press, Boca Raton, FL.

Drennan J and Steele BCH. 1991. Zirconia and hafnia. In: *Concise Encyclopedia of Advanced Ceramic Materials*. RJ Brook, Ed., pp. 525–528. Pergamon Press, Oxford.

Ducheyne P and McGuckin, JF Jr. 1990. Composite bioactive ceramic-metal materials. In: *Handbook of Bioactive Ceramics*, T Yamamuro, LL Hench, and J Wilson, Eds., pp. 75–86. CRC Press, Boca Raton, FL.

Ducheyne P. 1985. Bioglass coatings and bioglass composites as implant materials. *J. Biomed. Mater. Res.* 19:273–291.

Ely JL and Haubald AO. 1993. Static fatigue and stress corrosion in pyrolitic carbon. In: *Bioceramics*, Vol. 6, P Ducheyne and D Christiansen, Eds., pp. 199–204. Butterworth-Heinemann, Boston, MA.

Fanovich MA, Castro MS, and Porto Lopez JM. 1998. Improvement of the microstructure and micro-hardness of hydroxyapatite ceramics by addition of lithium. *Mat. Lett.* 33: 269–272.

Feenstra L and de Groot K. 1983. Medical use of calcium phosphate ceramics. In: *Bioceramics of Calcium Phosphate*, K de Groot, Ed., pp. 131–141. CRC Press, Boca Raton, FL.

Freeman MJ, McCullum DE, and Bajpai PK. 1981. Use of ALCAP ceramics for rebuilding maxillo-facial defects. *Trans. Soc. Biomat.* 4:109.

Fredette SA, Hanker JS, Terry BC, and Beverly L. 1989. Comparison of dense versus porous hydroxyapatite (HA) particles for rat mandibular defect repair. *Mat. Res. Soc. Symp. Proc.* 110:233–238.

Fulmer MT, Martin RI, and Brown PW. 1992. Formation of calcium deficient hydroxyapatite at near-physiological temperature, *J. Mat. Sci.: Mater. Med.* 3:299–305.

Fuski MP, Larrabee RA, and Bajpai PK. 1993. Effect of ferric calcium phosphorous oxide ceramic implant in bone on some parameters of blood. *Trends Biomater. Artif. Org.* 7:16–19.

Gheysen G, Ducheyne P, Hench LL, and de Meester P. 1983. Bioglass composites: a potential material for dental application. *Biomaterials.* 4:81–84.

Graves GA Jr, Hentrich RL Jr, Stein HG, and Bajpai PK. 1972. Resorbable ceramic implants in bioceramics. In: *Engineering and Medicine*, Part I, CW Hall, SF Hulbert, SN Levine, and FA Young, Eds., pp. 91–115. Wiley-Interscience, New York.

Grenoble DE, Katz JL, Dunn KL, Gilmore RS, and Murty KL. 1972. The elastic properties of hard tissues and apatites, *J. Biomed. Mater. Res.* 6:221–233.

Gromofsky JR, Arar H, and Bajpai PK. 1988. Development of zinc calcium phosphorous oxide ceramic-organic acid composites for repairing traumatized hard tissue. In: *Digest of Papers, Seventh Southern Biomedical Engineering Conference*, Greenville, SC, DD Moyle, Ed., pp. 20–23. McGregor and Werner, Washington, D.C.

Grote JJ. 1987. Reconstruction of the ossicular chain with hydroxyapatite prostheses. *Am. J. Otol.* 8:396–401.

Guillemin G, Meunier A, Dallant P, Christel P, Pouliquen JC, and Sedel L. 1989. Comparison of coral resorption and bone apposition with two natural corals of different porosities. *J. Biomed. Mat. Res.* 23:765–779.

Hammer J III, Reed O, and Greulich R. 1972. Ceramic root implantation in baboons. *J. Biomed. Mater. Res.* 6:1–13.

Heimke G. 1992. Use of alumina ceramics in medicine. In: *Bioceramics*, Vol. 3, JE Hulbert and SF Hulbert, Eds., pp. 19–30. Rose Hulman Institute of Technology, Terre Haute, IN.

Hench LL. 1991. Bioceramics: from concept to clinic. *J. Am. Ceram. Soc.* 74:1487–1510.

Hench LL. 1993. Bioceramics: from concept to clinic. *Am. Ceram. Soc. Bull.*, 72:93–98.

Hench LL and Ethridge EC. 1982. *Biomaterials: An Interfacial Approach*, p. 147. Academic Press, New York.

Hentrich RL Jr, Graves GA Jr, Stein HG, and Bajpai PK. 1971. An evaluation of inert and resorbable ceramics for future clinical applications. *J. Biomed. Mater. Res.* 5:25–51.

Hentrich RL Jr, Graves GA Jr, Stein HG, and Bajpai PK. 1969. An evaluation of inert and resorbable ceramics for future clinical applications. Fall Meeting, Ceramics–Metals Systems, Division of the American Ceramic Society, Cleveland, OH.

Holmes R, Mooney V, Bucholz R, and Tencer A. 1984. A coralline hydroxyapatite bone graft substitute. *Clin. Orthopaed. Related Res.* 188:252–262.

Hontsu S, Matsumoto T, Ishii J, Nakamori M, Tabata H, and Kawai T. 1997. Electrical properties of hydroxyapatite thin films grown by pulsed laser deposition. *Thin Solid Films* 295: 214–217.

Huaxia JI, Ponton CB, and Marquis PM. 1992. Microstructural characterization of hydroxyapatite coating on titanium, *J. Mat. Sci.: Mater. Med.* 3:283–287.

Hulbert SF. 1992. Use of ceramics in medicine. In: *Bioceramics*, Vol. 3, JE Hulbert and SF Hulbert, Eds., pp. 1–18. Rose Hulman Institute of Technology, Terre Haute, IN.

Hulbert SF and Klawitter JJ. 1971. Application of porous ceramics for the development of load-bearing internal orthopedic applications. *Biomed. Mater. Symp.* pp. 161–229.

Hulbert SF, Bokros JC, Hench LL, Wilson J, and Heimke G. 1987. Ceramics in clinical applications: past, present, and future. In: *High Tech Ceramics*, P Vincezini, Ed., pp. 189–213. Elsevier, Amsterdam.

Jarcho M, Salsbury RL, Thomas MB, and Doremus RH. 1979. Synthesis and fabrication of β-tricalcium phosphate (whitlockite) ceramics for potential prosthetic applications. *J. Mater. Sci.* 14:142–150.

Jenei SR, Bajpai PK, and Salsbury RL. Resorbability of commercial hydroxyapatite in lactate buffer. In: *Proceedings of the Second Annual Scientific Session of the Academy of Surgical Research, Clemson, SC*, DN Powers, Ed., pp. 13–16. Clemson University Press, Clemson, SC.

Kaae JL. 1971. Structure and mechanical properties of isotropic pyrolitic carbon deposited below 1600°C. *J. Nucl. Mater.* 38:42–50.

Kawahara H, Ed. 1989. *Oral Implantology and Biomaterials*, Elsevier, Amsterdam.

Kawashima N, Soetanto K, Watanabe K, Ono K, and Matsuno T. 1997. The surface characteristics of the sintered body of hydroxyapatite–zirconia composite particles. *Colloids Surfaces B: Biointerfaces* 10: 23–27.

Khavari F and Bajpai PK. 1993. Coralline-sulfate bone substitutes. *Biomed. Sci. Instrumen.* 29:65–69.

Kijima T and Tsutsumi M. 1979. Preparation and thermal properties of dense polycrystalline oxyhydroxyapatite, *J. Am. Cer. Soc.* 62:954–960.

Kingery WD, Bowen HK, and Uhlmann DR. 1976. *Introduction to Ceramics*, 2nd ed., p. 368. Wiley, New York.

Knowles JC and Bonfield W. 1993. Development of a glass reinforced hydroxyapatite with enhanced mechanical properties: the effect of glass composition on mechanical properties and its relationship to phase changes, *J. Biomed. Mater. Res.* 27:1591–1598.

Kokubo T, Kushitani H, Ohtsuki C, Sakka S, and Yamamuro T. 1992. Chemical reaction of bioactive glass and glass-ceramics with a simulated body fluid. *J. Mater. Sci.: Mater. Med.* 3:79–83.

Krainess FE and Knapp WJ. 1978. Strength of a dense alumina ceramic after aging *in vitro*. *J. Biomed. Mater. Res.* 12:241–246.

Kumar P, Shimizu K, Oka M, Kotoura Y, Nakayama Y, Yamamuro T, Yanagida T, and Makinouchi K. 1989. Biological reaction of zirconia ceramics. In: *Bioceramics, Proceedings of 1st International Symposium on Ceramics in Medicine*, H Oonishi, H Aoki, and K Sawai, Eds., pp. 341–346. Ishiyaku Euroamerica, Inc., Tokyo.

Larrabee RA, Fuski MP, and Bajpai PK. 1993. A ferric–calcium–phosphorous–oxide ceramic for rebuilding bone. *Biomed. Sci. Instrumen.* 29:59–64.

Lemons JE, Bajpai PK, Patka P, Bonel G, Starling LB, Rosenstiel T, Muschler G, Kampnier S, and Timmermans T. 1988. Significance of the porosity and physical chemistry of calcium phosphate ceramics orthopaedic uses. In: *Bioceramics: Material Characteristics Versus in Vivo Behavior. Ann. N.Y. Acad. Sci.* 523:190–197.

Lemons JE and Niemann KMW. 1979. *Porous Tricalcium Phosphate Ceramic for Bone Replacement.* 25th Annual ORS Meetings, San Francisco, CA, February 20–22, p. 162.

Li R, Clark AE, and Hench LL. 1991. An investigation of bioactive glass powders by sol-gel processing, *J. Appl. Biomater.* 2:231–239.

Lim GK, Wang J, Ng SC, Chew CH, and Gan LM. 1997. Processing of hydroxyapatite via microemulsion and emulsion routes. *Biomaterials* 18:1433–1439.

Liu D. 1996. Fabrication and chracterization of porous hydroxyapatite granules. *Biomaterials* 17:1955–1957.

Lyckfeldt O and Ferreira JMF. 1998. Processing of porous ceramics by 'starch consolidation.' *J. Eur. Cer. Soc.* 18:131–140.

Mattie DR and Bajpai PK. 1988. Analysis of the biocompatibility of ALCAP ceramics in rat femurs. *J. Biomed. Mater. Res.* 22:1101–1126.

Meenen NM, Osborn JF, Dallek M, and Donath K. 1992. Hydroxyapatite–ceramic for juxta-articular implantation, *J. Mater. Sci.: Mater. Med.* 3:345–351.

Metsger S, Driskell TD, and Paulsrud JR. 1982. Tricalcium phosphate ceramic—a resorbable bone implant: review and current status. *JADA,* 105:1035–1038.

Moldovan K and Bajpai PK. 1994. A ceramic system for continuous release of aspirin. *Biomed. Sci. Instrumen.* 30:175–180.

More RB and Silver MD. 1990. Pyrolitic carbon prosthetic heart valve occluder wear: *in vitro* results for the Bjork–Shiley prosthesis. *J. Appl. Biomater.* 1:267–278.

Morris LM and Bajpai PK. 1989. Development of a resorbable tricalcium phosphate (TCP) amine antibiotic composite. *Mater. Res. Soc. Symp.* 110:293–300.

Murakami T and Ohtsuki N. 1989. Friction and wear characteristics of sliding pairs of bioceramics and polyethylene. In: *Bioceramics, Proceedings of 1st International Symposium on Ceramics in Medicine,* H Oonishi, H Aoki, and K Sawai, Eds., pp. 225–230. Ishiyaku Euroamerica, Inc., Tokyo.

Nagy EA and Bajpai PK. 1994. Development of a ceramic matrix system for continuous delivery of azidothymidine. *Biomed. Sci. Instrumen.* 30:181–186.

Niwa S, Sawai K, Takahashie S, Tagai H, Ono M, and Fukuda Y. 1980. Experimental studies on the implantation of hydroxyapatite in the medullary canal of rabbits. In: *Trans. First World Biomaterials Congress,* Baden, Austria. p. 4.10.4.

Ogino M, Ohuchi F, and Hench LL. 1980. Compositional dependence of the formation of calcium phosphate film on bioglass, *J. Biomed. Mater. Res.* 12:55–64.

Ohashi T, Inoue S, Kajikawa K, Ibaragi K, Tada T, Oguchi M, Arai T, and Kondo K. 1988. The clinical wear rate of acetabular component accompanied with alumina ceramic head. In: *Bioceramics, Proceedings of 1st International Symposium on Ceramics in Medicine,* H Oonishi, H Aoki, and K Sawai, Eds., pp. 278–283. Ishiyaku EuroAmerica, Inc., Tokyo.

Ohtsuki C, Kokubo T, and Yamamuro T. 1992. Compositional dependence of bioactivity of glasses in the system $CaO-SiO_2-Al_2O_3$: its *in vitro* evaluation. *J. Mater. Sci.: Mater. Med.* 3:119—125.

Ohura K, Nakamura T, Yamamuro T, Ebisawa Y, Kokubo T, Kotoura Y, and Oka M. 1992. Bioactivity of $Cao-SiO_2$ glasses added with various ions, *J. Mater. Sci.: Mater. Med.* 3:95–100.

Oonishi H. 1992. Bioceramic in orthopaedic surgery—our clinical experiences. In: *Bioceramics,* Vol. 3, JE Hulbert and SF Hulbert, Eds., pp. 31–42. Rose Hulman Institute of Technology, Terre Haute, IN.

Park JB and Lakes RS. 1992. *Biomaterials—An Introduction,* 2nd ed., Plenum Press, New York.

Park JB. 1991. Aluminum oxides: biomedical applications. In: *Concise Encyclopedia of Advanced Ceramic Materials,* RJ Brook, Ed., pp. 13–16. Pergamon Press, Oxford.

Parker DR and Bajpai PK. 1993. Effect of locally delivered testosterone on bone healing. *Trans. Soc. Biomat.* 26: 293.

Peltier LF. 1961. The use of plaster of Paris to fill defects in bone. *Clin. Orthop.* 21:1–29.

Piattelli A and Trisi P. 1994. A light and laser scanning microscopy study of bone/hydroxyapatite-coated titanium implants interface: histochemical evidence of unmineralized material in humans. *J. Biomed. Mater. Res.* 28:529–536.

Pories WJ and Strain WH. 1970. Zinc and wound healing. In: *Zinc Metabolism,* AS Prasad, Ed., pp. 378–394. Charles C Thomas, Springfield, IL.

Posner AS, Perloff A, and Diorio AD. 1958. Refinement of hydroxyapatite structure, *Acta. Cryst.* 11:308–309.

Reck R, Störkel S, and Meyer A. 1988. Bioactive glass-ceramics in middle ear surgery: an eight-year review. In: *Bioceramics: Material Characteristics Versus in Vivo Behavior. Ann. N.Y. Acad. Sci.* 523:100–106.

Ricci JL, Bajpai PK, Berkman A, Alexander H, and Parsons JR. 1986. Development of a fast-setting ceramic-based grout material for filling bone defects. In: *Biomedical Engineering. V. Recent Developments, Proceedings of the Fifth Southern Biomedical Engineering Conference,* Shreveport, LA. S Saha, Ed., pp. 475–481. Pergamon Press, New York.

Ritter JE Jr, Greenspan DC, Palmer RA, and Hench LL. 1979. Use of fracture of an alumina and Bioglass coated alumina, *J. Biomed. Mater. Res.* 13:251–263.

Sartoris DJ, Gershuni DH, Akeson WH, Holmes RE, and Resnick D. 1986. Coralline hydroxyapatite bone graft substitutes: preliminary report of radiographic evaluation. *Radiology* 159:133–137.

Scheidler PA and Bajpai PK. 1992. Zinc sulfate calcium phosphate (ZSCAP) composite for repairing traumatized bone. *Biomed. Sci. Instrumen.* 28:183–188.

Schepers E, Ducheyne P, and De Clercq M. 1989. Interfacial analysis of fiber-reinforced bioactive dental root implants. *J. Biomed. Mater. Res.* 23:735–752.

Schepers E, De Clercq M, and Ducheyne P. 1988. Interfacial behavior of bulk bioactive glass and fiber-reinforced bioactive glass dental root implants. *Ann. N.Y. Acad. Sci.* 523:178–189.

Schepers EJG, Ducheyne P, Barbier L, and Schepers S. 1993. Bioactive glass particles of narrow size range: a new material for the repair of bone defects. *Impl. Dent.* 2:151–156.

Schwartz Z, Braun G, Kohave D, Brooks B, Amir D, Sela J, and Boyan B. 1993. Effects of hydroxyapatite implants on primary mineralization during rat tibial healing: biochemical and morphometric analysis. *J. Biomed. Mater. Res.* 27:1029–1038.

Sedel L, Meunier A, Nizard RS, and Witvoet J. 1991. Ten year survivorship of cemented ceramic-ceramic total hip replacement. In: *Bioceramics*, Vol. 4. *Proceedings of the 4th International Symposium on Ceramics in Medicine.* W Bonfield, GW Hastings, and KE Tanner, Eds., pp. 27–37. Butterworth-Heinemann, London.

Shackelford JF. 1988. *Introduction to Materials Science for Engineers*, 2nd ed. Macmillan, New York.

Shimm HS and Haubold AD. 1980. The fatigue behavior of vapor deposited carbon films. *Biomater. Med. Dev. Art. Org.* 8:333–344.

Shields JA, Shields CL, and De Potter P. 1993. Hydroxyapatite orbital implant after enucleation-experience with 200 cases. *Mayo Clinic Proc.* 68:1191–1195.

Shobert EI II. 1964. *Carbon and Graphite*, Academic Press, New York.

Stricker NJ, Larrabee RA, and Bajpai PK. 1992. Biocompatibility of ferric calcium phosphorous oxide ceramics. *Biomed. Sci. Instrumen.* 28:123–128.

Suchanek W, Yashima M, Kakihana M, and Yoshimura M. 1997. Hydroxyapatite ceramics with selected sintering additives. *Biomaterials* 18:923–933.

Sudanese A, Toni A, Cattaneo GL, Ciaroni D, Greggi T, Dallart D, Galli G, and Giunti A. 1989. In *Bioceramics. Proceedings of 1st International Symposium on Ceramics in Medicine*, H Oonishi, H Aoki, and K Sawai, Eds., pp. 237–240. Ishiyaku Euroamerica, Inc., Tokyo.

Takatsuko K, Yamamuro T, Kitsugi T, Nakamura T, Shibuya T, and Goto T. 1993. A new bioactive glass-ceramic as a coating material on titanium alloy. *J. Appl. Biomater.* 4:317–329.

Terry BC, Baker RD, Tucker MR, and Hanker JS. 1989. Alveolar ridge augmentation with composite implants of hydroxylapatite and plaster for correction of bony defects, deficiencies and related contour abnormalities. *Mat. Res. Soc. Symp.* 110:187–198.

Valiathan A, Randhawa GS, and Randhawa A. 1993. Biomaterial aspects of calcium hydroxyapatite, *Trends Biomater. Artif. Org.* 7:1–7.

Varma HK and Sivakumar R. 1996. Dense hydroxyapatite ceramics through gel casting technique. *Mat. Lett.* 29:57–61.

Whitehead RY, Lacefield WR, and Lucas LC. 1993. Structure and integrity of a plasma sprayed hydroxyapatite coating on titanium, *J. Biomed. Mater. Res.* 27:1501–1507.

Wolford LM, Wardrop RW, and Hartog JM. 1987. Coralline porous hydroxylapatite as a bone graft substitute in orthognathic surgery. *J. Oral. Maxillofacial Surg.* 45:1034–1042.

Wyatt DF, Bajpai PK, Graves GA Jr, and Stull PA. 1976. Remodelling of calcium aluminate phosphorous pentoxide ceramic implants in bone. *IRCS Med. Sci.*, 4:421.

Yamamuro T, Hench LL, and Wilson J. 1990. *Handbook of Bioactive Ceramics*, Vols. I and II. CRC Press, Boca Raton, FL.

Yamamuro T, Shikata J, Kakutani Y, Yoshii S, Kitsugi T, and Ono K. 1988. Novel methods for clinical applications of bioactive ceramics. In: *Bioceramics: Material Characteristics Versus in Vivo Behavior.* *Ann. N.Y. Acad. Sci.* 523:107–114.

Zimmerman MC, Alexander H, Parsons JR, and Bajpai PK. 1991. The design and analysis of laminated degradable composite bone plates for fracture fixation. In *High-Tech Textiles*, TL Vigo and AF Turbak, Eds., pp. 132–148. ACS Symposium Series 457, American Chemical Society, Washington, D.C.

Further Information

Bajpai PK. 1987. Surgical Cements. U.S. Patent No. 4,668,295.

Bajpai PK. 1988. ZCAP Ceramics. U.S. Patent No. 4,778,471.

Bonfield W, Hastings GW, and Tanner KE. 1991. *Bioceramics*, Vol. 4. *Proceedings of the 4th International Symposium on Ceramics in Medicine.* Butterworth-Heinemann, London.

Brook J. 1991. *Concise Encyclopedia of Advanced Ceramic Materials.* Pergamon Press, Oxford.

de Groot K. 1983. *Bioceramics of Calcium Phosphate.* CRC Press, Boca Raton, FL.

Ducheyne P and Lemons JE. 1988. *Bioceramics: Material characteristics versus in vivo behavior. Ann. N.Y. Acad. Sci.* 523.

Ducheyne P and Christiansen D. 1993. *Bioceramics*, Vol. 6. Butterworth-Heinemann, Boston.

Filgueiras MRT, LaTorre G, and Hench LL. 1993. Solution effects on the surface reactions of three bioactive glass compositions. *J. Biomed. Mater. Res.* 27:1485–1493.

Frank RM, Wiedemann P, Hemmerle J, and Freymann M. 1991. Pulp capping with synthetic hydroxyapatite in human premolars, *J. Appl. Biomater.* 2:243–250.

Fulmer MT and Brown PW. 1993. Effects of Na_2HPO_4 and NaH_2PO_4 on hydroxyapatite formation. *J. Biomed. Mater. Res.* 27:1095–1102.

Garcia R and Doremus RH. 1992. Electron microscopy of the bone-hydroxyapatite interface from a human dental implant, *J. Mater. Sci.: Mater. Med.* 3:154–156.

Hall CW, Hulbert SF, Levine SN, and Young FA. 1972. *Engineering and Medicine.* Wiley-Interscience, New York.

Hench LL. 1991. Bioceramics: from concept to clinic. *J. Am. Ceram. Soc.* 74:1487–1510.

Hench LL and Ethridge EC. 1982. *Biomaterials: An Interfacial Approach.* Academic Press, New York.

Hulbert JA and Hulbert SF. 1992. *Bioceramics*, Vol. 3. *Proceedings of the 3rd International Symposium on Ceramics in Medicine*, Rose Hulman Institute of Technology, Terre Haute, IN.

Kawahara H., Ed. 1989. *Oral Implantology and Biomaterials*, Elsevier, Amsterdam.

Kingery WD, Bowen HK, and Uhlmann DR. 1976. *Introduction to Ceramics*, 2nd ed., p. 368. Wiley, New York.

Lemons JE. 1988. *Quantitative Characterization and Performance of Porous Implants for Hard Tissue Applications*, ASTM STP 953. American Society for Testing and Materials, Philadelphia, PA.

Mattie DR and Bajpai PK. 1986. Biocompatibility testing of ALCAP ceramics. *IRCS. Med. Sci.* 14:641–643.

Neo M, Nakamura T, Ohtsuki C, Kokubo T, and Yamamuro T. 1993. Apatite formation on three kinds of bioactive material at an early stage *in vivo*: a comparative study by transmission electron microscopy. *J. Biomed. Mater. Res.* 27:999–1006.

Oonishi H, Aoki H, and Sawai K. 1988. *Bioceramics*, Vol. 1. *Proceedings of 1st International Symposium on Ceramics in Medicine.* Ishiyaku EuroAmerica, Inc., Tokyo.

Oonishi H and Ooi Y. 1981. *Orthopaedic Ceramic Implants*, Vol. I. *Proceedings of Japanese Society of Orthopaedic Ceramic Implants.*

Park JB and Lakes RS. 1992. *Biomaterials—An Introduction*, 2nd ed., Plenum Press, New York.

Ravaglioli A and Krajewski A. 1992. *Bioceramics and the Human Body.* Elsevier Applied Science, London.

Rubin LR. 1983. *Biomaterials in Reconstructive Surgery.* C.V. Mosby, St. Louis, MO.

Sharma CP and Szycher M. 1991. *Blood Compatible Materials and Devices: Perspectives Toward the 21st Century.* Technomic, Lancaster, PA.

Signs SA, Pantano CG, Driskell TD, and Bajpai PK. 1979. *In vitro* dissolution of synthos ceramics in an acellular physiological environment. *Biomater. Med. Dev. Art. Org.*, 7:183–190.

Stea S, Tarabusi C Ciapetti G, Pizzoferrato A, Toni A, and Sudanese A. 1992. Microhardness evaluations of the bone growing into porous implants. *J. Mater. Sci.: Mater. Med.* 3:252–254.

van Blitterswijk CA and Grote JJ. 1989. Biological performance of ceramics during inflammation and infection. *Crit. Rev. Biocompatibility* 5:13–43.

Wilson J and Low SB. 1992. Bioactive ceramics for periodontal treatment: comparative studies in the patus monkey. *J. Appl. Biomater.* 3:123–129.

Yamamuro T, Hench LL, and Wilson J. 1990. *Handbook of Bioactive Ceramics.* CRC Press, Boca Raton, FL.

Zhang X and Ikada Y. 1994. *Biomedical Materials Research in The Far East (I).* Kobunshi Kankokai, Inc., Kyoto, Japan.

3

Polymeric Biomaterials

Hai Bang Lee
Korea Research Institute of Chemical Technology

Gilson Khang
Chonbuk National University

Jin Ho Lee
Hannam University

3.1 Introduction

Synthetic polymeric materials have been widely used in medical disposable supplies, prosthetic materials, dental materials, implants, dressings, extracorporeal devices, encapsulants, polymeric drug delivery systems, tissue engineered products, and orthodoses like those of metal and ceramics substituents [Lee, 1989]. The main advantages of the polymeric biomaterials compared to metal or ceramic materials are ease of manufacturability to produce various shapes (latex, film, sheet, fibers, etc.), ease of secondary processability, reasonable cost, and availability with desired mechanical and physical properties. The required properties of polymeric biomaterials are similar to other biomaterials, that is, biocompatibility, sterilizability, adequate mechanical and physical properties, and manufacturability as given in Table 3.1.

The objectives of this chapter are to review (1) the basic chemical and physical properties of the synthetic polymers, (2) the sterilization of the polymeric biomaterials, (3) the importance of the surface treatment for improving biocompatability, and (4) the application of the chemogradient surface for the study on cell to polymer interactions.

3.2 Polymerization and Basic Structure

Polymerization

In order to link the small molecules one has to force them to lose their electrons by the chemical processes of condensation and addition. By controlling the reaction temperature, pressure, and time in the presence of catalyst(s), the degree to which repeating units are put together into chains can be manipulated.

TABLE 3.1   Requirements for Biomedical Polymers

Property	Description
Biocompatibility	Noncarcinogenesis, nonpyrogenicity, nontoxicity, and nonallergic response
Sterilizability	Autoclave, dry heating, ethylenoxide gas, and radiation
Physical property	Strength, elasticity, and durability
Manufacturability	Machining, molding, extruding, and fiber forming

Modified from Ikada [1989].

TABLE 3.2   Typical Condensation Polymers

Type	Interunit Linkage
Polyester	$\overset{O}{\overset{\|}{-C-O-}}$
Polyamide	$\overset{O\ \ H}{\overset{\|\ \ \|}{-C-N-}}$
Polyurea	$\overset{H\ \ O\ \ H}{\overset{\|\ \ \|\ \ \|}{-N-C-N-}}$
Polyurethane	$\overset{O\ \ H}{\overset{\|\ \ \|}{-O-C-N-}}$
Polysiloxane	$\overset{R}{\underset{R}{-Si-O-}}$
Protein	$\overset{O\ \ H}{\overset{\|\ \ \|}{-C-N-}}$

Condensation or Step Reaction Polymerization

During condensation polymerization a small molecule such as water will be condensed out by the chemical reaction. For example:

$$R-NH_2 + R'COOH \rightarrow R'CONHR + \quad H_2O \qquad (3.1)$$

$$\underset{(amine)}{} \quad \underset{(carboxylic\ acid)}{} \qquad \underset{(amide)}{} \quad \underset{(condensed\ molecule)}{}$$

This particular process is used to make polyamides (nylons). Nylon was the first commercial polymer, made in the 1930s.

Some typical condensation polymers and their interunit linkages are given in Table 3.2. One major drawback of condensation polymerization is the tendency for the reaction to cease before the chains grow to a sufficient length. This is due to the decreased mobility of the chains and reactant chemical species as polymerization progresses. This results in short chains. However, in the case of nylon the chains are polymerized to a sufficiently large extent before this occurs and the physical properties of the polymer are preserved.

Natural polymers, such as polysaccharides and proteins, are also made by condensation polymerization. The condensing molecule is always water (H_2O).

Addition or Free Radical Polymerization

Addition polymerization can be achieved by rearranging the bonds within each monomer. Since each "mer" has to share at least two covalent electrons with other mers the monomer should have at least one double bond. For example, in the case of ethylene:

TABLE 3.3 Monomers for Addition Polymerization and Suitable Processes

Monomer Name	Chemical Structure	Polymerization Mechanism[a]			
		Radical	Cationic	Anionic	Coordination
Acrylonitrile	$CH_2=CH$ $\quad\ \ C\equiv N$	+	−	+	+
Ethylene	$CH_2=CH_2$	+	+	−	−
Methacrylate	$CH_2=CH$ $\quad\ \ COOCH_3$	+	−	+	+
Methylmethacrylate	$CH_2=CCH_3$ $\quad\ \ COOCH_3$	+	−	+	+
Propylene	$CH_2=CH$ $\quad\ \ CH_3$	−	−	−	+
Styrene	$CH_2=CH$ $\quad\ \ C_6H_5$	+	+	+	+
Vinylchloride	$CH_2=CH$ $\quad\ \ Cl$	+	−	−	+
Vinylidenechloride	$\quad\ \ Cl$ $CH_2=C$ $\quad\ \ Cl$	+	−	+	−

[a] +: high polymer formed; −: no reaction or oligomers only.
Modified from Billmeyer [1984].

$$n \ \{ \overset{\overset{\displaystyle H}{|}}{\underset{\underset{\displaystyle H}{|}}{C}} = \overset{\overset{\displaystyle H}{|}}{\underset{\underset{\displaystyle H}{|}}{C} } \} \rightarrow - \overset{\overset{\displaystyle H}{|}}{\underset{\underset{\displaystyle H}{|}}{C}} \Big[\overset{\overset{\displaystyle H}{|}}{\underset{\underset{\displaystyle H}{|}}{C}} - \overset{\overset{\displaystyle H}{|}}{\underset{\underset{\displaystyle H}{|}}{C}} \Big] \overset{\overset{\displaystyle H}{|}}{\underset{\underset{\displaystyle H}{|}}{C}} - \tag{3.2}$$

The breaking of a double bond can be done with an initiator. This is usually a free radical such as benzoyl peroxide ($H_5C_6COO–OOCC_6H_5$). The initiation can be activated by heat, ultraviolet light, and other chemicals. The free radicals (initiators) can react with monomers and this free radical can react with another monomer and the process can continue on. This process is called *propagation*. The propagation process can be terminated by combining two free radicals, by transfer, or by disproportionate processes. Some of the free radical polymers are given in Table 3.3. There are three more types of initiating species for addition polymerization besides free radicals: cations, anions, and coordination (stereospecific) catalysts. Some monomers can use two or more of the initiation processes but others can use only one process as given in Table 3.3.

Basic Structure

Polymers have very long chain molecules which are formed by covalent bonding along the backbone chain. The long chains are held together either by secondary bonding forces such as van der Waals and hydrogen bonds or primary covalent bonding forces through cross links between chains. The long chains are very flexible and can be tangled easily. In addition, each chain can have side groups, branches, and copolymeric chains or blocks which can also interfere with the long-range ordering of chains. For example, paraffin wax has the same chemical formula as polyethylene (PE) $[(CH_2CH_2)_n]$, but will crystallize almost completely because of its much shorter chain lengths. However, when the chains become extremely long (from 40 to 50 repeating units $[–CH_2CH_2–]$ to several thousands as in linear PE) they cannot be crystallized completely (up to 80 to 90% crystallization is possible). Also, branched PE in which side chains are attached to the main backbone chain at positions normally occupied by a hydrogen atom will not crystallize easily due to the steric hindrance of side chains resulting in a more noncrystalline structure. The partially crystallized structure is called *semicrystalline* which is the most commonly occurring structure for linear polymers. The semicrystalline structure is represented by disordered

Crystalline(folded & extended chains)
Amorphous(uncoordinated chains)

FIGURE 3.1 Fringed-micelle model of a linear polymer with semicrystalline structure.

noncrystalline (amorphous) regions and ordered crystalline regions which may contain folded chains as shown in Fig. 3.1.

The degree of polymerization (DP) is defined as an average number of mers, or repeating units, per molecule, i.e., chain. Each chain may have a different number of mers depending on the condition of polymerization. Also, the length of each chain may be different. Therefore, it is assumed there is an average degree of polymerization or average molecular weight (MW). The relationship between molecular weight and degree of polymerization can be expressed as:

$$\text{MW of polymer} = \text{DP} \times \text{MW of mer (or repeating unit)} \tag{3.3}$$

The two average molecular weights most commonly used are defined in terms of the numbers of molecules, Ni, having molecular weight, Mi; or wi, the weight of species with molecular weights Mi as follows:

1. The number-average molecular weight, Mn, is defined by the equation,

$$Mn = \frac{\Sigma WiMi}{\Sigma NiWi} = \Sigma niMi = \frac{\Sigma wi}{\Sigma\left(wi/Mi\right)} = \frac{1}{\Sigma\left(wi/Mi\right)} \tag{3.4}$$

2. The weight-average molecular weight, Mw, is defined by the equation,

$$Mw = \frac{\Sigma wiMi}{\Sigma wi} = \Sigma wiMi = \frac{\Sigma NiMi^{2}}{\Sigma NiMi} \tag{3.5}$$

An absolute method of measuring the molecular weight is one that depends on theoretical considerations, counting molecules and their weight directly. The relative methods require calibration based on an absolute method and include intrinsic viscosity and gel permeation chromatography (GPC). Absolute methods of determining the number-average molecular weight (Mn) include osmometry and other colligative methods and end group analysis. Light-scattering yields an absolute weight-average molecular weight (Mw).

As the molecular chains become longer by the progress of polymerization, their relative mobility decreases. The chain mobility is also related to the physical properties of the final polymer. Generally, the higher the molecular weight, the less the mobility of chains which results in higher strength and greater thermal stability. The polymer chains can be arranged in three ways; linear, branched, and a cross-linked (or three-dimensional) network as shown in Fig. 3.2. Linear polymers such as polyvinyls, polyamides, and polyesters are much easier to crystallize than the cross-linked or branched polymers. However, they cannot be crystallized 100% as with metals. Instead they become semicrystalline polymers. The arrangement of chains in crystalline regions is believed to be a combination of folded and extended chains. The chain folds, which are seemingly more difficult to form, are necessary to explain observed single crystal structures in which the crystal thickness is too small to accommodate the length of the

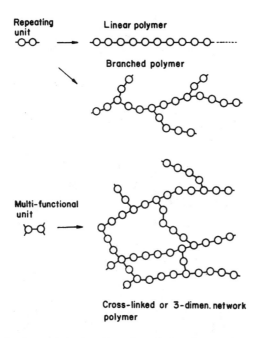

Repeating unit → Linear polymer

Branched polymer

Multi-functional unit →

Cross-linked or 3-dimen. network polymer

FIGURE 3.2 Arrangement of polymer chains into linear, branched, and network structure depending on the functionality of the repeating units.

chain as determined by electron and x-ray diffraction studies. The classical "fringed-micelle" model in which the amorphous and crystalline regions coexist has been modified to include chain folds in the crystalline regions. The cross-linked or three-dimensional network polymers such as polyphenolform-aldehyde cannot be crystallized at all and they become noncrystalline, amorphous polymers.

Vinyl polymers have a repeating unit $-CH_2-CHX-$ where X is some monovalent side group. There are three possible arrangements of side groups (X): (1) atactic, (2) isotactic, and (3) syndiotactic. In atactic arrangements the side groups are randomly distributed while in syndiotactic and isotactic arrangements they are either in alternating positions or on one side of the main chain. If side groups are small like polyethylene (X=H) and the chains are linear, the polymer crystallizes easily. However, if the side groups are large as in polyvinyl chloride (X=Cl) and polystyrene (X=C_6H_5, benzene ring) and are randomly distributed along the chains (atactic), then a noncrystalline structure will be formed. The isotactic and syndiotactic polymers usually crystallize even when the side groups are large.

Copolymerization, in which two or more homopolymers (one type of repeating unit throughout its structure) are chemically combined, always disrupts the regularity of polymer chains thus promoting the formation of a noncrystalline structure. Possible arrangement of the different copolymerization is shown in Fig. 3.3. The addition of plasticizers to prevent crystallization by keeping the chains separated from one another will result in more flexible polymers, a noncrystalline version of a polymer which normally crystallizes. An example is celluloid which is normally made of crystalline nitrocellulose plasticized with camphor. Plasticizers are also used to make rigid noncrystalline polymers like polyvinylchloride (PVC) into a more flexible solid (a good example is Tygon® tubing).

Elastomers, or rubbers, are polymers which exhibit large stretchability at room temperature and can snap back to their original dimensions when the load is released. The elastomers are noncrystalline polymers which have an intermediate structure consisting of long chain molecules in three-dimensional networks (see next section for more details). The chains also have "kinks" or "bends" in them which straighten when a load is applied. For example, the chains of *cis*-polyisoprene (natural rubber) are bent at the double bond due to the methyl group interfering with the neighboring hydrogen in the repeating unit $[-CH_2-C(CH_3)=CH-CH_2-]$. If the methyl group is on the opposite side of the hydrogen then it becomes *trans*-polyisoprene which will crystallize due to the absence of the steric hindrance present in

FIGURE 3.3   Possible arrangements of copolymers.

the *cis* form. The resulting polymer is a very rigid solid called *gutta percha* which is not an elastomer. Below the glass transition temperature (T_g; second order transition temperature between viscous liquid and solid) natural rubber loses its compliance and becomes a glass-like material. Therefore, to be flexible, all elastomers should have T_g well below room temperature. What makes the elastomers not behave like liquids above T_g is in fact due to the cross links between chains which act as pinning points. Without cross links the polymer would deform permanently. An example is latex, which behaves as a viscous liquid. Latex can be cross-linked with sulfur (vulcanization) by breaking double bonds (C=C) and forming C–S–S–C bonds between the chains. The more cross links are introduced, the more rigid the structure becomes. If all the chains are cross-linked together, the material will become a three-dimensional rigid polymer.

Effect of Structural Modification on Properties

The physical properties of polymers can be affected in many ways. In particular, the chemical composition and arrangement of chains will have a great effect on the final properties. By such means the polymers can be tailored to meet the end use.

Effect of Molecular Weight and Composition

The molecular weight and its distribution have a great effect on the properties of a polymer since its rigidity is primarily due to the immobilization or entanglement of the chains. This is because the chains are arranged like cooked spaghetti strands in a bowl. By increasing the molecular weight the polymer chains become longer and less mobile and a more rigid material results as shown in Fig. 3.4. Equally important is that all chains should be equal in length since if there are short chains they will act as plasticizers. Another obvious way of changing properties is to change the chemical composition of the backbone or side chains. Substituting the backbone carbon of a polyethylene with divalent oxygen or sulfur will decrease the melting and glass transition temperatures since the chain becomes more flexible

FIGURE 3.4 Approximate relations among molecular weight, T_g, T_m, and polymer properties.

due to the increased rotational freedom. On the other hand if the backbone chains can be made more rigid then a stiffer polymer will result.

Effect of Side Chain Substitution, Cross-Linking, and Branching

Increasing the size of side groups in linear polymers such as polyethylene will decrease the melting temperature due to the lesser perfection of molecular packing, i.e., decreased crystallinity. This effect is seen until the side group itself becomes large enough to hinder the movement of the main chain as shown in Table 3.4. Very long side groups can be thought of as being branches.

Cross-linking of the main chains is in effect similar to the side chain substitution with a small molecule, i.e., it lowers the melting temperature. This is due to the interference of the cross-linking which causes decreased mobility of the chains, resulting in further retardation of the crystallization rate. In fact, a large degree of cross-linking can prevent crystallization completely. However, when the cross-linking density increases for a rubber, the material becomes harder and the glass transition temperature also increases.

TABLE 3.4 Effect of Side Chain Substitution on Melting Temperature in Polyethylene

Side Chain	T_m (°C)
$-H$	140
$-CH_3$	165
$-CH_2CH_3$	124
$-CH_2CH_2CH_3$	75
$-CH_2CH_2CH_2CH_3$	−55
$-CH_2CHCH_2CH_3$ $\quad\quad CH_3$	196
$\quad\quad CH_3$ $-CH_2CCH_2CH_3$ $\quad\quad CH_3$	350

Effect of Temperature on Properties

Amorphous polymers undergo a substantial change in their properties as a function of temperature. The glass transition temperature, T_g, is a boundary between the glassy region of behavior in which the polymer is relatively stiff and the rubbery region in which it is very compliant. T_g can also be defined as the temperature at which the slope of volume change vs. temperature has a discontinuity in slope as shown in Fig. 3.5. Since polymers are noncrystalline or at most semicrystalline, the value obtained in this measurement depends on how fast it is taken.

3.3 Polymers Used as Biomaterials

Although hundreds of polymers are easily synthesized and could be used as biomaterials only 10 to 20 polymers are mainly used in medical device fabrications from disposable to long-term implants as given in Table 3.5. In this section, the general information of the characteristics, properties, and applications of the most commonly used polymers will be discussed [Billmeyer, 1984; Park, 1984; Leininger and Bigg, 1986; Shalaby, 1988; Brandrup and Immergut, 1989; Sharma and Szycher, 1991; Park and Lakes, 1992; Dumitriu, 1993; Lee and Lee, 1995; Ratner et al., 1996].

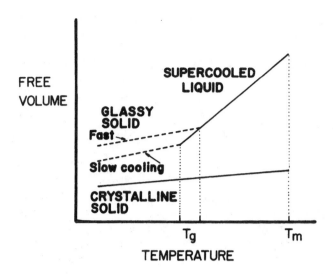

FIGURE 3.5 Change of volume vs. temperature of a solid. The glass transition temperature (T_g) depends on the rate of cooling and below (T_g) the material behaves as a solid like a window glass.

TABLE 3.5 Biomedical Application of Polymeric Biomaterials

Synthetic Polymers	Applications
Polyvinylchloride (PVC)	Blood and solution bag, surgical packaging, IV sets, dialysis devices, catheter bottles, connectors, and cannulae
Polyethylene (PE)	Pharmaceutical bottle, nonwoven fabric, catheter, pouch, flexible container, and orthopedic implants
Polypropylene (PP)	Disposable syringes, blood oxygenator membrane, suture, nonwoven fabric, and artificial vascular grafts
Polymethylmetacrylate (PMMA)	Blood pump and reservoirs, membrane for blood dialyzer, implantable ocular lens, and bone cement
Polystyrene (PS)	Tissue culture flasks, roller bottles, and filterwares
Polyethylenterephthalate (PET)	Implantable suture, mesh, artificial vascular grafts, and heart valve
Polytetrafluoroethylene (PTFE)	Catheter and artificial vascular grafts
Polyurethane (PU)	Film, tubing, and components
Polyamide (nylon)	Packaging film, catheters, sutures, and mold parts

Polyvinylchloride (PVC)

PVC is an amorphous, rigid polymer due to the large side group (Cl, chloride) with a T_g of 75~105°C. It has a high melt viscosity, hence it is difficult to process. To prevent the thermal degradation of the polymer (HCl could be released), thermal stabilizers such as metallic soaps or salts are incorporated. Lubricants are formulated on PVC compounds to prevent adhesion to metal surfaces and facilitate the melt flow during processing. Plasticizers are used in the range of 10 to 100 parts per 100 parts of PVC resin to make it flexible. Di-2-ethylhexylphthalate (DEHP or DOP) is used in medical PVC formulation. However, the plasticizers of trioctyltrimellitate (TOTM), polyester, azelate, and phosphate ester are also used to prevent extraction by blood, aqueous solution, and hot water during autoclaving sterilization.

PVC sheets and films are used in blood and solution storage bags and surgical packaging. PVC tubing is commonly used in intravenous (IV) administration, dialysis devices, catheters, and cannulae.

Polyethylene (PE)

PE is available commercially in five major grades: (1) high density (HDPE), (2) low density (LDPE), (3) linear low density (LLDPE), (4) very low density (VLDPE), and (5) ultra high molecular weight

(UHMWPE). HDPE is polymerized in a low temperature (60~80°C), and at a low pressure (~10 kg/cm^2) using metal catalysts. A highly crystalline, linear polymer with a density ranging from 0.94 to 0.965 g/cm^3 is obtained. LDPE is derived from a high temperature (150~300°C) and pressures (1000~3000 kg/cm^2) using free radical initiators. A highly branched polymer with lower crystallinity and densities ranging from 0.915 to 0.935 g/cm^3 is obtained. LLDPE (density: 0.91~0.94 g/cm^3) and VLDPE (density: 0.88~0.89 g/cm^3), which are linear polymers, are polymerized under low pressures and temperatures using metal catalysts with comonomers such as 1-butene, 1-hexene, or 1-octene to obtain the desired physical properties and density ranges.

HDPE is used in pharmaceutical bottles, nonwoven fabrics, and caps. LDPE is found in flexible container applications, nonwoven disposable and laminated (or coextruded with paper) foil, and polymers for packaging. LLDPE is frequently employed in pouches and bags due to its excellent puncture resistance and VLDPE is used in extruded tubes. UHMWPE (MW > 2 × 10^6 g/mol) has been used for orthopedic implant fabrications, especially for load-bearing applications such as an acetabular cup of total hip and the tibial plateau and patellar surfaces of knee joints. Biocompatability tests for PE are given by ASTM standards in F981, F639, and F755.

Polypropylene (PP)

PP can be polymerized by a Ziegler–Natta stereospecific catalyst which controls the isotactic position of the methyl group. Thermal (T_g: –12°C, T_m: 125~167°C), density (0.85~0.98 g/cm^3), and physical properties of PP are similar to PE. The average molecular weight of commercial PP ranges from 2.2~7.0 × 10^5 g/mol and has a wide molecular weight distribution (polydispersity) which is from 2.6 to 12. Additives for PP such as antioxidants, light stabilizer, nucleating agents, lubricants, mold release agents, antiblock, and slip agents are formulated to improve the physical properties and processability. PP has an exceptionally high flex life and excellent environment stress-cracking resistance, hence it had been tried for finger joint prostheses with an integrally molded hinge design [Park, 1984]. The gas and water vapor permeability of PP are in-between those of LDPE and HDPE. PP is used to make disposable hypothermic syringes; blood oxygenator membrane; packaging for devices, solutions, and drugs; suture; artificial vascular grafts; nonwoven fabrics; etc.

Polymethylmetacrylate (PMMA)

Commercial PMMA is an amorphous (T_g: 105°C and density: 1.15~1.195 g/cm^3) material with good resistance to dilute alkalis and other inorganic solutions. PMMA is best known for its exceptional light transparency (92% transmission), high refractive index (1.49), and good weathering properties and as one of the most biocompatible polymers. PMMA can be easily machined with conventional tools, molded, surface coated, and plasma etched with glow or corona discharge. PMMA is used broadly in medical applications such as a blood pump and reservoir, an IV system, membranes for blood dialyzer, and in *in vitro* diagnostics. It is also found in contact lenses and implantable ocular lenses due to excellent optical properties, dentures, and maxillofacial prostheses due to good physical and coloring properties, and bone cement for joint prostheses fixation (ASTM standard F451).

Other acrylic polymers such as polymethylacrylate (PMA), polyhydroxyethyl-methacrylate (PHEMA), and polyacrylamide (PAAm) are also used in medical applications. PHEMA and PAAm are hydrogels, lightly cross-linked by ethyleneglycoldimethylacrylate (EGDM) to increase their mechanical strength. The extended wear soft contact lenses are synthesized from PMMA and *N*-vinylpyrollidone or PHEMA, which have high water content (above 70%) and a high oxygen permeability.

Polystyrene (PS) and Its Co-Polymers

PS is polymerized by free radical polymerization and is usually atactic. Three grades are available: unmodified general purpose PS (GPPS, T_g: 100°C), high impact PS (HIPS), and PS foam. GPPS has good transparency, lack of color, ease of fabrication, thermal stability, low specific gravity (1.04~1.12 g/cm^3), and relatively high modulus. HIPS contains a rubbery modifier which forms chemical bonding with the growing PS chains. Hence, the ductility and impact strength are increased and the resistance to environmental stress cracking is also improved. PS is mainly processed by injection molding at 180~250°C. To improve processability additives such as stabilizers, lubricants, and mold-releasing agents are formulated. GPPS is commonly used in tissue culture flasks, roller bottles, vacuum canisters, and filterware.

Acrylonitrile-butadiene-styrene (ABS) copolymers are produced by three monomers; acrylonitrile, butadiene, and styrene. The desired physical and chemical properties of ABS polymers with a wide range of functional characteristics can be controlled by changing the ratio of these monomers. They are resistant to the common inorganic solutions and have good surface properties and dimensional stability. ABS is used for IV sets, clamps, blood dialyzers, diagnostic test kits, and so on.

Polyesters

Polyesters such as polyethyleneterephthalate (PET) are frequently found in medical applications due to their unique chemical and physical properties. PET is so far the most important of this group of polymers in terms of biomedical applications such as artificial vascular graft, sutures, and meshes. It is highly crystalline with a high melting temperature (T_m: 265°C), hydrophobic, and resistant to hydrolysis in dilute acids. In addition, PET can be converted by conventional techniques into molded articles such as Luer filters, check valves, and catheter housings. Polycaprolactone is crystalline and has a low melting temperature (T_m: 64°C). Its use as a soft matrix or coating for conventional polyester fibers was proposed by Leininger and Bigg [1986].

Polyamides (Nylons)

Polyamides are known as nylons and are designated by the number of carbon atoms in the repeating units. Nylons can be polymerized by step reaction (or condensation) and ring scission polymerization. They have excellent fiber-forming ability due to interchain hydrogen bonding and a high degree of crystallinity, which increases strength in the fiber direction.

The presence of –CONH– groups in polyamides attracts the chains strongly toward one another by hydrogen bonding. Since the hydrogen bond plays a major role in determining properties, the number and distribution of –CONH– groups are important factors. For example, T_g can be decreased by decreasing the number of –CONH– groups. On the other hand, an increase in the number of –CONH– groups improves physical properties such as strength as one can see that nylon 66 is stronger than nylon 610 and nylon 6 is stronger than nylon 11.

In addition to the higher nylons (610 and 11) there are aromatic polyamides named *aramids*. One of them is poly(*p*-phenylene terephthalate), commonly known as Kevlar®, made by DuPont. This material can be made into fibers. The specific strength of such fibers is five times that of steel; therefore, it is most suitable for making composites.

Nylons are hygroscopic and lose their strength *in vivo* when implanted. The water molecules serve as plasticizers which attack the amorphous region. Proteolytic enzymes also aid in hydrolyzing by attacking the amide group. This is probably due to the fact that the proteins also contain the amide group along their molecular chains which the proteolytic enzymes could attack.

Fluorocarbon Polymers

The best known fluorocarbon polymer is polytetrafluoroethylene (PTFE), commonly known as Teflon® (DuPont). Other polymers containing fluorine are polytrifluorochloroethylene (PTFCE), polyvinylfluoride (PVF), and fluorinated ethylene propylene (FEP). Only PTFE will be discussed here since the others have rather inferior chemical and physical properties and are rarely used for implant fabrication.

PTFE is made from tetrafluoroethylene under pressure with a peroxide catalyst in the presence of excess water for removal of heat. The polymer is highly crystalline (over 94% crystallinity) with an average molecular weight of $0.5~5 \times 10^6$ g/mol. This polymer has a very high density (2.15~2.2 g/cm^3) and low modulus of elasticity (0.5 GPa) and tensile strength (14 MPa). It also has a very low surface tension (18.5 erg/cm^2) and friction coefficient (0.1).

Standard specifications for the implantable PTFE are given by ASTM F754. PTFE also has an unusual property of being able to expand on a microscopic scale into a microporous material which is an excellent thermal insulator. PTFE cannot be injection molded or melt extruded because of its very high melt viscosity and it cannot be plasticized. Usually the powders are sintered to above 327°C under pressure to produce implants.

Rubbers

Silicone, natural, and synthetic rubbers have been used for the fabrication of implants. Natural rubber is made mostly from the latex of the *Hevea brasiliensis* tree and the chemical formula is the same as that of *cis*-1,4 polyisoprene. Natural rubber was found to be compatible with blood in its pure form. Also, cross-linking by x-ray and organic peroxides produces rubber with superior blood compatibility compared with rubbers made by the conventional sulfur vulcanization.

Synthetic rubbers were developed to substitute for natural rubber. The Ziegler–Natta types of stereospecific polymerization techniques have made this variety possible. The synthetic rubbers have rarely been used to make implants. The physical properties vary widely due to the wide variations in preparation recipes of these rubbers.

Silicone rubber, developed by Dow Corning company, is one of the few polymers developed for medical use. The repeating unit is dimethyl siloxane which is polymerized by a condensation polymerization. Low molecular weight polymers have low viscosity and can be cross-linked to make a higher molecular weight, rubber-like material. Medical grade silicone rubbers contain stannous octate as a catalyst and can be mixed with a base polymer at the time of implant fabrication.

Polyurethanes

Polyurethanes are usually thermosetting polymers: they are widely used to coat implants. Polyurethane rubbers are produced by reacting a prepared prepolymer chain with an aromatic di-isocyanate to make very long chains possessing active isocyanate groups for cross-linking. The polyurethane rubber is quite strong and has good resistance to oil and chemicals.

Polyacetal, Polysulfone, and Polycarbonate

These polymers have excellent mechanical, thermal, and chemical properties due to their stiffened main backbone chains. Polyacetals and polysulfones are being tested as implant materials, while polycarbonates have found their applications in heart/lung assist devices, food packaging, etc.

Polyacetals are produced by reacting formaldehyde. These are also sometimes called polyoxymethylene (POM) and known widely as Delrin® (DuPont). These polymers have a reasonably high molecular weight ($>2 \times 10^4$ g/mol) and have excellent mechanical properties. More importantly, they display an excellent resistance to most chemicals and to water over wide temperature ranges.

Polysulfones were developed by Union Carbide in the 1960s. These polymers have a high thermal stability due to the bulky side groups (therefore, they are amorphous) and rigid main backbone chains. They are also highly stable to most chemicals but are not so stable in the presence of polar organic solvents such as ketones and chlorinated hydrocarbons.

Polycarbonates are tough, amorphous, and transparent polymers made by reacting bisphenol A and diphenyl carbonate. It is noted for its excellent mechanical and thermal properties (high T_g: 150°C), hydrophobicity, and antioxidative properties.

Biodegradable Polymers

Several biodegradable polymers such as polylactide (PLA), polyglycolide (PGA), poly(glycolide-*co*-lactide) (PLGA), poly(dioxanone), poly(trimethylene carbonate), poly(carbonate), and so on have been used extensively or tested on a wide range of medical applications due to their good biocompatibility, controllable biodegradability, and relatively good processability [Khang et al., 1997a]. PLA, PGA, and PLGA are bioresorbable polyesters belonging to the group of poly α-hydroxy acids. These polymers degrade by nonspecific hydrolytic scission of their ester bonds. The hydrolysis of PLA yields lactic acid, which is a normal byproduct of anaerobic metabolism in the human body and is incorporated in the tricarboxylic acid (TCA) cycle to be finally excreted by the body as carbon dioxide and water. PGA biodegrades by a combination of hydrolytic scission and enzymatic (esterase) action producing glycolic acid which either can enter the TCA cycle or is excreted in urine and can be eliminated as carbon dioxide and water. The degradation time of PLGA can be controlled from weeks to over a year by varying the ratio of monomers and the processing conditions. It might be a suitable biomaterial for use in tissue engineered repair systems in which cells are implanted within PLGA films or scaffolds and in drug delivery systems in which drugs are loaded within PLGA microspheres. PGA (T_m: 225–230°C, T_g: 35–40°C) can be melt spun into fibers which can be converted into bioresorbable sutures, meshes, and surgical products. PLA (T_m: 173–178°C, T_g: 60–65°C) exhibits high tensile strength and low elongation resulting in a high modulus suitable for load-bearing applications such as in bone fracture fixation. Poly-p-dioxanone (T_m: 107–112°C, T_g: ~10°C) is a bioabsorbable polymer that can be fabricated into flexible monofilament surgical sutures.

3.4 Sterilization

Sterilizability of biomedical polymers is an important aspect of the properties because polymers have lower thermal and chemical stability than other materials such as ceramics and metals, consequently, they are also more difficult to sterilize using conventional techniques. Commonly used sterilization techniques are dry heat, autoclaving, radiation, and ethylene oxide gas [Block, 1977].

In dry heat sterilization, the temperature varies between 160 and 190°C. This is above the melting and softening temperatures of many linear polymers such as polyethylene and PMMA. In the case of polyamide (nylon), oxidation will occur at the dry sterilization temperature although this is below its melting temperature. The only polymers which can safely be dry sterilized are PTFE and silicone rubber.

Steam sterilization (autoclaving) is performed under high steam pressure at relatively low temperature (125–130°C). However, if the polymer is subjected to attack by water vapor, this method cannot be employed. PVC, polyacetals, PE (low-density variety), and polyamides belong to this category.

Chemical agents such as ethylene and propylene oxide gases [Glaser, 1979] and phenolic and hypochloride solutions are widely used for sterilizing polymers since they can be used at low temperatures. Chemical agents sometimes cause polymer deterioration even when sterilization takes place at room temperature. However, the time of exposure is relatively short (overnight), and most polymeric implants can be sterilized with this method.

Radiation sterilization [Sato, 1983] using the isotopic ^{60}Co can also deteriorate polymers since at high dosage the polymer chains can be dissociated or cross-linked according to the characteristics of the chemical structures, as shown in Table 3.6. In the case of PE, at high dosage (above 10^6 Gy) it becomes a brittle and hard material. This is due to a combination of random chain scission cross-linking. PP articles will often discolor during irradiation giving the product an undesirable color tint but the more severe problem is the embrittlement resulting in flange breakage, Luer cracking, and tip breakage. The physical properties continue to deteriorate with time, following irradiation. These problems of coloration and changing physical properties are best resolved by avoiding the use of any additives that discolor at the sterilizing dose of radiation [Khang et al., 1996c].

3.5 Surface Modifications for Improving Biocompatability

Prevention of thrombus formation is important in clinical applications where blood is in contact such as hemodialysis membranes and tubes, artificial heart and heart–lung machines, prosthetic valves, and

TABLE 3.6 Effect of Gamma Irradiation on Polymers
That Could Be Cross-Linked or Degraded

Cross-Linking Polymers	Degradable Polymers
Polyethylene	Polyisobutylene
Polypropylene	Poly-α–methylstyrene
Polystyrene	Polymethylmetacrylate
Polyarylates	Polymethacrylamide
Polyacrylamide	Polyvinylidenechloride
Polyvinylchloride	Cellulose and derivatives
Polyamides	Polytetrafluoroethylene
Polyesters	Polytrifluorochloroethylene
Polyvinylpyrrolidone	
Polymethacrylamide	
Rubbers	
Polysiloxanes	
Polyvinylalcohol	
Polyacroleine	

artificial vascular grafts. In spite of the use of anticoagulants, considerable platelet deposition and thrombus formation take place on the artificial surfaces [Branger, 1990].

Heparin, one of the complex carbohydrates known as mucopolysaccharides or glycosaminoglycan, is currently used to prevent formation of clots. In general, heparin is well tolerated and devoid of serious consequences. However, it allows platelet adhesion to foreign surfaces and may cause hemorrhagic complications such as subdural hematoma, retroperitoneal hematoma, gastrointestinal bleeding, hemorrage into joints, ocular and retinal bleeding, and bleeding at surgical sites [Lazarus, 1980]. These difficulties give rise to an interest in developing new methods of hemocompatible materials.

Many different groups have studied immobilization of heparin [Kim and Feijen, 1985; Park et al., 1988] on the polymeric surfaces, heparin analogs and heparin–prostaglandin or heparin–fibrinolytic enzyme conjugates [Jozefowicz and Jozefowicz, 1985]. The major drawback of these surfaces is that they are not stable in the blood environment. It has not been firmly established that a slow leakage of heparin is needed for it to be effective as an immobilized antithrombogenic agent; if not, its effectiveness could be hindered by being "coated over" with an adsorbed layer of more common proteins such as albumin and fibrinogen. Fibrinolytic enzymes, urokinase, and various prostaglandins have also been immobilized by themselves in order to take advantage of their unique fibrin dissolution or antiplatelet aggregation actions [Ohshiro, 1983].

Albumin-coated surfaces have been studied because surfaces that resisted platelet adhesion *in vitro* were noted to adsorb albumin preferentially [Keogh et al., 1992]. Fibronectin coatings have been used in *in vitro* endothelial cell seeding to prepare a surface similar to the natural blood vessel lumen [Lee et al., 1989]. Also, algin-coated surfaces have been studied due to their good biocompatibility and biodegradability [Lee et al., 1990b; Lee et al., 1997b].

Recently, plasma gas discharge [Khang et al., 1997a] and corona treatment [Khang et al., 1996d] with reactive groups introduced on the polymeric surfaces have emerged as other ways to modify biomaterial surfaces [Lee et al., 1991; Lee et al., 1992].

Hydrophobic coatings composed of silicon- and fluorine-containing polymeric materials as well as polyurethanes have been studied because of the relatively good clinical performances of Silastic®, Teflon®, and polyurethane polymers in cardiovascular implants and devices. Polymeric fluorocarbon coatings deposited from a tetrafluoroethylene gas discharge have been found to greatly enhance resistance to both acute thrombotic occlusion and embolization in small diameter Dacron® grafts.

Hydrophilic coatings have also been popular because of their low interfacial tension in biological environments [Hoffman, 1981]. Hydrogels as well as various combinations of hydrophilic and hydrophobic monomers have been studied on the premise that there will be an optimum polar-dispersion force ratio which could be matched on the surfaces of the most passivating proteins. The passive surface

TABLE 3.7   Physical and Chemical Surface Modification Methods for Polymeric Biomaterials

To modify blood compatibility	Octadecyl group attachment to surface
	Silicon containing block copolymer additive
	Plasma fluoropolymer deposition
	Plasma siloxane polymer deposition
	Radiation-grafted hydrogels
	Chemically modified polystyrene for heparin-like activity
To influence cell adhesion and growth	Oxidized polystyrene surface
	Ammonia plasma-treated surface
	Plasma-deposited acetone or methanol film
	Plasma fluoropolymer deposition
To control protein adsorption	Surface with immobilized polyethyelenglycol
	Treated ELISA dish surface
	Affinity chromatography particulates
	Surface cross-linked contact lens
To improve lubricity	Plasma treatment
	Radiation-grafted hydrogels
	Interpenetrating polymeric networks
To improve wear resistance and corrosion resistance	Ion implantation
	Diamond deposition
	Anodization
To alter transport properties	Plasma deposition (methane, fluoropolymer, siloxane)
To modify electrical characteristics	Plasma deposition
	Solvent coatings
	Parylene coatings

Source: Ratner et al. [1996], p. 106.

may induce less clot formation. Polyethylene oxide coated surfaces have been found to resist protein adsorption and cell adhesion and have therefore been proposed as potential "blood compatible" coatings [Lee et al., 1990a]. General physical and chemical methods to modify the surfaces of polymeric biomaterials are listed in Table 3.7 [Ratner et al., 1996].

Another way of making antithrombogenic surfaces is the saline perfusion method, which is designed to prevent direct contacts between blood and the surface of biomaterials by means of perfusing saline solution through the porous wall which is in contact with blood [Park and Kim, 1993; Khang et al., 1996a; Khang et al., 1996b]. It has been demonstrated that the adhesion of the blood cells could be prevented by the saline perfusion through PE, alumina, sulfonated/nonsulfonated PS/SBR, ePTFE (expanded polytetrafluoroethylene), and polysulfone porous tubes.

3.6   Chemogradient Surfaces for Cell and Protein Interaction

The behavior of the adsorption and desorption of blood proteins or adhesion and proliferation of different types of mammalian cells on polymeric materials depends on the surface characteristics such as wettability, hydrophilicity/hydrophobicity ratio, bulk chemistry, surface charge and charge distribution, surface roughness, and rigidity.

Many research groups have studied the effect of the surface wettability on the interactions of biological species with polymeric materials. Some have studied the interactions of different types of cultured cells or blood proteins with various polymers with different wettabilities to correlate the surface wettability and blood or tissue compatibility [Baier et al., 1984]. One problem encountered from the study using different kinds of polymers is that the surfaces were heterogeneous, both chemically and physically (different surface chemistry, roughness, rigidity, crystallinity, etc.), which caused widely varying results. Some others have studied the interactions of different types of cells or proteins with a range of methacrylate copolymers with different wettabilities and have the same kind of chemistry but are still physically

FIGURE 3.6 Schematic diagram showing corona discharge apparatus for the preparation of wettability chemogradient surfaces.

heterogeneous [van Wachem et al., 1987]. Another methodological problem is that such studies are often tedious, laborious, and time consuming because a large number of samples must be prepared to characterize the complete range of the desired surface properties.

Many studies have been focused on the preparation of surfaces whose properties are changed gradually along the material length. Such chemogradient surfaces are of particular interest in basic studies of the interactions between biological species and synthetic materials surfaces since the affect of a selected property can be examined in a single experiment on one surface preparation. A chemogradient of methyl groups was formed by diffusion of dimethyldichlorosilane through xylene on flat hydrophilic siliconedioxide surfaces [Elwing et al., 1989]. The wettability chemogradient surfaces were made to investigate hydrophilicity-induced changes of adsorbed proteins.

Recently, a method for preparing wettability chemogradients on various polymer surfaces was developed [Lee et al., 1989 and 1990; Khang et al., 1997b]. The wettability chemogradients were produced via radio frequency (RF) and plasma discharge treatment by exposing the polymer sheets continuously to the plasma [Lee et al., 1991]. The polymer surfaces oxidized gradually along the sample length with increasing plasma exposure time and thus the wettability chemogradient was created. Another method for preparing a wettability chemogradient on polymer surfaces using corona discharge treatment has been developed as shown in Fig. 3.6 [Lee et al., 1992]. The wettability chemogradient was produced by treating the polymer sheets with corona from a knife-type electrode whose power was gradually changed along the sample length. The polymer surface gradually oxidized with the increasing power and the wettability chemogradient was created. Chemogradient surfaces with different functional gruops such as $-COOH$, $-CH_2OH$, $-CONH_2$, and $-CH_2NH_2$ were produced on PE surfaces by the above corona treatment followed by vinyl monomer grafting and substitution reactions [Kim et al., 1993; Lee et al.,1994a; Lee et al.,1994b]. We have also prepared chargeable functional groups [Lee et al., 1997c; Lee et al., 1997d; Lee et al., 1998a], comb-like polyethyleneoxide (PEO) [Jeong et al., 1996; Lee et al., 1997a], and phospholipid polymer chemogradient surfaces [Iwasaki et al., 1997] by the corona discharge treatment, followed by graft copolymerization with subsequent substitution reaction of functional vinyl monomers as acrylic acid, sodium *p*-sulfonic styrene, and *N, N*-dimethyl aminopropyl acrylamide, poly(ethyleneglycol) mono-methacrylate, and ω-methacryloyloxyalkyl phosphorylcholine (MAPC), respectively.

The water contact angles of the corona-treated PE surfaces gradually decrease along the sample length with increasing corona power (from about 95° to about 45°) as shown in Fig. 3.7. The decrease in contact angles, i.e., the increase in wettability along the sample length, was due to the oxygen-based polar functionalities incorporated on the surface by the corona treatment. It was also confirmed also by Fourier-transform infrared spectroscopy in the attenuated total reflectance mode and electron spectroscopy for chemical analysis (ESCA).

FIGURE 3.7 Changes in water contact angle of corona-treated PE surface along the sample length. Sample number $n = 3$.

In order to investigate the interaction of different types of cells in terms of the surface hydrophilicity/hydrophobicity of polymeric materials, Chinese hamster ovaries (CHOs), fibroblasts, and bovine aortic endothelial cells (ECs) were cultured for 1 and 2 days on the PE wettability chemogradient surfaces. The maximum adhesion and growth of the cells appeared around a water contact angle of 50–55° as shown in Fig. 3.8. The observation of scanning electron microscopy (SEM) also verified that the cells are more adhered, spread, and grown onto the sections with moderate hydrophilicity as shown in Fig. 3.9.

FIGURE 3.8 CHO, fibroblast, and endothelial cell growth on wettability chemogradient PE surfaces after 2 days of culture (number of seeded cells, $4 \times 10^4/cm^2$); $n = 3$.

FIGURE 3.9 SEM microphotographs of CHO, fibroblast, and endothelial cells grown on PE wettability chemogradient surface along the sample length after 2 days culture (original magnification: 400×).

To determine the cell proliferation rates, the migration of fibroblasts on PE wettability chemogradient surfaces was observed [Khang et al., 1998b]. After the change of culture media at 24 h, cell growth morphology was recorded for 1- or 2-h intervals at the position of 0.5, 1.5, 2.5, and 4.5 cm for the counting of grown cells and the observation of cell morphology with a video tape recorder. The proliferation rates of fibroblast cells were calculated from the slopes of Fig. 3.10 as given in Table 3.8. The proliferation rates on the PE surfaces with wettability chemogradient showed that as the surface wettability increased, the adsorption of nitrogen increased and then decreased (see Fig. 3.11). The maximum proliferation rate of the cells as 1111 cells/h·cm² appeared at around the position 2.5 cm.

To observe the effect of serum proteins on the cell adhesion and growth behaviors, fetal bovine serum (FBS), which contains more than 200 kinds of different proteins, was adsorbed onto the wettability gradient PE surfaces for 1 h at 37°C. Figure 3.11 shows the relative adsorbed amount of serum proteins on the wettability gradient surfaces determined by ESCA. The maximum adsorption of the proteins appeared at around the 2.5-cm position, which is the same trend as the cell adhesion, growth, and migration behaviors. It can be explained that preferential adsorption of some serum proteins, such as fibronectin and vitronectin from culture medium, onto the moderately wettable surfaces may be a reason for better cell adhesion, spreading, and growth. Proteins such as fibronectin and vitronectin are well known as cell-adhesive proteins. Cells attached on surfaces are spread only when they are compatible on the surfaces. It seems that surface wettability plays an important role for cell adhesion, spreading, and migration.

Also investigated were: (1) platelet adhesion on wettability chemogradient [Lee and Lee, 1998], (2) cell interaction on microgrooved PE surfaces (groove depth, 0.5 μm; groove width, 0.45 μm; and pitch, 0.9 μm) with wettability chemogradient [Khang et al., 1997c], (3) detachment of human endothelial

FIGURE 3.10   Fibroblast cell proliferation rates on wettability chemogradient PE surfaces (24- to 60-h culture).

TABLE 3.8. Proliferation Rates of Fibroblast Cells on Wettability Gradient
PE Surfaces

Position (cm)	Contact Angle (°)	Cell Proliferation Rate (cells/h·cm²)
2.5	55	1,111
4.5	45	924
1.5	67	838
0.5	85	734

Note: 24- to 60-h culture.

FIGURE 3.11   Serum protein adsorption on PE wettability chemogradient surface (1-h adsorption); $n = 3$.

under flow from wettability gradient surface with different functional groups [Ruardy et al., 1997], (4) cell interaction on microporous polycarbonate membrane with wettability chemogradient [Lee et al., 1999], and (5) cell interaction on poly(lactide-*co*-glycolide) surface with wettability chemogradient [Khang et al., 1998a].

During the last several years, "chemogradient surfaces" have evolved into easier-to-use and more popular tools for the study of protein adsorption and platelet or cell interactions continuously which relate to the surface properties such as wettability, chemistry and charge, or dynamics of polymeric materials. In many studies, different kinds of polymeric materials with widely varying surface chemistries are used and the explanation of the results is often controversial due to the surface heterogeneity. In addition, these studies are tedious, laborious, and time consuming, and biological variations are more likely to occur. The application of chemogradient surfaces for these studies can reduce these discomforts and problems and eventually save time and money. Also, chemogradient surfaces are valuable in investigating the basic mechanisms by which complicated systems such as proteins or cells interact with surfaces, since a continuum of selected and controlled physical–chemical properties can be studied in one experiment on the polymeric surface.

The possible applications of chemogradient surfaces in the near future are: (1) separation devices of cells and/or biological species by different surface properties, (2) column packing materials for separation, and (3) biosensoring.

Acknowledgments

This work was supported by grants from the Korea Ministry of Health and Welfare (grant nos. HMP-95-G-2-33 and HMP-97-E-0016) and the Korea Ministry of Science and Technology (grant no. 97-N1-02-05-A-02).

Defining Terms

Acetabulum: The socket portion of the hip joint.

Addition (or free radical) polymerization: Polymerization in which monomers are added to the growing chains, initiated by free radical agents.

Biocompatibility: Acceptance of an artificial implant by the surrounding tissues and as a whole. The implant should be compatible with tissues in terms of mechanical, chemical, surface, and pharmacological properties.

Biomaterials: Synthetic materials used to replace part of a living system or to function in intimate contact with living tissue.

Bone cement: Mixture of polymethylmethacrylate powder and methylmethacrylate monomer liquid to be used as a grouting material for the fixation of orthopedic joint implants.

Branching: Chains grown from the sides of the main backbone chains.

Chemogradient surface: The surface whose properties such as wettability, surface charge, and hydrophilicity/hydrophobicity ratio are changed gradually along the material length.

Condensation (step reaction) polymerization: Polymerization in which two or more chemicals are reacted to form a polymer by condensing out small molecules such as water and alcohol.

Copolymers: Polymers made from two or more monomers which can be obtained by grafting, block, alternating, or random attachment of the other polymer segment.

Covalent bonding: Bonding of atoms or molecules by sharing valence electrons.

Dacron®:   Polyethyleneterephthalate polyester that is made into fiber. If the same polymer is made into a film, it is called Mylar®.

Delrin®:   Polyacetal made by Union Carbide.

Elastomers: Rubbery materials. The restoring force comes from uncoiling or unkinking of coiled or kinked molecular chains. They can be highly stretched.

Embolus: Any foreign matter, as a blood clot or air bubble, carried in the blood stream.

Fibrinogen: A plasma protein of high molecular weight that is converted to fibrin through the action of thrombin. This material is used to make (absorbable) tissue adhesives.

Filler: Materials added as a powder to a rubber to improve its mechanical properties.

Free volume: The difference in volume occupied by the crystalline state (minimum) and noncrystalline state of a material for a given temperature and a pressure.

Glass transition temperature: Temperature at which solidification without crystallization takes place from viscous liquid.

Grafts: A transplant.

Heparin: A substance found in various body tissues, especially in the liver, that prevents the clotting of blood.

Hydrogel: Polymer which can absorb 30% or more of its weight in water.

Hydrogen bonding: A secondary bonding through dipole interactions in which the hydrogen ion is one of the dipoles.

Hydroquinone: Chemical inhibitor added to the bone cement liquid monomer to prevent accidental polymerization during storage.

Initiator: Chemical used to initiate the addition polymerization by becoming a free radical which in turn reacts with a monomer.

Ionic bonding: Bonding of atoms or molecules through electrostatic interaction of positive and negative ions.

Kevlar®:   Aromatic polyamides made by DuPont.

Lexan®:   Polycarbonate made by General Electric.

Oxygenator: An apparatus by which oxygen is introduced into blood during circulation outside the body, as during open-heart surgery.

Plasticizer: Substance made of small molecules, mixed with (amorphous) polymers to make the chains slide more easily past each other, making the polymer less rigid.

Refractive index: Ratio of speed of light in vacuum to speed of light in a material. It is a measure of the ability of a material to refract (bend) a beam of light.

Repeating unit: Basic molecular unit that can represent a polymer backbone chain. The average number of repeating units is called the degree of polymerization.

Semicrystalline solid: Solid which contains both crystalline and noncrystalline regions and usually occurs in polymers due to their long chain molecules.

Side group: Chemical group attached to the main backbone chain. It is usually shorter than the branches and exists before polymerization.

Steric hindrance: Geometrical interference which restrains movements of molecular groups such as side chains and main chains of a polymer.

Suture: Material used in closing a wound with stitches.

Tacticity: Arrangement of asymmetrical side groups along the backbone chain of polymers. Groups could be distributed at random (atactic), on one side (isotactic), or alternating (syndiotactic).

Teflon®:   Polytetrafluoroethylene made by DuPont.

Thrombus: The fibrinous clot attached at the site of thrombosis.

Udel®:   Polysulfone made by General Electric.

Valence electrons: The outermost (shell) electrons of an atom.

van der Waals bonding: A secondary bonding arising through the fluctuating dipole–dipole interactions.

Vinyl polymers: Thermoplastic linear polymers synthesized by free radical polymerization of vinyl monomers having a common structure of $CH_2=CHR$.

Vulcanization: Cross-linking of a (natural) rubber by adding sulfur.

Ziegler–Natta catalyst: Organometallic compounds which have the remarkable capacity of polymerizing a wide variety of monomers to linear and stereoregular polymers.

References

Baier, R.E., Meyer, A.E., Natiella, J.R., Natiella, R.R., and Carter, J.M. 1984. Surface properties determine bioadhesive outcomes: methods and results, *J. Biomed. Mater. Res.*, 18:337–355

Billmeyer, F.W. Jr. 1984. *Textbook of Polymer Science*, 3rd ed., John Wiley & Sons, New York.

Block, S.S., Ed. 1977. *Disinfection, Sterilization, and Preservation*, 2nd ed., Lea & Febiger, Philadelphia, PA.

Bloch, B. and Hastings, G.W. 1972. *Plastic Materials in Surgery*, 2nd ed., Charles C Thomas, Springfield, IL.

Brandrup, J. and Immergut, E.H., Eds. 1989. *Polymer Handbook*, 3rd ed., Wiley-Interscience, New York.

Branger, B., Garreau, M., Baudin, G., and Gris, J.C. 1990. Biocompatibility of blood tubings, *Int. J. Artif. Organs*, 13(10):697–703.

Dumitriu, S., Ed. 1993. *Polymeric Biomaterials*, Marcel Dekker, New York.

Elwing, E., Askendal, A., and Lundstorm, I. 1989. Desorption of fibrinogen and γ-globulin from solid surfaces induced by a nonionic detergent, *J. Colloid Interface Sci.*, 128:296–300.

Glaser, Z.R. 1979. Ethylene oxide: toxicology review and field study results of hospital use, *J. Environ. Pathol. Toxicol.*, 2:173–208.

Hoffman, A.S. 1981. Radiation processing in biomaterials: a review, *Radiat. Phys. Chem.*, 18(1):323–340.

Ikada, Y., Ed. 1989. Bioresorbable fibers for medical use. In: *High Technology Fiber*, Part B, Marcel Dekker, New York.

Iwasaki, Y., Ishihara, K., Nakabayashi, N., Khang, G., Jeon, J.H., Lee, J.W., and Lee, H.B. 1997. Preparation of gradient surfaces grafted with phospholipid polymers and evaluation of their blood compatibility. In: *Advances in Biomaterials Science*, Vol. 1, T. Akaike, T. Okano, M. Akashi, M. Terano, and N. Yui, Eds., pp. 91–100. CMC, Tokyo.

Jeong, B.J., Lee, J.H., and Lee, H.B. 1996. Preparation and characterization of comb-like PEO gradient surfaces, *J. Colloid Interface Sci.*, 178:757–763.

Jozefowicz, M. and Jozefowicz, J. 1985. New approaches to anticoagulation: heparin-like biomaterials, *J. Am. Soc. Art. Intern. Org.* 8:218–222.

Keogh, J.R., Valender, F.F., and Eaton J.W. 1992. Albumin-binding surfaces for implantable devices, *J. Biomed. Mater. Res.*, 26:357–372.

Khang, G., Park J.B., and Lee, H.B. 1996a. Prevention of platelet adhesion on the polysulfone porous catheter by saline perfusion. I. *In vitro* investigation, *Bio-Med. Mater. Eng.*, 6(1):47–66.

Khang, G., Park, J.B., and Lee, H.B. 1996b. Prevention of platelet adhesion on the polysulfone porous catheter by saline perfusion. II. *Ex vivo* and *in vivo* investigation, *Bio-Med. Mater. Eng.*, 6(2):123–134.

Khang, G., Lee, H.B., and Park, J.B. 1996c. Radiation effects on polypropylene for sterilization, *Bio-Med. Mater. Eng.*, 6(5):323–334.

Khang, G., Kang, Y.H., Park, J.B., and Lee, H.B. 1996d. Improved bonding strength of polyethylene/polymethylmetacrylate bone cement—a preliminary study, *Bio-Med. Mater. Eng.*, 6(5):335–344.

Khang, G., Jeon, J.H., Lee, J.W., Cho, S.C., and Lee, H.B. 1997a. Cell and platelet adhesion on plasma glow discharge-treated poly(lactide-*co*-glycolide), *Bio-Med. Mater. Eng.*, 7(6):357–368.

Khang, G., Lee, J.H., and Lee, H.B. 1997b. Cell and platelet adhesion on gradient surfaces. In: *Advances in Biomaterials Science*, Vol. 1, T. Akaike, T. Okano, M. Akashi, Terano, and N. Yui, Eds., pp. 63–70. CMC, Tokyo.

Khang, G., Lee, J.W., Jeon, J.H., Lee, J.H., and Lee, H.B. 1997c. Interaction of fibroblasts on microgrooved polyethylene surfaces with wettabililty gradient, *Biomater. Res.*, 1(1):1–6.

Khang, G., Cho, S.Y., Lee, J.H., Rhee, J.M., and Lee, H.B. 1998a. Interactions of fibroblast, osteoblast, hepatoma, and endothelial cells on poly(lactide-*co*-glycolide) surface with chemogradient, 2nd Ann. Meeting Tissue Eng. Soc., Orlando, FL.

Khang, G., Jeon, J.H., and Lee, H.B. 1998b. Fibroblast cell migration on polyethylene wettability chemogradient surfaces, 24th Ann. Meeting Soc. for Biomaterials, San Diego, CA.

Kim, H.G., Lee, J.H., Lee, H.B., and Jhon, M.S. 1993. Dissociation behavior of surface-grafted poly(acrylic acid): effects of surface density and counterion size, *J. Colloid Interface Sci.*, 157(1):82–87.

Kim, S.W. and Feijen, J. 1985. Surface modification of polymers for improved blood biocompatibility, *CRC Crit. Rev. Biocompat.*, 1(3):229–260.

Lazarus, J.M. 1980. Complications in hemodialysis: an overview, *Kidney Int.*, 18:783–796.

Lee, H.B. 1989. Application of synthetic polymers in implants. In: *Frontiers of Macromolecular Science*, T. Seagusa, T., Higashimura, and A. Abe, Eds., pp. 579–584. Blackwell Scientific, Oxford.

Lee, H.B. and Lee, J.H. 1995. Biocompatibility of solid substrates based on surface wettability, In: *Encyclopedic Handbook of Biomaterials and Bioengineering: Materials*, Vol. 1, D.L. Wise, D.J. Trantolo, D.E. Altobelli, M.J. Yasemski, J.D. Gresser, and E.R. Schwartz, Eds., pp. 371–398. Marcel Dekker, New York.

Lee, J.H. and Lee, H.B. 1998. Platelet adhesion onto wettability gradient surfaces in the absence and presence of plasma protein, *J. Biomed. Mater. Res.*, 41:304–311.

Lee, J.H., Khang, G., Park, K.H., Lee, H.B., and Andrade, J.D. 1989. Polymer surfaces for cell adhesion: I. Surface modification of polymers and ESCA analysis, *J. Korea Soc. Med. Biolog. Eng.*, 10(1):43–51.

Lee, J.H., Khang, G., Park, J.W., and Lee, H.B. 1990a. Plasma protein adsorption on polyethyleneoxide gradient surfaces, 33rd IUPAC Inter. Symp. on Macromolecules, July 8–13, Montreal, Canada.

Lee, J.H., Shin, B.C., Khang, G., and Lee, H.B. 1990b. Algin impregnated vascular graft: I. *In vitro* investigation, *J. Korea Soc. Med. Biolog. Eng.*, 11(1):97–104.

Lee, J.H., Park, J.W., and Lee, H.B. 1991. Cell adhesion and growth on polymer surfaces with hydroxyl groups prepared by water vapor plasma treatment, *Biomaterials*, 12:443–448.

Lee, J.H., Kim, H.G., Khang, G., Lee, H.B., and Jhon, M.S. 1992. Characterization of wettability gradient surfaces prepared by corona discharge treatment, *J. Colloid Interface Sci.*, 151(2):563–570.

Lee, J.H., Kim, H.W., Pak, P.K., and Lee, H.B. 1994a. Preparation and characterization of functional group gradient surfaces, *J. Polym. Sci., Part A, Polym. Chem.*, 32:1569–1579.

Lee, J.H., Jung, H.W., Kang, I.K., and Lee, H.B. 1994b. Cell behavior on polymer surfaces with different functional groups, *Biomaterials*, 15:705–711.

Lee, J.H., Jeong, B.J., and Lee, H.B. 1997a. Plasma protein adsorption and platelet adhesion onto comb-like PEO gradient surface, *J. Biomed. Mater. Res.*, 34:105–114.

Lee, J.H., Kim W.G., Kim, S.S., Lee, J.H., and Lee, H.B. 1997b. Development and characterization of an alginate-impregnated polyester vascular graft, *J. Biomed. Mater. Res.*, 36:200–208.

Lee, J.H., Khang, G., Lee, J.H., and Lee, H.B. 1997c. Interactions of protein and cells on functional group gradient surfaces, *Macromol. Symp.*, 118:571–576.

Lee, J.H., Khang, G., Lee, J.H., and Lee, H.B. 1997d. Interactions of cells on chargeable functional group gradient surfaces, *Biomaterials*, 18(4):351–358.

Lee, J.H., Khang, G., Lee, J.H., and Lee, H.B. 1998. Platelet adhesion onto chargeable functional group gradient surfaces, *J. Biomed. Mater. Res.*, 40:180–186.

Lee, J.H., Lee, S.J., Khang, G., and Lee, H.B. 1999. Interactions of cells onto microporous polycarbonate membrane with wettability gradient surfaces, *J. Biomat. Sci., Polm. Edn.*, 10:283–294.

Leininger, R.I. and Bigg, D.M. 1986. Polymers. In: *Handbook of Biomaterials Evaluation*, pp. 24–37. Macmillan, New York.

Oshiro, T. 1983. Thrombosis, antithrombogenic characteristics of immobilized urokinase on synthetic polymers. In: *Biocompatible Polymers, Metals, and Composites*, M. Szycher, Ed., pp. 275–299. Technomic, Lancaster, PA.

Park, J.B. 1984. *Biomaterials Science and Engineering*, Plenum Press, New York.

Park, J.B. and Kim S.S. 1993. Prevention of mural thrombus in porous inner tube of double-layered tube by saline perfusion, *Bio-Medical Mater. Eng.*, 3:101–116.

Park, J.B. and Lakes, R. 1992. *Biomaterials: An Introduction*, 2nd ed., pp. 141–168. Plenum Press, New York.

Park, K.D., Okano, T., Nojiri, C., and Kim S.W. 1988. Heparin immobilized onto segmented polyurethane effect of hydrophillic spacers, *J. Biomed. Mater. Res.*, 22:977–992.

Ratner, B.D., Hoffman, A.S., Schoen, F.J., and Lemons, J.E. 1996. *Biomaterials Science: An Introduction to Materials in Medicine*, Academic Press, New York.

Raurdy, T.G., Moorlag, H.E., Schkenraad, J.M., van der Mei, H.C., and Busscher, H.J. 1997. Detachment of human endothelial under flow from wettability gradient surface with different functional groups, *Cell Mater.*, 7:123–133.

Sato, K. 1983. Radiation sterilization of medical products, *Radioisotopes*, 32:431–439.

Shalaby, W.S. 1988. Polymeric materials. In: *Encyclopedia of Medical Devices and Instruments*, J.G. Webster, Ed., pp. 2324–2335, Wiley-Interscience, New York.

Sharma, C.P. and Szycher, M. Eds. 1991. *Blood Compatible Materials and Devices: Perspectives Toward the 21st Century*, Technomic, Lancaster, PA.

van Wachem, P.B., Beugeling. T., Feijen, J., Bantjes, A., Detmers, J.P., and van Aken, W.G. 1985. Interaction of cultured human endothelial cells with polymeric surfaces of different wettabilities, *Biomaterials*, 6:403–408.

4

Composite Biomaterials

Roderic S. Lakes
University of Wisconsin-Madison

Composite materials are solids which contain two or more distinct constituent materials or phases on a scale larger than the atomic. The term "composite" is usually reserved for those materials in which the distinct phases are separated on a scale larger than the atomic, and in which properties such as the elastic modulus are significantly altered in comparison with those of a homogeneous material. Accordingly, reinforced plastics such as fiberglass as well as natural materials such as bone are viewed as composite materials, but alloys such as brass are not. A foam is a composite in which one phase is empty space. Natural biological materials tend to be composites. Natural composites include bone, wood, dentin, cartilage, and skin. Natural foams include lung, cancellous bone, and wood. Natural composites often exhibit hierarchical structures in which particulate, porous, and fibrous structural features are seen on different micro-scales [Katz, 1980; Lakes, 1993]. In this chapter, composite material fundamentals and applications in biomaterials [Park and Lakes, 1988] are explored. Composite materials offer a variety of advantages in comparison with homogeneous materials. These include the ability for the scientist or engineer to exercise considerable control over material properties. There is the potential for stiff, strong, lightweight materials as well as for highly resilient and compliant materials. In biomaterials, it is important that each constituent of the composite be biocompatible. Moreover, the interface between constituents should not be degraded by the body environment. Some applications of composites in biomaterial applications are: (1) dental filling composites, (2) reinforced methyl methacrylate bone cement and ultra-high-molecular-weight polyethylene, and (3) orthopedic implants with porous surfaces.

4.1 Structure

The properties of composite materials depend very much upon *structure*. Composites differ from homogeneous materials in that considerable control can be exerted over the larger scale structure, and hence over the desired properties. In particular, the properties of a composite material depend upon the *shape* of the heterogeneities, upon the *volume fraction* occupied by them, and upon the *interface* among the constituents. The shape of the heterogeneities in a composite material is classified as follows. The principal inclusion shape categories are (1) the particle, with no long dimension; (2) the fiber, with one long dimension; and (3) the platelet or lamina, with two long dimensions, as shown in Fig. 4.1. The inclusions may vary in size and shape within a category. For example, particulate inclusions may be

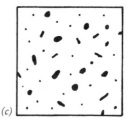

FIGURE 4.1   Morphology of basic composite inclusions. (a) particle, (b) fiber, (c) platelet.

spherical, ellipsoidal, polyhedral, or irregular. If one phase consists of voids, filled with air or liquid, the material is known as a cellular solid. If the cells are polygonal, the material is a honeycomb; if the cells are polyhedral, it is a foam. It is necessary in the context of biomaterials to distinguish the above structural cells from biological cells, which occur only in living organisms. In each composite structure, we may moreover make the distinction between random orientation and preferred orientation.

4.2   Bounds on Properties

Mechanical properties in many composite materials depend on structure in a complex way; however, for some structures, the prediction of properties is relatively simple. The simplest composite structures are the idealized Voigt and Reuss models, shown in Fig. 4.2. The dark and light areas in these diagrams represent the two constituent materials in the composite. In contrast to most composite structures, it is easy to calculate the stiffness of materials with the Voigt and Reuss structures, since in the Voigt structure the strain is the same in both constituents; in the Reuss structure the stress is the same. The Young's modulus, E, of the Voigt composite is:

$$E = E_i V_i + W_m \left[1 - V_i \right]$$ (4.1)

in which E_i is the Young's modulus of the inclusions, V_i is the volume fraction of inclusions, and E_m is the Young's modulus of the matrix. The Voigt relation for the stiffness is referred to as the rule of mixtures.

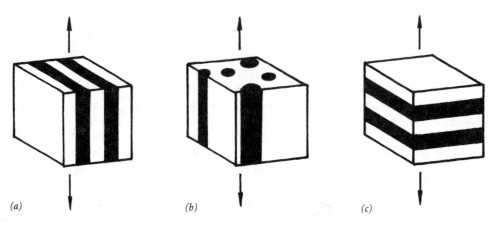

(a)   *(b)*   *(c)*

FIGURE 4.2   Voigt (a, laminar; b, fibrous) and Reuss (c) composite models, subjected to tension force indicated by arrows.

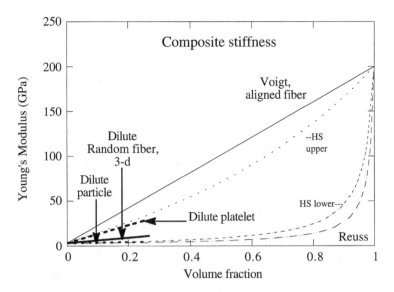

FIGURE 4.3 Stiffness vs. volume fraction for Voigt and Reuss models, as well as for dilute isotropic suspensions of platelets, fibers, and spherical particles embedded in a matrix. Phase moduli are 200 GPa and 3 GPa.

The Reuss stiffness, E:

$$E = \left[\frac{V_i}{E_i} + \frac{\left(1-V_i\right)}{E_m} \right]^{-1}$$

(4.2)

is less than that of the Voigt model. The Voigt and Reuss models impose upper and lower bounds, respectively, upon the stiffness of a composite of arbitrary phase geometry [Paul, 1960]. The bounds are far apart if, as is commonplace, the phase moduli differ a great deal, as shown in Fig. 4.3. For composite materials which are isotropic, the more complex relations of Hashin and Shtrikman (1963) provide tighter bounds upon the moduli (Fig. 4.3); both the Young's and shear moduli must be known for each constituent to calculate these bounds.

4.3 Anisotropy of Composites

Observe that the Reuss laminate is identical to the Voigt laminate, except for a rotation with respect to the direction of load. Therefore, the stiffness of the laminate is *anisotropic*, that is, dependent on direction [Agarwal and Broutman, 1980; Nye, 1976; Lekhnitskii, 1963]. Anisotropy is characteristic of composite materials. The relationship between stress σ_{ij} and strain ε_{kl} in anisotropic materials is given by the tensorial form of Hooke's law as follows:

$$\sigma_{ij} = \sum_{k=1}^{3} \sum_{l=1}^{3} C_{ijkl} \varepsilon_{kl}$$

(4.3)

Here, C_{ijkl} is the elastic modulus tensor. It has $3^4 = 81$ elements; however, since the stress and strain are represented by symmetric matrices with six independent elements each, the number of independent modulus tensor elements is reduced to 36. An additional reduction to 21 is achieved by considering elastic materials for which a strain energy function exists. Physically, C_{2323} represents a shear modulus since it couples a shear stress with a shear strain. C_{1111} couples axial stress and strain in the 1 or x direction, but it is not the same as Young's modulus. The reason is that Young's modulus is measured with the lateral strains free to occur via the Poisson effect, while C_{1111} is the ratio of axial stress to strain when there is only one non-zero strain value; there is no lateral strain. A modulus tensor with 21 independent elements describes a *triclinic* crystal, which is the least symmetric crystal form. The unit cell has three different oblique angles and three different side lengths. A triclinic composite could be made with groups of fibers of three different spacings, oriented in three different oblique directions. Triclinic modulus elements such as C_{2311}, known as cross-coupling constants, have the effect of producing a shear stress in response to a uniaxial strain; this is undesirable in many applications. An *orthorhombic* crystal or an *orthotropic* composite has a unit cell with orthogonal angles. There are nine independent elastic moduli. The associated engineering constants are three Young's moduli, three Poisson's ratios, and three shear moduli; the cross-coupling constants are zero when stresses are aligned to the symmetry directions. An example of such a composite is a unidirectional fibrous material with a rectangular pattern of fibers in the cross-section. Bovine bone, which has a laminated structure, exhibits orthotropic symmetry, as does wood. In a material with *hexagonal* symmetry, out of the nine C elements, there are five independent elastic constants. For directions in the transverse plane the elastic constants are the same, hence the alternate name transverse isotropy. A unidirectional fiber composite with a hexagonal or random fiber pattern has this symmetry, as does human Haversian bone. In *cubic* symmetry, there are three independent elastic constants, a Young's modulus, E, a shear modulus, G, and an independent Poisson's ratio, ν. Cross-weave fabrics have cubic symmetry. Finally, an *isotropic* material has the same material properties in any direction. There are only two independent elastic constants, hence E, G, ν, and also the bulk modulus B are related in an isotropic material. Isotropic materials include amorphous solids, polycrystalline metals in which the grains are randomly oriented, and composite materials in which the constituents are randomly oriented.

Anisotropic composites offer superior strength and stiffness in comparison with isotropic ones. Material properties in one direction are gained at the expense of properties in other directions. It is sensible, therefore, to use anisotropic composite materials only if the direction of application of the stress is known in advance.

4.4 Particulate Composites

It is often convenient to stiffen or harden a material, commonly a polymer, by the incorporation of particulate inclusions. The shape of the particles is important [see, e.g., Christensen, 1979]. In isotropic systems, stiff platelet (or flake) inclusions are the most effective in creating a stiff composite, followed by fibers; the least effective geometry for stiff inclusions is the spherical particle, as shown in Fig. 4.3. A dilute concentration of spherical particulate inclusions of stiffness E_i and volume fraction V_i, in a matrix (with Poisson's ratio assumed to be 0.5) denoted by the subscript m, gives rise to a composite with a stiffness E:

$$E = \frac{5\left(E_i - E_m\right)V_i}{3 + 2\dfrac{E_i}{E_m}} + E_m \tag{4.4}$$

The stiffness of such a composite is close to the Hashin–Shtrikman lower bound for isotropic composites. Even if the spherical particles are perfectly rigid compared with the matrix, their stiffening effect at low concentrations is modest. Conversely, when the inclusions are more compliant than the matrix, spherical ones reduce the stiffness the least and platelet ones reduce it the most. Indeed, soft platelets are suggestive of crack-like defects. Soft platelets, therefore, result not only in a compliant composite, but also a weak

FIGURE 4.4 Microstructure of a dental composite, Miradapt® (Johnson & Johnson), 50% by volume; filler: barium glass and colloidal silica [Park and Lakes, 1992].

one. Soft spherical inclusions are used intentionally as crack stoppers to enhance the toughness of polymers such as polystyrene [high-impact polystyrene], with a small sacrifice in stiffness.

Particle reinforcement has been used to improve the properties of bone cement. For example, inclusion of bone particles in PMMA cement somewhat improves the stiffness and improves the fatigue life considerably [Park et al., 1986]. Moreover, the bone particles at the interface with the patient's bone are ultimately resorbed and are replaced by ingrown new bone tissue. This approach is in the experimental stages.

Rubber used in catheters, rubber gloves, etc. is usually reinforced with very fine particles of silica (SiO_2) to make the rubber stronger and tougher.

Teeth with decayed regions have traditionally been restored with metals such as silver amalgam. Metallic restorations are not considered desirable for anterior teeth for cosmetic reasons. Acrylic resins and silicate cements had been used for anterior teeth, but their poor material properties led to short service life and clinical failures. Dental composite resins have virtually replaced these materials and are very commonly used to restore posterior teeth as well as anterior teeth [Cannon, 1988].

The dental composite resins consist of a polymer matrix and stiff inorganic inclusions [Craig, 1981]. A representative structure is shown in Fig. 4.4. The particles are very angular in shape. The inorganic inclusions confer a relatively high stiffness and high wear resistance on the material. Moreover, since they are translucent and their index of refraction is similar to that of dental enamel, they are cosmetically acceptable. Available dental composite resins use quartz, barium glass, and colloidal silica as fillers. Fillers have particle size from 0.04 to 13 μm, and concentrations from 33 to 78% by weight. In view of the greater density of the inorganic filler phase, a 77% weight percent of filler corresponds to a volume percent of about 55%. The matrix consists of a polymer, typically BIS-GMA. In restoring a cavity, the dentist mixes several constituents, then places them in the prepared cavity to polymerize. For this procedure to be successful the viscosity of the mixed paste must be sufficiently low and the polymerization must be controllable. Low viscosity liquids such as triethylene glycol dimethacrylate are used to lower

TABLE 4.1 Properties of Bone, Teeth, and Biomaterials

Material	Young's Modulus E (GPa)	Density ρ (g/cm³)	Strength (MPa)	Ref.
Hard tissue Tooth, bone, human compact bone, longitudinal direction	17	1.8	130 (tension)	Craig, and Peyton, 1958; Peters et al., 1984; Park and Lakes, 1992; Reilly and Burstein, 1975
Tooth dentin	18	2.1	138 (compression)	
Tooth enamel	50	2.9		
Polymers				Park and Lakes, 1992
Polyethylene (UHMW)	1	0.94	30 (tension)	
Polymethyl methacrylate, PMMA	3	1.1	65 (tension)	
PMMA bone cement	2	1.18	30 (tension)	
Metals				Park and Lakes, 1992
316L Stainless steel (wrought)	200	7.9	1000 (tension)	
Co–Cr–Mo (cast)	230	8.3	660 (tension)	
Co–Ni–Cr–Mo (wrought)	230	9.2	1800 (tension)	
Ti6Al4V	110	4.5	900 (tension)	
Composites				
Graphite-epoxy (unidirectional fibrous, high modulus)	215	1.63	1240 (tension)	Schwartz, 1997
Graphite-epoxy (quasi-isotropic fibrous)	46	1.55	579 (tension)	Schwartz, 1997
Dental composite resins (particulate)	10–16		170–260 (compression)	Cannon, 1988
Foams				Gibson and Ashby, 1988
Polymer foams	10^{-4}–1	0.002–0.8	0.01–1 (tension)	

the viscosity and inhibitors such as BHT (butylated trioxytoluene) are used to prevent premature polymerization. Polymerization can be initiated by a thermochemical initiator such as benzoyl peroxide, or by a photochemical initiator (benzoin alkyl ether) which generates free radicals when subjected to ultraviolet light from a lamp used by the dentist.

Dental composites have a Young's modulus in the range 10 to 16 GPa, and the compressive strength from 170 to 260 MPa [Cannon, 1988]. As shown in Table 4.1, these composites are still considerably less stiff than dental enamel, which contains about 99% mineral. Similar high concentrations of mineral particles in synthetic composites cannot easily be achieved, in part because the particles do not pack densely. Moreover, an excessive concentration of particles raises the viscosity of the unpolymerized paste. An excessively high viscosity is problematical since it prevents the dentist from adequately packing the paste into the prepared cavity; the material will then fill in crevices less effectively.

The thermal expansion of dental composites, as with other dental materials, exceeds that of tooth structure. Moreover, there is a contraction during polymerization of 1.2 to 1.6%. These effects are thought to contribute to leakage of saliva, bacteria, etc. at the interface margins. Such leakage in some cases can cause further decay of the tooth.

Use of colloidal silica in the so-called "microfilled" composites allows these resins to be polished, so that less wear occurs and less plaque accumulates. It is more difficult, however, to make these with a high fraction of filler. All the dental composites exhibit creep. The stiffness changes by a factor of 2.5 to 4 (depending on the particular material) over a time period from 10 sec to 3 h under steady load [Papadogianis et al., 1985]. This creep may result in indentation of the restoration, but wear seems to be a greater problem.

Dental composite resins have become established as restorative materials for both anterior and posterior teeth. The use of these materials is likely to increase as improved compositions are developed and in response to concern over long-term toxicity of silver–mercury amalgam fillings.

4.5 Fibrous Composites

Fibers incorporated in a polymer matrix increase the stiffness, strength, fatigue life, and other properties [Agarwal and Broutman, 1980; Schwartz, 1992]. Fibers are mechanically more effective in achieving a stiff, strong composite than are particles. Materials can be prepared in fiber form with very few defects which concentrate stress. Fibers such as graphite are stiff (Young's modulus is 200 to 800 GPa) and strong (the tensile strength is 2.7 to 5.5 GPa). Composites made from them can be as strong as steel but much lighter, as shown in Table 4.1. The stiffness of a composite with aligned fibers, if it is loaded along the fibers, is equivalent to the Voigt upper bound, Eq. (4.1). Unidirectional fibrous composites, when loaded along the fibers, can have strengths and stiffnesses comparable to that of steel, but with much less weight (Table 4.1). However if it is loaded transversly to the fibers, such a composite will be compliant, with a stiffness not much greater than that of the matrix alone. While unidirectional fiber composites can be made very strong in the longitudinal direction, they are weaker than the matrix alone when loaded transversely, as a result of stress concentration around the fibers. If stiffness and strength are needed in all directions, the fibers may be oriented randomly. For such a three-dimensional isotropic composite, for a low concentration of fibers,

$$E = \frac{E_i V_i}{6} + E_m,$$ (4.5)

so the stiffness is reduced by about a factor of six in comparison with an aligned composite as illustrated in Fig. 4.3. However if the fibers are aligned randomly in a plane, the reduction in stiffness is only a factor of three. The degree of anisotropy in fibrous composites can be very well controlled by forming laminates consisting of layers of fibers embedded in a matrix. Each layer can have fibers oriented in a different direction. One can achieve quasi-isotropic behavior in the laminate plane; such a laminate is not as strong or as stiff as a unidirectional one, as illustrated in Table 4.1. Strength of composites depends on such particulars as the brittleness or ductility of the inclusions and the matrix. In fibrous composites failure may occur by (1) fiber breakage, buckling, or pullout; (2) matrix cracking; or (3) debonding of fiber from matrix.

Short fiber composites are used in many applications. They are not as stiff or as strong as composites with continuous fibers, but they can be formed economically by injection molding or by *in situ* polymerization. Choice of an optimal fiber length can result in improved toughness, due to the predominance of fiber pull-out as a fracture mechanism.

Carbon fibers have been incorporated in the high-density polyethylene used in total knee replacements (Fig. 4.5). The standard ultra-high-molecular-weight polyethylene (UHMWPE) used in these implants is considered adequate for most purposes for implantation in older patients. A longer wear-free implant lifetime is desirable for use in younger patients. It is considered desirable to improve the resistance to creep of the polymeric component, since excessive creep results in an indentation of that component after long-term use. Representative properties of carbon-reinforced, ultra-high-molecular-weight polyethylene are shown in Fig. 4.6 [Sclippa and Piekarski, 1973]. Enhancements of various properties by a factor of two are feasible.

Polymethyl methacrylate (PMMA) used in bone cement is compliant and weak in comparison with bone; therefore, several reinforcement methods have been attempted. Metal wires have been used clinically as macroscopic "fibers" to reinforce PMMA cement used in spinal stabilization surgery [Fishbane and Pond, 1977]. The wires are made of a biocompatible alloy such as cobalt–chromium alloy or stainless steel. Such wires are not currently used in joint replacements owing to the limited space available. Graphite fibers have been incorporated in bone cement [Knoell et al., 1975] on an experimental basis. Significant improvements in the mechanical properties have been achieved. Moreover, the fibers have an added beneficial effect of reducing the rise in temperature which occurs during the polymerization of

FIGURE 4.5   Knee prostheses with polyethylene tibial components reinforced with carbon fiber.

the PMMA in the body. Such high temperature can cause problems such as necrosis of a portion of the bone into which it is implanted. Thin, short titanium fibers have been embedded in PMMA cement [Topoleski et al., 1992]; a toughness increase of 51% was observed with a 5% volumetric fiber content. Fiber reinforcement of PMMA cement has not found much acceptance since the fibers also increase the viscosity of the unpolymerized material. It is consequently difficult for the surgeon to form and shape the polymerizing cement during the surgical procedure.

Metals are currently used in bone plates for immobilizing fractures and in the femoral component of total hip replacements. A problem with currently used implant metals is that they are much stiffer than bone, so they shield the nearby bone from mechanical stress. Stress shielding results in a kind of disuse atrophy: the bone resorbs [Engh and Bobyn, 1988]. Therefore, composite materials have been investigated as alternatives [Bradley et al., 1980; Skinner, 1988]. Fibrous composites can deform to higher strains (to about 0.01) than metals (0.001 for a mild steel) without damage. This resilience is an attractive characteristic for more flexible bone plates and femoral stems. Flexible composite bone plates are effective

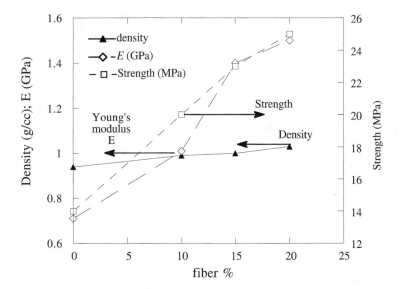

FIGURE 4.6 Properties of carbon-fiber-reinforced ultra-high-molecular-weight polyethylene. Replotted from Sclippa and Piekarski [1973].

in promoting healing [Jockish, 1992]. Composite hip replacement prostheses have been made with carbon fibers in a matrix of polysulfone and polyetherether ketone (PEEK). These prostheses experience heavy load with a static component. Structural metals such as stainless steel and cobalt–chromium alloys do not creep significantly at room or body temperature. In composites which contain a polymer constituent, creep behavior is a matter of concern. The carbon fibers exhibit negligible creep, but polymer constituents tend to creep. Prototype composite femoral components were found to exhibit fiber dominated creep of small magnitude and are not expected to limit the life of the implant [Maharaj and Jamison, 1993].

Fibrous composites have also been used in external medical devices such as knee braces [Yeaple, 1989], in which biocompatibility is not a concern but light weight is crucial.

4.6 Porous Materials

The presence of voids in porous or cellular solids will reduce the stiffness of the material. For some purposes, that is both acceptable and desirable. Porous solids are used for many purposes: flexible structures such as (1) seat cushions, (2) thermal insulation, (3) filters, (4) cores for stiff and lightweight sandwich panels, (5) flotation devices, and (6) to protect objects from mechanical shock and vibration; and in biomaterials, as coatings to encourage tissue ingrowth. Representative cellular solid structures are shown in Fig. 4.7.

The stiffness of an open-cell foam is given by Gibson and Ashby [1988]:

$$E = E_s \left[V_s \right]^2 \tag{4.6}$$

in which E_s is the Young's modulus and V_s is the volume fraction of the solid phase of the foam; V_s is also called the relative density.

The strength for crushing of a brittle foam and the elastic collapse of an elastomeric foam are given, respectively, by

$$\sigma_{crush} = 0.65 \, \sigma_{f,s} \left[V_s \right]^{3/2} \tag{4.7}$$

FIGURE 4.7   Cellular solids structures, after Gibson and Ashby [1988]. Left: Synthetic cellular solids: (a) open-cell polyurethane, (b) closed-cell polyethylene, (c) foamed nickel, (d) foamed copper, (e) foamed zirconia, (f) foamed mullite, (g) foamed glass, (h) polyester foam with both open and closed cells. Right: Natural cellular solids: (a) cork, (b) balsa wood, (c) sponge, (d) cancellous bone, (e) coral, (f) cuttlefish bone, (g) iris leaf, (h) plant stalk.

$$\sigma_{coll} = 0.05 \, E_s \left[V_s \right]^2 \qquad\qquad (4.8)$$

Here, $\sigma_{f,s}$ is the fracture strength of the solid phase. These strength relations are valid for relatively small density. Their derivation is based on the concept of *bending* of the cell ribs and is presented by Gibson and Ashby [1988]. Most man-made closed cell foams tend to have a concentration of material at the cell edges, so that they behave mechanically as open cell foams. The salient point in the relations for the mechanical properties of cellular solids is that the *relative density* dramatically influences the stiffness and the strength. As for the relationship between stress and strain, a representative stress strain curve is shown in Fig. 4.8. The physical mechanism for the deformation mode beyond the elastic limit depends on the material from which the foam is made. Trabecular bone, for example, is a natural cellular solid, which tends to fail in compression by crushing. Many kinds of trabecular bone appear to behave mechanically as an open cell foam. For trabecular bone of unspecified orientation, the stiffness is proportional to the cube of the density and the strength as the square of the density [Gibson and Ashby, 1988], which indicates behavior dominated by bending of the trabeculae. For bone with oriented trabeculae, both stiffness and strength in the trabecular direction are proportional to the density, a fact which indicates behavior dominated by axial deformation of the trabeculae.

Porous materials have a high ratio of surface area to volume. When porous materials are used in biomaterial applications, the demands upon the inertness and biocompatibility are likely to be greater than for a homogeneous material.

Porous materials, when used in implants, allow tissue ingrowth [Spector et al., 1988a,b]. The ingrowth is considered desirable in many contexts, since it allows a relatively permanent anchorage of the implant to the surrounding tissues. There are actually two composites to be considered in porous implants: (1) the implant prior to ingrowth, in which the pores are filled with tissue fluid which is ordinarily of no

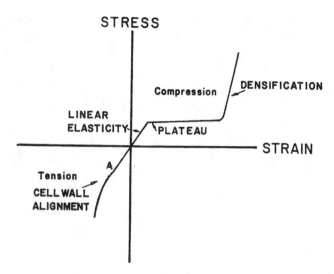

FIGURE 4.8 Representative stress–strain curve for a cellular solid. The plateau region for compression in the case of elastomeric foam (a rubbery polymer) represents elastic buckling; for an elastic-plastic foam (such as metallic foam) it represents plastic yield, and for an elastic-brittle foam (such as ceramic) it represents crushing. On the tension side, point A represents the transition between cell wall bending and cell wall alignment. In elastomeric foam, the alignment occurs elastically, in elastic plastic foam it occurs plastically, and an elastic-brittle foam fractures at A.

mechanical consequence; and (2) the implant filled with tissue. In the case of the implant prior to ingrowth, it must be recognized that the stiffness and strength of the porous solid are much less than in the case of the solid from which it is derived.

Porous layers are used on bone compatible implants to encourage bony ingrowth [Galante et al., 1971; Ducheyne, 1984]. The pore size of a cellular solid has no influence on its stiffness or strength (though it does influence the toughness); however, pore size can be of considerable biological importance. Specifically, in orthopedic implants with pores larger than about 150 μm, bony ingrowth into the pores occurs and this is useful to anchor the implant. This minimum pore size is on the order of the diameter of osteons in normal Haversian bone. It was found experimentally that pores <75 μm in size did not permit the ingrowth of bone tissue. Moreover, it was difficult to maintain fully viable osteons within pores in the 75- to 150-μm size range. Representative structure of such a porous surface layer is shown in Fig. 4.9. Porous coatings are also under study for application in anchoring the artificial roots of dental implants to the underlying jawbone. Porous hydroxyapatite has been studied for use in repairing large defects in bone [Holmes et al., 1986; Meffert et al., 1985]. Hydroxyapatite is the mineral constituent of bone, and it has the nominal composition $Ca_{10}(PO_4)_6(OH)_2$. Implanted hydroxyapatite is slowly resorbed by the body over several years and replaced by bone. Tricalcium phosphate is resorbed more quickly and has been considered as an implant constituent to speed healing.

When a porous material is implanted in bone, the pores become filled first with blood which clots, then with osteoprogenitor mesenchymal cells, then, after about 4 weeks, with bony trabeculae. The ingrown bone then becomes remodeled in response to mechanical stress. The bony ingrowth process depends on a degree of mechanical stability in the early stages of healing. If too much motion occurs, the ingrown tissue will be collagenous scar tissue, not bone.

Porous materials used in soft tissue applications include polyurethane, polyamide, and polyester velours used in percutaneous devices. Porous reconstituted collagen has been used in artificial skin, and braided polypropylene has been used in artificial ligaments. As in the case of bone implants, the porosity encourages tissue ingrowth which anchors the device.

Blood vessel replacements are made with porous materials which encourage soft tissue to grow in, eventually forming a new lining, or neointima. The new lining consists of the patient's own cells. It is a

FIGURE 4.9   Irregular pore structure of porous coating in Ti5Al4V alloy for bony ingrowth, from Park and Lakes [1992]. The top scanning electron microscopic picture is a 5× magnification of the rectangular region of the bottom picture (200×).

natural nonthrombogenic surface resembling the lining of the original blood vessel. This is a further example of the biological role of porous materials as contrasted with the mechanical role.

Ingrowth of tissue into implant pores is not always desirable. For example, sponge (polyvinyl alcohol) implants used in early mammary augmentation surgery underwent ingrowth of fibrous tissue and contracture and calcification of that tissue, resulting in hardened, calcified breasts. Current mammary implants make use of a balloon-like nonporous silicone rubber layer enclosing silicone oil or gel, or perhaps a saline solution in water. A porous layer of polyester felt or velour attached to the balloon is provided at the back surface of the implant so that limited tissue ingrowth will anchor it to the chest wall and prevent it from migrating.

Foams are also used externally to protect the human body from injury. Examples include knee pads, elbow pads, wrestling mats, and wheelchair cushions. Since these foams are only in contact with skin rather than any internal organs, they are not subject to rigorous biocompatibility requirements. They are therefore designed based on mechanical considerations. Foam used in sports equipment must have the correct compliance to limit impact force without bottoming out. Foam used in wheelchair cushions is intended to prevent pressure sores in people who suffer limited mobility. The properties of cushions are crucial in reducing illness and suffering in people who are confined to wheelchairs or hospital beds for long periods. Prolonged pressure on body parts can obstruct circulation in the capillaries. If this lasts too long it may cause a sore or ulcer called a pressure sore, also called a bed sore. In its most severe manifestation, a pressure sore can form a deep crater-like ulcer in which underlying muscle or bone is exposed [Dinsdale, 1974]. A variety of flexible cushion materials have been tried to minimize the incidence and severity of pressure sores [Garber, 1985]. Viscoelastic foam allows the cushion to progressively conform to the body shape. However, progressive densification of the foam due to creep results in a stiffer cushion which must be periodically replaced.

Porous materials are produced in a variety of ways. For example, in the case of bone compatible surfaces they are formed by sintering of beads or wires. Vascular and soft tissue implants are produced by weaving or braiding fibers as well as by nonwoven "felting" methods. Protective foams for use outside the body are usually produced by use of a "blowing agent" which is a chemical which evolves gas during the polymerization of the foam. An interesting approach to producing micro-porous materials is the replication of structures found in biological materials: the *replamineform* process [White et al., 1976]. The rationale is that the unique structure of communicating pores is thought to offer advantages in the induction of tissue ingrowth. The skeletal structure of coral or echinoderms (such as sea urchins) is replicated by a casting process in metals and polymers; these have been tried in vascular and tracheal prostheses as well as in bone substitutes.

4.7 Biocompatibility

Carbon itself has been successfully used as a biomaterial. Carbon based fibers used in composites are known to be inert in aqueous (even seawater) environments; however, they do not have a track record in the biomaterials setting. *In vitro* studies by Kovacs [1993] disclose substantial electrochemical activity of carbon fiber composites in an aqueous environment. If such composites are placed near a metallic implant, galvanic corrosion is a possibility. Composite materials with a polymer matrix absorb water when placed in a hydrated environment such as the body. Moisture acts as a plasticizer of the matrix and shifts the glass transition temperature towards lower values [DeIasi and Whiteside, 1978], hence a reduction in stiffness and an increase in mechanical damping. Water immersion of a graphite epoxy cross-ply composite [Gopalan et al., 1989] for 20 days reduced the strength by 13% and the stiffness by 9%. Moisture absorption by polymer constituents also causes swelling. Such swelling can be beneficial in dental composites since it offsets some of the shrinkage due to polymerization.

Flexible composite bone plates are effective in promoting healing [Jockish, 1992], but particulate debris from composite bone plates gives rise to a foreign body reaction similar to that caused by ultra-high-molecular-weight polyethylene.

Summary

Composite materials are a relatively recent addition to the class of materials used in structural applications. In the biomaterials field, the ingress of composites has been even more recent. In view of their potential for high performance, composite materials are likely to find increasing use as biomaterials.

References

Agarwal, A. G. and Broutman, L. J. 1980. *Analysis and Performance of Fiber Composites,* John Wiley & Sons, New York.

Bradley, J. S., Hastings, G. W., and Johnson-Hurse, C. 1980. Carbon fiber reinforced epoxy as a high strength, low modulus material for internal fixation plates, *Biomaterials,* 1, 38–40.

Cannon, M. L. 1988. Composite resins. In: *Encyclopedia of Medical Devices and Instrumentation,* J. G. Webster, Ed., John Wiley & Sons, New York.

Christensen, R. M. 1979. *Mechanics of Composite Materials,* John Wiley & Sons, New York.

Craig, R. 1981. Chemistry, composition, and properties of composite resins. In: *Dental Clinics of North America,* H. Horn, Ed., W.B. Saunders, Philadelphia, PA.

Craig, R. G. and Peyton, F. A. 1958. Elastic and mechanical properties of human dentin, *J. Dental Res.*, 37, 710–718.

DeIasi, R. and Whiteside, J. B. 1978. Effect of moisture on epoxy resins and composites. In: *Advanced Composite Materials—Environmental Effects*, J. R. Vinson, Ed., ASTM STP 658, American Society for Testing and Materials, Philadelphia, PA.

Dinsdale, S. M. 1974. Decubitus ulcers: role of pressure and friction in causation, *Arch. Phys. Med. Rehab.*, 55, 147–152.

Ducheyne, P. 1984. Biological fixation of implants. In: *Functional Behavior of Orthopaedic Biomaterials*, G. W. Hastings and P. Ducheyne, Eds., CRC Press, Boca Raton, FL.

Engh, C. A. and Bobyn, J. D. 1988. Results of porous coated hip replacement using the AML prosthesis. In: *Non-Cemented Total Hip Arthroplasty*, Raven Press, New York.

Fishbane, B. M. and Pond, R. B. 1977. Stainless steel fiber reinforcement of polymethylmethacrylate, *Clin. Orthop.*, 128, 490–498.

Galante, J., Rostoker, W., Lueck, R., and Ray, R. D. 1971. Sintered fiber metal composites as a basis for attachment of implants to bone, *J. Bone Joint Surg.*, 53A, 101–114.

Garber, S. L. 1985. Wheelchair cushions: a historical review, *Am. J. Occup. Ther.*, 39, 453–459.

Gibson, L.J. and Ashby, M. F. 1988. *Cellular Solids*, Cambridge, U.K.

Gopalan, R., Somashekar, B. R., and Dattaguru, B. 1989. Environmental effects on fiber-polymer composites, *Polymer Degradation Stability*, 24, 361–371.

Hashin Z. and Shtrikman, S. 1963. A variational approach to the theory of the elastic behavior of multiphase materials, *J. Mech. Phys. Solids*, 11, 127–140.

Holmes, D. E., Bucholz, R. W., and Mooney, V. 1986. Porous hydroxyapatite as a bone graft substitute in metaphyseal defects, *J. Bone Joint Surg.*, 68, 904–911.

Jockish, K. A., Brown, S. A., Bauer, T. W., and Merritt, K. 1992. Biological response to chopped carbon reinforced PEEK, *J. Biomed. Mater. Res.*, 26, 133–146.

Katz, J. L. 1980. Anisotropy of Young's modulus of bone, *Nature*, 283, 106–107.

Knoell, A., Maxwell, H., and Bechtol, C. 1975. Graphite fiber reinforced bone cement, *Ann. Biomed. Eng.*, 3, 225–229.

Kovacs, P. 1993. In vitro studies of the electrochemical behavior of carbon-fiber composites. In: *Composite Materials for Implant Applications in the Human Body: Characterization and Testing*, R. D. Jamison and L. N. Gilbertson, Eds., ASTM STP 1178, American Society for Testing and Materials, Philadelphia, PA, pp. 41–52.

Lakes, R. S. 1993. Materials with structural hierarchy, *Nature*, 361, 511–515.

Lekhniitski, S. 1977. *Theory of Elasticity of an Anisotropic Body*, Mir Publishers, Moscow.

Maharaj, G. R. and Jamison, R. D. 1993. Creep testing of a composite material human hip prosthesis, In: *Composite Materials for Implant Applications in the Human Body: Characterization and Testing*, R. D. Jamison and L. N. Gilbertson, Eds., ASTM STP 1178, American Society for Testing and Materials, Philadelphia, PA, 86–97.

Meffert, R. M., Thomas, J. R., Hamilton, K. M., and Brownstein, C. N. 1985. Hydroxylapatite as allopathic graft in the treatment of periodontal osseous defects, *J. Periodontol.*, 56, 63–73.

Nye, J. F. 1976. *Physical Properties of Crystals*, Oxford University Press, Oxford.

Papadogianis, Y., Boyer, D. B., and Lakes, R. S. 1985. Creep of posterior dental composites, *J. Biomed. Mater. Res.*, 19, 85–95.

Park, H. C., Liu, Y. K., and Lakes, R. S. 1986. The material properties of bone-particle impregnated PMMA, *J. Biomech. Eng.*, 108, 141–148.

Park, J. B. and Lakes, R. S. 1992. *Biomaterials*, Plenum Press, New York.

Paul, B. 1960. Prediction of elastic constants of multiphase materials, *Trans. AIME*, 218, 36–41.

Peters, M. C., Poort, H.W., Farah, J. W., and Graig, R. G. 1983. Stress analysis of a tooth restored with a post and a core, *J. Dental Res.*, 62, 760–763.

Reilly, D. T. and Burstein, A. H. 1975. The elastic and ultimate properties of compact bone tissue, *J. Biomech.*, 8, 393–405.

Schwartz, M. M. 1992. *Composite Materials Handbook,* 2nd ed., McGraw-Hill, New York.

Sclippa, E. and Piekarski, K. 1973. Carbon fiber reinforced polyethylene for possible orthopaedic usage, *J. Biomed. Mater. Res.,* 7, 59–70.

Skinner, H. B. 1988. Composite technology for total hip arthroplasty, *Clin. Orthop. Rel. Res.,* 235, 224–236.

Spector, M., Miller, M., Beals, N. 1988a. Porous materials. In: *Encyclopedia of Medical Devices and Instrumentation,* J. G. Webster, Ed., John Wiley & Sons, New York.

Spector, M., Heyligers, I., and Robertson, J. R. 1988b. Porous polymers for biological fixation, *Clin. Orthop. Rel. Res.,* 235, 207–219.

Topoleski, L. D. T., Ducheyne, P., and Cackler, J. M. 1992. The fracture toughness of titanium fiber reinforced bone cement, *J. Biomed. Mater. Res.,* 26, 1599–1617.

White, R. A., Weber, J. N., and White, E. W. 1976. Replamineform: a new process for preparing porous ceramic, metal, and polymer prosthetic materials, *Science,* 176, 922.

Yeaple, F. 1989. Composite knee brace returns stability to joint, *Design News,* 46, 116, Oct. 23.

5

Biodegradable Polymeric Biomaterials: An Updated Overview

Chih-Chang Chu
Cornell University

5.1 Introduction

The term *biodegradation* is loosely associated with materials that could be broken down by nature either through hydrolytic mechanisms without the help of enzymes and/or enzymatic mechanism. Other terms such as *absorbable*, *erodible*, and *resorbable* have also been used in the literature to indicate biodegradation. Interest in biodegradable polymeric biomaterials for biomedical engineering use has increased dramatically during the past decade. This is because this class of biomaterials has two major advantages that non-biodegradable biomaterials do not have. First, they do not elicit permanent chronic foreign-body reactions due to the fact that they are gradually absorbed by the human body and do not permanently leave traces of residual in the implantation sites. Second, some of them have recently been found to be able to regenerate tissues, so-called *tissue engineering*, through the interaction of their biodegradation with immunologic cells like macrophages. Hence, surgical implants made from biodegradable biomaterials could be used as a temporary scaffold for tissue regeneration. This approach toward the reconstruction of injured, diseased, or aged tissues is one of the most promising fields in the 21st century.

TABLE 5.1   Properties of Commercially Important Synthetic Absorbable Polymers

Polymer	Crystallinity	T_m (°C)	T_g (°C)	T_{dec} (°C)	Fiber Strength (MPa)	Fiber Modulus (GPa)	Fiber Elongation (%)
PGA	High	230	36	260	890	8.4	30
PLLA	High	170	56	240	900	8.5	25
PLA	None	—	57	—	—	—	—
Polyglactin910[a]	High[c]	200	40	250	850	8.6	24
Polydioxanone	High	106	<20	190	490	2.1	35
Polyglyconate[b]	High[c]	213	<20	260	550	2.4	45
Poliglecaprone25[d]	—	<220	−36~15		91,100[e]	113,000[e]	39

  [a] Glycolide per lactide = 9/1.
  [b] Glycolide per trimethylene carbonate = 9/1.
  [c] Depending on the copolymer composition.
  [d] 2/0 size Monocryl (glycolide-ε-caprolactone copolymer).
  [e] PSI unit.
  Source: Kimura, Y., 1993. *Biodegradable Polymers.* In: *Biomedical Applications of Polymeric Materials,* T. Tsuruta, T. Hayashi, K. Kataoka, K. Ishihara, and Y. Kimura, Eds., CRC Press, Boca Raton, FL; Chu, C.C., von Fraunhofer, J.A., and Greisler, H.P., 1996. *Wound Closure Biomaterials and Devices.* CRC Press, Boca Raton, FL.

Although the earliest and most commercially significant biodegradable polymeric biomaterials originated from linear aliphatic polyesters like polyglycolide and polylactide from poly(α-hydroxyacetic acids), recent introduction of several new synthetic and natural biodegradable polymeric biomaterials extends the domain beyond this family of simple polyesters. These new commercially significant biodegradable polymeric biomaterials include poly(orthoesters), polyanhydrides, polysaccharides, poly(ester-amides), tyrosine-based polyarylates or polyiminocarbonates or polycarbonates, poly(D,L-lactide-urethane), poly(β-hydroxybutyrate), poly(ε-caprolactone), poly[*bis*(carboxylatophenoxy) phosphazene], poly(amino acids), pseudo-poly(amino acids), and copolymers derived from amino acids and non-amino acids.

All the above biodegradable polymeric biomaterials could be generally divided into eight groups based on their chemical origin: (1) biodegradable linear aliphatic polyesters (e.g., polyglycolide, polylactide, polycaprolactone, polyhydroxybutyrate) and their copolymers within the aliphatic polyester family like poly(glycolide-L-lactide) copolymer and poly(glycolide-ε-caprolactone) copolymer; (2) biodegradable copolymers between linear aliphatic polyesters in group 1 and monomers other than linear aliphatic polyesters like poly(glycolide-trimethylene carbonate) copolymer, poly(L-lactic acid-L-lysine) copolymer, Tyrosine-based polyarylates or polyiminocarbonates or polycarbonates, poly(D,L-lactide-urethane), and poly(ester-amide); (3) polyanhydrides; (4) poly(orthoesters); (5) Poly(ester-ethers) like poly-*p*-dioxanone; (6) biodegradable polysaccharides like hyaluronic acid, chitin and chitson; (7) polyamino acids like poly-L-glutamic acid and poly-L-lysine; (8) inorganic biodegradable polymers like polyphosphazene and poly[*bis*(carboxylatophenoxy)phosphazene] which have a nitrogen-phosphorus backbone instead of ester linkage. Recently, there is a new approach of making new biodegradable polymers through melt-blending of highly accepted biodegradable polymers like those of glycolide and lactide base [Shalaby, 1994].

The earliest, most successful, and frequent biomedical applications of biodegradable polymeric bio-materials have been in wound closure [Chu et al., 1996]. All biodegradable wound closure biomaterials are based upon the glycolide and lactide families. For example, polyglycolide (Dexon from American Cyanamid), poly(glycolide-L-lactide) random copolymer with 90 to 10 molar ratio (Vicryl from Ethicon), poly(ester-ether) (PDS from Ethicon), poly(glycolide-trimethylene carbonate) random block copolymer (Maxon from American Cyanamid), and poly(glycolide-ε-caprolactone) copolymer (Monocryl from Ethicon). This class of biodegradable polymeric biomaterials is also the one most studied for their chemical, physical, mechanical, morphological, and biological properties and their changes with degra-dation time and environment. Some of the above materials like Vicryl have been commercially used as surgical meshes for repair of a hernia or the body wall.

The next largest biomedical application of biodegradable polymeric biomaterials that are commercially satisfactory is drug control/release devices. Some well-known examples in this application are polyanhydrides and poly(ortho-ester). Biodegradable polymeric biomaterials, particularly totally resorbable composites, have also been experimentally used in the field of orthopedics, mainly as components for internal bone fracture fixation like PDS pins. However, their wide acceptance in other parts of orthopedic implants may be limited due to their inherent mechanical properties and their biodegradation rate. Besides the commercial uses described above, biodegradable polymeric biomaterials have been experimented with as (1) vascular grafts, (2) vascular stents, (3) vascular couplers for vessel anastomosis, (4) nerve growth conduits, (5) augmentation of defected bone, (6) ligament/tendon prostheses, (7) intramedullary plug during total hip replacement, (8) anastomosis ring for intestinal surgery, and (9) stents in ureterostomies for accurate suture placement.

Due to space limitation, the emphasis of this chapter will be on the commercially most significant and successful biomedical biodegradable polymers based on (1) linear aliphatic polyesters, (2) some very recent research and development of important classes of synthetic biodegradable polymers, (3) a new theoretical approach to modeling the hydrolytic degradation of glycolide/lactide-based biodegradable polymers, (4) the effects of some new extrinsic factors on the degradation of the most commercially significant biodegradable polymers, and (5) the new biomedical applications of this class of synthetic biodegradable polymers in tissue engineering and regeneration. The details of the applications of this family and other biodegradable polymeric biomaterials and their chemical, physical, mechanical, biological, and biodegradation properties can be found in other reviews [Barrows, 1986; Kimura, 1993; Shalaby, 1994; Chu et al., 1996; Hollinger, 1995; Vert et al., 1992; Park et al., 1993].

5.2 Glycolide/Lactide-Based Biodegradable Linear Aliphatic Polyesters

This class of biodegradable polymers includes the most successful, important, and commercially widely used biodegradable biomaterials in surgery. It is also the class of biodegradable biomaterials that were most extensively studied in terms of degradation mechanisms and structure–property relationships. Among them, polyglycolide or polyglycolic acid (PGA) is the most important one because most other biodegradable polymers are derived from PGA either through copolymerization, e.g., poly(glycolide-L-lactide) copolymer, or modified glycolide monomer, e.g., poly-p-dioxanone.

Glycolide-Based Biodegradable Homopolymer Polyesters

PGA can be polymerized either directly or indirectly from glycolic acid. The direct polycondensation produces a polymer of M_n less than 10,000 because of the requirement of a very high degree of dehydration (99.28% up) and the absence of monofunctional impurities. For PGA of molecular weight higher than 10,000 it is necessary to proceed through the ring-opening polymerization of the cyclic dimers of glycolic acid. Numerous catalysts are available for this ring-opening polymerization. They include organometallic compounds and Lewis acids [Chujo et al., 1967; Wise et al., 1979]. For biomedical applications, stannous chloride dihydrate or trialkyl aluminum are preferred. PGA was found to exhibit an orthorhombic unit cell with dimensions $a = 5.22$ Å, $b = 6.19$ Å, and c (fiber axis) = 7.02 Å. The planar zigzag-chain molecules form a sheet structure parallel to the ac plane and do not have the polyethylene type arrangement [Chatani et al., 1968]. The molecules between two adjacent sheets orient in opposite directions. The tight molecular packing and the close approach of the ester groups might stabilize the crystal lattice and contribute to the high melting point, T_m, of PGA (224–230°C). The glass transition temperature, T_g, ranges from 36 to 40°C. The specific gravities of PGA are 1.707 for a perfect crystal and 1.50 in a completely amorphous state [Chujo et al., 1967a]. The heat of fusion of 100% crystallized PGA is reported to be 12 kJ/mole (45.7 cal/g) [Brandrup et al., 1975]. A recent study of injection-molded PGA disks reveals their IR spectroscopic characteristics [Chu et al., 1995]. As shown in Fig. 5.1, the four bands at 850, 753, 713, and 560 cm^{-1} are associated with the amorphous regions of the PGA disks and could be used to assess

FIGURE 5.1   FTIR spectra of polyglycolic acid disks as a function of *in vitro* hydrolysis time in phosphate buffer of pH 7.44 at 37°C. (a): 0 day; (b) 55 h; (c) 7 days; (d) 21 days.

the extent of hydrolysis. Peaks associated with the crystalline phase included those at 972, 901, 806, 627, and 590 cm^{-1}. Two broad, intense peaks at 1142 and 1077 cm^{-1} can be assigned to C–O stretching modes in the ester and oxymethylene groups, respectively. These two peaks are associated mainly with ester and oxymethylene groups originating in the amorphous domains. Hydrolysis could cause both of these C–O stretching modes to substantially decrease in intensity.

Glycolide-Based Biodegradable Copolyesters Having Aliphatic Polyester-Based Co-Monomers

Other commercially successful glycolide-based biodegradable polymeric biomaterials are the copolymers of glycolide with other monomers within linear aliphatic polyesters like lactides, carbonates, and ε-capro-lactone. The glycolide-lactide random copolymers are the most studied and have a wide range of properties and applications, depending on the composition ratio of glycolide to lactide. Figure 5.2 illustrates the dependence of biodegradation rate on the composition of glycolide to lactide in the copolymer. For wound closure purposes, a high concentration of glycolide monomer is required for achieving proper mechanical and degradation properties. Vicryl sutures, sometime called polyglactin 910, contain a 90/10 molar ratio of glycolic to L-lactide and this molar ratio is important for the Vicryl suture to retain crystalline characteristics. For biomedical use, Lewis acid catalysts are preferred for the copol-ymers [Wise et al., 1979]. If DL- instead of L-lactide is used as the co-monomer, the U-shape relationship between the level of crystallinity and glycolide composition disappears. This is because polylactide from 100% DL-lactide composition is totally amorphous. IR bands associated with Vicryl molecules in the amorphous domains are 560, 710, 850, and 888 cm^{-1}, while 590, 626, 808, 900, and 972 cm^{-1} are associated with the crystalline domains [Frederick et al., 1984]. Like PGA, these IR bands could be used to assess the extent of hydrolysis.

A relatively new block copolymer of glycolide and carbonates, such as trimethylene carbonate, has been commercialized. Maxon is made from a block copolymer of glycolide and 1,3-dioxan-2-one (trimethylene carbonate or GTMC) and consists of 32.5% by weight (or 36 mol%) trimethylene carbonate

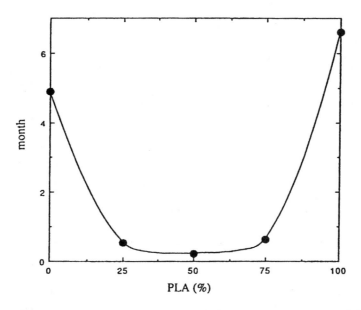

FIGURE 5.2 The effect of poly(L-lactide) composition in polyglycolide on the time required for 50% mass loss implanted under the dorsal skin of rat. (*Source:* Miller, R.A., Brady, J.M., and Cutright, D.E., 1977. *J. Biomed. Mater. Res.*, 11(5):711. With permission.)

[Katz et al., 1985; Casey et al., 1984]. Maxon is a poly(ester-carbonate). The polymerization process of Maxon is divided into two stages. The first stage is the formation of a middle block which is a random copolymer of glycolide and 1,3-dioxan-2-one. Diethylene glycol is used as an initiator and stannous chloride dihydrate ($SnCl_2 \cdot 2H_2O$) serves as the catalyst. The polymerization is conducted at about 180°C. The weight ratio of glycolide to trimethylene carbonate in the middle block is 15:85. After the synthesis of the middle block, the temperature of the reactive bath is raised to about 220°C to prevent the crystallization of the copolymer and additional glycolide monomers as the end blocks are added into the reaction bath to form the final triblock copolymer.

The latest glycolide-based copolymer that has become commercially successful is Monocryl suture. It is a segmented block copolymer consisting of both soft and hard segments. The purpose of having soft segments in the copolymer is to provide good handling properties like pliability, while the hard segments are used to provide adequate strength. The generic copolymerization process between glycolic acid and ε-caprolactone was reported by Fukuzaki et al. in Japan [1989, 1991]. The resulting copolymers were low molecular weight biodegradable copolymers of glycolic acid and various lactones for potential drug delivery purposes. The composition of lactone ranged from as low as 15 to as high as 50 mol% and the average for molecular weight ranged from 4510 to 16,500. The glass transition temperature ranged from 18 to −43°C, depending on the copolymer composition and molecular weight.

Monocryl is made from two stages of the polymerization process [Bezwada et al., 1995]. In the first stage, soft segments of prepolymer of glycolide and ε-caprolactone are made. This soft segmented prepolymer is further polymerized with glycolides to provide hard segments of polyglycolide. Monocryl has a composition of 75% glycolide and 25% ε-caprolactone and should have a higher molecular weight than those glycolide/ε-caprolactone copolymers reported by Fukuzaki et al. for adequate mechanical properties required by sutures. The most unique aspect of Monocryl monofilament suture is its pliability as claimed by Ethicon [Bezwada et al., 1995]. The force required to bend a 2/0 suture is only about 2.8×10^4 lb-in.[2] for Monocryl, while the same size PDSII and Maxon monofilament sutures require about 3.9 and 11.6×10^4 lb-in.[2] force, respectively. This inherent pliability of Monocryl is due to the presence of soft segments and T_g resulting from the ε-caprolactone co-monomer unit. Its T_g is expected to be between 15 and −36°C.

Glycolide-Based Biodegradable Copolyesters with Non-Aliphatic Polyester-Based Co-Monomers

In this category, the most important one is the glycolide copolymer consisting of poly(ethylene 1,4-phenylene-*bis*-oxyacetate) (PEPBO) [Jamiokowski and Shalaby, 1991]. The development of this type of glycolide-based copolymer was initiated because of the adverse effect of γ-irradiation on the mechanical properties of glycolide-based synthetic absorbable sutures. There is a great desire to develop γ-irradiation sterilizable, synthetic, absorbable polymers to take advantage of the highly convenient and reliable method of sterilization. Shalaby et al. recently reported that the incorporation of about 10 mol% of a polymeric radiostabilizer like PEPBO into PGA backbone chains would make the copolymer sterilizable by γ-irradiation without a significant accelerated loss of mechanical properties upon hydrolysis when compared with the unirradiated copolymer control (MPG) [Jamiokowski et al., 1991]. The changes in tensile breaking force of both MPG and PGA sutures implanted intramuscularly and subcutaneously in rats for various periods show the great advantage of such copolymers. MPG fibers γ-irradiated at 2.89 Mrads did not show any loss in tensile breaking force during the first 14 days postimplantation when compared with unimplanted samples. On the contrary, PGA sutures γ-irradiated at 2.75 Mrads lost 62% of the tensile breaking force of their unimplanted samples. There was no tensile breaking force remaining for the irradiated PGA at the end of 21 days, while both 2.89 and 5 Mrads irradiated MPG retained 72 and 55% of their corresponding 0 day controls, respectively. The inherent more hydrolytic resistance of MPG must be attributed to the presence of an aromatic group in the backbone chains. This aromatic polyester component is also responsible for the observed γ-irradiation stability. It is not known at this time whether the new γ-irradiation-resistant MPG is biocompatible with biologic tissues due to the lack of published histologic data.

Glycolide-Derived Biodegradable Polymers Having Ether Linkage

Poly-*p*-dioxanone (PDS) is derived from the glycolide family with better flexibility. It is polymerized from ether-containing lactones, 1,4-dioxane-2,5-dione (i.e., *p*-dioxanone) monomers with a hydroxylic initiator, and tin catalyst [Shalaby, 1994]. The resulting polymer is semi-crystalline with T_m about 106 to 115°C and T_g −10 to 0°C. The improved flexibility of PDS relative to PGA as evidenced in its lower T_g is due to the incorporation of an ether segment in the repeating unit which reduces the density of ester linkages for intermolecular hydrogen bonds. Because of the less dense ester linkages in PDS when compared with PGA or glycolide-L-lactide copolymers, PDS is expected and has been shown to degrade at a slower rate *in vitro* and *in vivo*. PDS having an inherent viscosity of 2.0 dL/g in hexafluoroisopropanol is adequate for making monofilament sutures. Recently, an advanced version of PDS, PDSII, was introduced. PDSII was achieved by subjecting the melt-spun fibers to a high temperature (128°C) for a short period of time. This additional treatment partially melts the outermost surface layer of PDS fibers and leads to a distinctive skin-core morphology. The heat employed also results in larger crystallites in the core of the fiber than the untreated PDS fiber. The tensile strength-loss profile of PDSII sutures is better than that of PDS sutures.

A variety of copolymers having high molar ratios of PDS compared to other monomers within the same linear aliphatic polyester family have been reported for the purpose of improving the mechanical and biodegradation properties [Shalaby, 1994]. For example, copolymer of PDS (80%) and PGA (up to 20%) has an absorption profile similar to Dexon and Vicryl sutures but it has compliance similar to PDS. Copolymer of PDS (85%) and PLLA (up to 15%) results in a more compliant (low modulus) suture than homopolymer PDS but with absorption profiles similar to PDS [Bezwada et al., 1990].

Copolymer fibers made from PDS and monomers other than linear aliphatic polyester like morpholine-2,5-dione (MD) exhibit rather interesting biodegradation properties. This copolymer fiber was absorbed 10 to 25% earlier than PDS. The copolymer, however, retained a tensile breaking strength profile similar to PDS with a slightly faster strength loss during the earlier stage, i.e., the first 14 days [Shalaby, 1994]. This ability to break the inherent fiber structure–property relationship through copolymerization is a major improvement in biodegradation properties of absorbable sutures. It is interesting to recognize that a small percentage (3%) of MD in the copolymer suture is sufficient to result in a faster mass loss profile without the expense of its tensile strength-loss profile. The ability to achieve this ideal biodegradation property might be attributed to both an increasing hydrophilicity of the copolymer and the disruption of crystalline domains due to MD moiety. As described later, the loss of suture mass is mainly due to the destruction of crystalline domains, while the loss of tensile breaking strength is chiefly due to the scission of tie-chain segments located in the amorphous domains. The question is why MD-PDS copolymeric suture retains its strength loss similar to PDS. The possible explanation is that the amide functional groups in MD could form stronger intermolecular hydrogen bonds than ester functional groups. This stronger hydrogen bond contributes to the strength retention of the copolymer of PDS and MD during *in vivo* biodegradation. The incorporation of MD moiety into PDS also lowers the unknot and knot strength of unhydrolyzed specimens, but increases elongation at break. This suggests that the copolymer of PDS and MD should have a lower level of crystallinity than PDS which is consistent with its observed faster mass loss *in vivo*.

To improve γ-irradiation stability of PDS, radiostabilizers like PEPBO have been copolymerized with PDS to form segmented copolymers the same way as PEPBO with glycolide described above [Shabaly, 1994; Koelmel et al., 1991]. The incorporation of 5 to 10% of such stabilizer in PDS has been shown not only to improve γ-irradiation resistance considerably but also to increase the compliance of the material. For example, PEPBO–PDS copolymer retained 79, 72, and 57% of its original tensile breaking strength at 2, 3, and 4 weeks in *in vivo* implantation, while PDS homopolymer retained only 43, 30, and 25% at the corresponding periods. It appears that an increasing (CH_2) group between the two ester functional groups of the radiation stabilizers improves the copolymer resistance toward γ-irradiation.

Lactide Biodegradable Homopolymers and Copolymers

Polylactides, particularly poly-L-lactide (PLLA), and copolymers having >50% L- or DL-lactide have been explored for medical use without much success mainly due to their much slower absorption and difficulty in melt processing. PLLAs are prepared in solid state through ring-opening polymerization due to their thermal instability and should be melt-processed at the lowest possible temperature [Shalaby, 1994]. Other methods like solution spinning, particularly for high molecular weight, and suspension polymerization have been reported as better alternatives. PLLA is a semi-crystalline polymer with $T_m = 170°C$ and $T_g = 56°C$. This high T_g is mainly responsible for the extremely slow biodegradation rate reported in the literature. The molecular weight of lactide-based biodegradable polymers suitable for medical use ranges from 1.5 to 5.0 dL/g inherent viscosity in chloroform. Ultra high molecular weight of polylactides has been reported [Tunc, 1983; Leenslag et al., 1984]. For example, an intrinsic viscosity as high as 13 dL/g was reported by Leenslag et al. High strength PLLA fibers from this ultra-high-molecular-weight polylactide was made by hot-drawing fibers from solutions of good solvents. The resulting fibers had tensile breaking strength close to 1.2 GPa [Gogolewski et al., 1983]. Due to a dissymmetric nature of lactic acid, the polymer made from the optically inactive racemic mixture of D and L enantiomers, poly-DL-lactide, however, is an amorphous polymer.

Lactide-based copolymers having a high percentage of lactide have recently been reported, particularly those copolymerized with aliphatic polycarbonates like trimethylene carbonate (TMC) or 3,3-dimethyl-trimethylene carbonate (DMTMC) [Shieh et al., 1990]. The major advantage of incorporating TMC or DMTMC units into lactide is that the degradation products from TMC or DMTMC are largely neutral pH and hence are considered to be advantageous. Both *in vitro* toxicity and *in vivo* non-specific foreign body reactions like sterile sinuses have been reported in orthopedic implants made from PGA and/or PLLA [Bostman et al., 1990; Daniels et al., 1992; Eitenmuller et al., 1989; Winet et al., 1993; Hofmann, 1992]. Several investigators indicated that the glycolic or lactic-acid rich-degradation products have the potential to significantly lower the local pH in a closed and less body-fluid-buffered regions surrounded by bone [Sugnuma et al., 1992]. This is particularly true if the degradation process proceeds with a burst mode (i.e., a sudden and rapid release of degradation products). This acidity tends to cause abnormal bone resorption and/or demineralization. The resulting environment may be cytotoxic [Daniels et al., 1992]. Indeed, inflammatory foreign body reactions with a discharging sinus and osteolytic foci visible on x-ray have been encountered in clinical studies [Eitenmuller et al., 1989]. Hollinger et al. recently confirmed the problem associated with PGA and/or PLLA orthopedic implants [Winet et al., 1993]. A rapid degradation of a 50:50 ratio of glycolide-lactide copolymer in bone chambers of rabbit tibias has been found to inhibit bone regeneration. However, emphasis has been placed on the fact that extrapolation of *in vitro* toxicity to *in vivo* biocompatibility must consider microcirculatory capacity. The increase in the local acidity due to a faster accumulation of the highly acidic degradation products is also known to lead to an accelerated acid-catalyzed hydrolysis in the immediate vicinity of the biodegradable device. This acceleration in hydrolysis could lead to a faster loss of mechanical property of the device than we expect. This finding suggests the need to use components in totally biodegradable composites so that degradation products with less acidity would be released into the surrounding area. A controlled slow release rather than a burst release of degradation products at a level that the surrounding tissue could timely metabolize them would also be helpful in dealing with the acidity problem. Copolymers of composition ratio of 10DMTMC/90LLA or 10TMC/90LLA appear to be a promising absorbable orthopaedic device. Other applications of this type of copolymers include nerve growth conduits, tendon prostheses, and coating materials for biodegradable devices.

Another unique example of L-lactide copolymer is the copolymer of L-lactide and 3-(S)[(alkyloxycarbonyl) methyl]-1,4-dioxane-2,5-dione, a cyclic diester [Kimura, 1993]. The most unique aspect of this new biodegradable copolymer is the carboxyl acid pendant group which obviously would make the new polymer not only more hydrophilic and lead to faster biodegradation but also more reactive toward future chemical modification through the pendant carboxyl group. The availability of these carboxyl-reactive pendant sites could be used to chemically bond antimicrobial agents or other biochemicals like growth factors for making future wound closure biomaterials having new and important biological functions. Unfortunately, there are no reported data to evaluate the performance of this new absorbable polymer for biomedical engineering use up to the present time.

Block copolymers of PLLA with poly(amino acids) have also been reported as a potential controlled drug delivery system [Nathan et al., 1994]. This new class of copolymers consists of both ester and amide linkages in the backbone molecules and is sometimes referred as poly(depsipeptides) or poly(esters-amides). Poly(depsipeptides) could also be synthesized from ring-opening polymerization of morpholine-2,5-dione and its derivatives [Helder et al., 1986]. Barrows has also made a series of poly(ester-amides) from polyesterification of diols that contain preformed amide linkages, such as amidediols [Barrows, 1994]. Katsarava and Chu et al. reported the synthesis of high-molecular-weight poly(ester-amides) of M_w from 24,000 to 167,000 with narrow polydispersity (M_w/M_n = 1.20–1.81) via solution polycondensation of di-*p*-toluenesulfonic acid salts of *bis*-(α-amino acid) α,ω-alkylene diesters and di-*p*-nitrophenyl esters of diacids [Katsarava et al., 1999]. These poly(ester-amide)s consisted of naturally occurring and non-toxic building blocks and had excellent film forming properties. These polymers were mostly amorphous materials with T_g from 11 to 59°C. The rationale for making poly(ester-amides) is to combine the well-known absorbability and biocompatibility of linear aliphatic polyesters with the high performance and the flexibility of potential chemical reactive sites of amide of polyamides. Poly(ester-amides) could be degraded either by enzyme and/or nonenzymatic mechanisms. There is no commercial use of this class of copolymers at the present time.

The introduction of poly(ethylene oxide) (PEO) into PLLA in order to modulate the hydrophilicity and degradability of PLLA for drug control/release biomaterials has been reported and an example is the triblock copolymer of PLA/PEO/PLA [Li et al., 1998a]. Biomaterials having an appropriate PLLA and PEO block length were found to have a hydrogel property that could deliver hydrophilic drugs as well as hydrophobic ones like steroids and hormones. Another unique biodegradable biomaterial consisting of a star-block copolymer of PLLA, PGA, and PEO was also reported for protein drug delivery devices [Li et al., 1998b]. This star-shaped copolymer has 4 or 8 arms made of PEO, PLLA, and PGA. The glass transition temperature and the crystallinity of this star-shaped block copolymer were significantly lower than the corresponding linear PLLA and PGA.

Because of the characteristic of very slow biodegradation rate of PLLA and the copolymers having a high composition ratio of PLLA, their biomedical applications have been mainly limited to (1) orthopedic surgery, (2) drug control/release devices, (3) coating materials for suture, (4) vascular grafts, and (5) surgical meshes to facilitate wound healing after dental extraction.

5.3 Non-Glycolide/Lactide-Based Linear Aliphatic Polyesters

All glycolide/lactide-based linear aliphatic polyesters are based on poly(α-hydroxy acids). There are two unique groups of linear aliphatic polyesters based on poly(ω-hydroxy acids): the most famous ones are poly(ε-caprolactone) [Kimura, 1993], poly(β-hydroxybutyrate) (PHB), poly(β-hydroxyvalerate) (PHV), and the copolymers of PHB/PHV [Gross, 1994]. Poly(ε-caprolactone) has been used as a co-monomer with a variety of glycolide/lactide-based linear aliphatic polyesters described earlier. PHB and PHV belong to the family of poly(hydroxyalkanoates) and are mainly produced by prokaryotic types of microorganisms like *Pseudomonas olevorans* or *Alcaligenes eutrophus* through biotechnology. PHB and PHV are the principal energy and carbon storage compounds for these microorganisms and are produced when there are excessive nutrients in the environment. These naturally produced PHB and PHV are stereochemically pure and are isotactic. They could also be synthesized in labs, but the characteristics of steroregularity is lost.

This family of biodegradable polyesters is considered to be environmentally friendly because they are produced from propionic acid and glucose and could be completely degraded to water, biogas, biomass, and humic materials [Gross, 1994]. Their biodegradation requires enzymes. Hence, PHB, PHV, and their copolymers are probably the most important biodegradable polymers for environmental use. However, the biodegradability of this class of linear aliphatic polyesters in human or animal tissues has been questionable. For example, high molecular weight PHB or PHB/PHV fibers do not degrade in tissues or simulated environments over periods of up to 6 months [Williams, 1990]. The degradability of PHB could be accelerated by γ-irradiation or copolymerization with PHV.

An interesting derivative of PHB, poly(β-malic acid) (PMA), has been synthesized from β-benzyl malolactonate followed by catalytic hydrogenolysis. PMA differs from PHB in that the β-(CH_3) substituent is replaced by $-COOH$ [Kimura, 1993]. The introduction of pendant carboxylic acid group would make PMA more hydrophilic and easier to be absorbed.

5.4 Non-Aliphatic Polyesters Type Biodegradable Polymers

Aliphatic and Aromatic Polycarbonates

The most significant aliphatic polycarbonates are based upon DMTMC and TMC. They are made by the same ring-opening polymerization as glycolide-based biodegradable polyesters. The homopolymers are biocompatible with a controllable rate of biodegradation. Pellets of poly(ethylene carbonate) were absorbed completely in 2 weeks in the peritoneal cavity of rats. A slight variation of this polycarbonate, i.e., poly(propylene carbonate), however, did not show any sign of absorption after 2 months [Barrows, 1986]. Copolymers of DMTMC/ε-caprolactone and DMTMC/TMC have been reported to have adequate properties for wound closure, tendon prostheses, and vascular grafts. The most important advantage of aliphatic polycarbonates is the neutral pH of the degradation products.

Poly(BPA-carbonates) made from bisphenol A (BPA) and phosgene is non-biodegradable, but an analog of poly(BPA-carbonate) like poly(iminocarbonates) has been shown to degrade in about 200 days [Barrows, 1986]. In general, this class of aromatic polycarbonates takes an undesirably long period to degrade, presumably due to the presence of an aromatic ring which could protect adjacent ester bonds to be hydrolyzed by water or enzymes. Different types of degradation products of this polymer under different pH environments are produced. At pH > 7.0, the degradation products of this polymer are BPA, and ammonia and CO_2, while insoluble poly(BPA-carbonate) oligomers were produced with pH < 7.0

[Barrows, 1986]. The polymer had good mechanical properties and acceptable tissue biocompatibility. Unfortunately, there is currently no commercial use of this class of polymer in surgery.

Poly(alkylene oxalates) and Copolymers

This class of high crystalline biodegradable polymers was initially developed [Shalaby, 1994] for absorbable sutures and their coating. They consist of $[-ROOC-COO-]_n$ repeating unit where R is $(CH_2)_x$ with x ranging from 4 to 12. R could also be cyclic (1,4-*trans*-cyclohexanedimethanol) or aromatic (1,4-benzene, 1,3-benzene dimethanol) for achieving higher melting temperature. The biodegradation properties depend on the number of (CH_2) groups, x, and the type of R group (i.e., acyclic vs. cyclic or aromatic). In general, a higher number of methylene groups and/or the incorporation of cyclic or aromatic R groups would retard the biodegradation rate and hence make the polymer be absorbed slower. For example, there was no mass of the polymer with $x = 4$ remaining *in vivo* (rats) after 28 days, while the polymer with $x = 6$ retained 80% of its mass after 42 days *in vivo*. An isomorphic copolyoxalate consisting of 80% cyclic R group like 1,4-*trans*-cyclohexanedimethanol and 20% acyclic R group like 1,6-hexanediol retained 56% of its original mass after 180 days *in vivo*. By varying the ratio of cyclic to acyclic monomers, copolymers with a wide range of melting temperatures could be made; e.g.,copolymer of 95/5 ratio of cyclic (i.e., 1,4-*trans*-cyclohexanedimethanol)/acyclic (i.e., 1,6-hexanediol) monomers had a $T_m = 210°C$, while the copolymer with 5/95 ratio had a $T_m = 69°C$. Poly(alkylene oxalates) with $x = 3$ or 6 had been experimented with as drug control/release devices. The tissue reaction to this class of biodegradable polymers has been minimal.

5.5   Biodegradation Properties of Synthetic Biodegradable Polymers

The reported biodegradation studies of a variety of biodegradable polymeric biomaterials have mainly focused on their tissue biocompatibility, the rate of drug release, or loss of strength and mass. The degradation mechanisms and the effects of intrinsic and extrinsic factors have been reviewed, including pH [Chu, 1981, 1982], enzymes [Chu et al., 1983; Williams, 1979; Williams et al., 1977, 1984], γ-irradiation [Chu et al., 1982, 1983; Campbell et al., 1981; Williams et al., 1984; Zhang et al., 1993], electrolytes [Pratt et al., 1993a], cell medium [Chu et al., 1992], annealing treatment [Chu et al., 1988], plasma surface treatment [Loh et al., 1992], external stress [Chu, 1985a; Miller et al., 1984], and polymer morphology [Chu et al., 1989]. A chemical means to examine the degradation of PGA fibers [Chu et al., 1985] has been systemically examined and the subject has been reviewed [Chu, 1985b, 1991, 1995a, 1995b; Chu et al., 1996; Hollinger, 1995]. Table 5.2 is an illustration of structural factors of polymers that could control their degradation [Kimura, 1993]. Besides these series of experimental studies of a variety of factors that could affect the degradation of biodegradable polymeric biomaterials, two new areas broaden the above traditional study of biodegradation properties of biodegradable polymers into the frontier of science: theoretical modeling and the role of free radicals.

TABLE 5.2   Structural Factors To Control the Polymer Degradability

Factor	Method of Control
Chemical structure of main chain and side groups	Selection of chemical bonds and functional groups
Aggregation state	Processing, copolymerization
Crystalline state	Polymer blend
Hydrophilic/hydrophobic balance	Copolymerization, introduction of functional groups
Surface area	Micropores
Shape and morphology	Fiber, film, composite

Source: Kimura, Y., 1993, In: *Biomedical Applications of Polymeric Materials*, T. Tsuruta, T. Hayashi, K. Kataoka, K. Ishihara, and Y. Kimura, Eds., pp. 164–190. CRC Press, Boca Raton, FL. With permission.

Theoretical Modeling of Degradation Properties

The most systematic theoretical modeling study of degradation properties of biodegradable biomaterials was reported by Pratt and Chu who used computational chemistry to theoretically model the effects of a variety of substituents which could exert either steric effect and/or inductive effect on the degradation properties of glycolide/lactide-based biodegradable polymers [Pratt et al., 1993; Pratt and Chu, 1994a and b]. This new approach could provide scientists with a better understanding of the relationship between the chemical structure of biodegradable polymers and their degradation behavior at a molecular level. It also could help the future research and development of this class of polymers through the intelligent prediction of structure–property relationships. In those studies, Pratt and Chu examined the affect of various derivatives of linear aliphatic polyester (PGA) and a naturally occurring linear polysaccharide (hyaluronic acid) on their hydrolytic degradation phenomena and mechanisms.

The data showed a decrease in the rate of hydrolysis by about a factor of 10^6 with isopropyl α-substituents, but nearly a six-fold increase with *t*-butyl α-substituents [Pratt and Chu, 1993]. The role of electron donating and electron withdrawing groups on the rate of hydrolytic degradation of linear aliphatic polyesters was also theoretically modeled by Pratt and Chu [Pratt and Chu, 1994a]. Electron withdrawing substituents α to the carbonyl group would be expected to stabilize the tetrahedral intermediate resulting from hydroxide attack, i.e., favoring hydroxide attack but disfavoring alkoxide elimination. Electron releasing groups would be expected to show the opposite effect. Similarly, electronegative substituents on the alkyl portion of the ester would stabilize the forming alkoxide ion and favor the elimination step. Pratt and Chu found that the rate of ester hydrolysis is greatly affected by halogen substituents due primarily to charge delocalization. The data suggest that the magnitude of the inductive effect on the hydrolysis of glycolic esters decreases significantly as the location of the substituent is moved further away from the α-carbon because the inductive effect is very distance sensitive. In all three locations of substitutions (α, β, and γ), Cl and Br substituents exhibited the largest inductive effect compared to other halogen elements.

Therefore, Pratt and Chu concluded that the rate of ester hydrolysis is greatly affected by both alkyl and halogen substituents due primarily to either steric hindrance or charge delocalization. In the steric effect, alkyl substituents on the glycolic esters cause an increase in activation enthalpies, and a corresponding decrease in reaction rate, up to about three carbon sizes, while bulkier alkyl substituents other than isopropyl make the rate-determining elimination step more facile. It appears that aliphatic polyesters containing α isopropyl groups, or slightly larger linear alkyl groups, such as *n*-butyl, *n*-pentyl, etc., would be expected to show a longer strength retention, given the same fiber morphology. In the inductive effect, α-substituents on the acyl portion of the ester favor the formation of the tetrahedral intermediate through charge delocalization, with the largest effect seen with Cl substitution, but retard the rate-determining alkoxide elimination step by stabilizing the tetrahedral intermediate. The largest degree of stabilization is caused by the very electronegative *F* substituent.

The Role of Free Radicals in Degradation Properties

Salthouse et al. demonstrated that the biodegradation of synthetic absorbable sutures is closely related to macrophage activity through the close adhesion of macrophage onto the surface of the absorbable sutures [Matlaga et al., 1980]. It is also known that inflammatory cells, particularly leukocytes and macrophages, are able to produce highly reactive oxygen species like superoxide ($\cdot O_2^-$) and hydrogen peroxide during inflammatory reactions toward foreign materials [Badwey et al., 1980; Devereux et al., 1991]. These highly reactive oxygen species participate in the biochemical reaction, frequently referred to as a respiratory burst, which is characterized by the one electron reduction of O_2 into superoxide via either NADPH or NADH oxidase as shown below. The reduction of O_2 results in an increase in O_2 uptake and the consumption of glucose:

$$2O_2 + NADPH \xrightarrow{\text{(NADPH Oxidase)}} 2\cdot O_2^- + NADP^+ + H^+ \quad (5.1)$$

The resulting superoxide radicals are then neutralized to H_2O_2 via cytoplasmic enzyme superoxide dismutase (SOD):

$$2 \cdot O_2^- + 2H^+ \xrightarrow{\text{(SOD)}} H_2O_2 + O_2 \qquad (5.2)$$

Williams et al. suggested that these reactive oxygen species may be harmful to polymeric implant surfaces through their production of highly reactive, potent, and harmful hydroxyl radicals $\cdot OH$ in the presence of metals like iron as shown in the following series of redox reactions [Ali et al., 1993; Zhong et al., 1994; Williams et al., 1991]:

$$\bullet O_2 + M^{+n} \rightarrow O_2 + M^{+(n-1)} \qquad (5.3)$$

$$H_2O_2 + M^{+(n-1)} \rightarrow \bullet OH + HO^- + M^{+n} \qquad (5.4)$$

The net reaction will be:

$$\bullet O_2^- + H_2O_2 \rightarrow \bullet OH + HO^- + O_2 \qquad (5.5)$$

and is often referred to as the metal-catalyzed Haber–Weiss reaction [Haber et al., 1934].

Although the role of free radicals in the hydrolytic degradation of synthetic biodegradable polymers is largely unknown, a very recent study using absorbable sutures like Vicryl in the presence of an aqueous free radical solution prepared from H_2O_2 and ferrous sulfate, $FeSO_4$, raised the possibility of the role of free radicals in the biodegradation of synthetic absorbable sutures [Williams et al., 1991; Zhong et al., 1994]. As shown below, both $\cdot OH$ radicals and OH^- are formed in the process of oxidation of Fe^{+2} by H_2O_2 and could exert some influence on the subsequent hydrolytic degradation of Vicryl sutures:

$$Fe^{+2} + H_2O_2 \rightarrow Fe^{+3} + \cdot OH + OH^-$$

SEM results indicated that Vicryl sutures in the presence of free radical solutions exhibited many irregular surface cracks at both 7 and 14 days *in vitro*, while the same sutures in the two controls (H_2O_2 or $FeSO_4$ solutions) did not have these surface cracks. Surprisingly, the presence of surface cracks of Vicryl sutures treated in the free radical solutions did not accelerate the tensile breaking strength loss as would be expected. Thermal properties of Vicryl sutures under the free radical and 3% H_2O_2 media showed the classical well-known maximum pattern of the change of the level of crystallinity with hydrolysis time. The level of crystallinity of Vicryl sutures peaked at 7 days in both media (free radical and 3% H_2O_2). The time for peak appearance in these two media was considerably earlier than Vicryl sutures in conventional physiological buffer media. Based on Chu's suggestion of using the time of the appearance of the crystallinity peak as an indicator of degradation rate, it appears that these two media accelerated the degradation of Vicryl sutures when compared with regular physiological buffer solution. Based on their findings, Williams et al. proposed the possible routes of the role of $\cdot OH$ radicals in the hydrolytic degradation of Vicryl sutures [Zhong et al., 1994]. Unfortunately, the possible role of OH^-, one of the byproducts of Fenton reagents ($H_2O_2/FeSO_4$), was not considered in the interpretation of their findings. OH^- species could be more potent than $\cdot OH$ toward hydrolytic degradation of synthetic absorbable sutures. This is because hydroxyl anions are the sole species which attack carbonyl carbon of the ester linkages during alkaline hydrolysis. Since an equal amount of $\cdot OH$ and OH^- are generated in Fenton reagents, the observed changes in morphological, mechanical, and thermal properties could be partially attributed to OH^- ions as well as $\cdot OH$ radicals.

Besides hydroxyl radicals, the production of superoxide ions and singlet oxygen during phagocytosis has been well documented [Babior et al., 1973]. Although the role of superoxide in simple organic ester hydrolysis has been known since the 1970s [Forrester et al., 1984, 1987; Johnson, 1976; Mango et al.,

1976; San Fillipo et al., 1976], its role in the hydrolytic degradation of synthetic biodegradable polyester-based biomaterials has remained largely unknown. Such an understanding of the superoxide ion role during the biodegradation of foreign materials has become increasing desirable because of the advanced understanding of how the human immune system reacts to foreign materials and the increasing use of synthetic biomaterials for human body repair.

Lee and Chu examined the reactivity of the superoxide ion toward biodegradable biomaterials having an aliphatic polyester structure at different reaction conditions such as temperature, time, and superoxide ion concentration [Lee and Chu, 1996]. Due to the extreme reactivity of the superoxide ion, it has been observed that the effect of superoxide ion-induced hydrolytic degradation of PDLLA and PLLA was significant in terms of changes in molecular weights and thermal properties. The superoxide ion-induced fragmentation of PDLLA would result in a mixture of various species with different chain lengths. A combined GPC method with a chemical tagging method revealed that the structure of oligomer species formed during the superoxide-induced degradation of PDLLA and PLLA was linear. The significant reduction in molecular weight of PDLLA by superoxide ion was also evident in the change of thermal properties like T_g. The linear low molecular weight species (oligomer, trimers, and dimers) in the reaction mixture could act as an internal plasticizer to provide the synergetic effects of lowering T_g by increasing free volume. The effect of the superoxide ion-induced hydrolytic degradation on molecular weight of PLLA was similar to PDLLA but with a much smaller magnitude. The mechanism of simple hydrolysis of ester by superoxide ion proposed by Forrester et al. was subsequently modified to interpret the data obtained from the synthetic biodegradable polymers.

In addition to the PDLLA and PLLA, superoxide ions also have a significant adverse effect on the hydrolytic degradation of synthetic absorbable sutures [Lee et al., 1996b]. A significant reduction in molecular weight has been found along with mechanical and thermal properties of these sutures over a wide range of superoxide ion concentrations, particularly during the first few hours of contact with superoxide ions. For example, the PGA suture lost almost all of its mass at the end of 24-h contact with superoxide ions at 25°C, while the same suture would take at least 50 days in an *in vitro* buffer for a complete mass loss. The surface morphology of these sutures was also altered drastically. The exact mechanism, however, is not fully known yet; Lee et al. suggested the possibility of simultaneous occurrence of several main-chain scissions by three different nucleophilic species.

Lee and Chu also reported that the addition of Fenton agent or hydrogen peroxide to the degradation medium would retard the well-known adverse effect of the conventional γ-irradiation sterilization of synthetic absorbable sutures [Lee and Chu, 1996]. They found that these γ-irradiated sutures retained better tensile breaking strength in the Fenton medium than in the regular buffer media. Chu et al. postulated that the γ-irradiation-induced α-carbon radicals in these sutures react with the hydroxyl radicals from the Fenton agent medium and hence neutralize the adverse effect of α-carbon radicals on the backbone chain scission. This mechanism is supported by the observed gradual loss of ESR signal of the sutures in the presence of the Fenton agent in the medium.

Instead of the adverse effect of free radicals on the degradation properties of synthetic biodegradable polyesters, Lee and Chu described an innovative approach of covalent bonding nitroxyl radicals onto these biodegradable polymers so that the nitroxyl radical attached polymers would have biological functions similar to nitric oxide [Lee et al., 1996a; Lee and Chu, 1998]. A preliminary *in vitro* cell culture study of these new biologically active biodegradable polymers indicated that they could retard the proliferation of human smooth muscle cells as native nitric oxide. The full potential of this new class of biologically active biodegradable polymers is currently under investigation by Chu for a variety of therapeutic applications.

5.6 The Role of Linear Aliphatic Biodegradable Polyesters in Tissue Engineering and Regeneration

The use of biodegradable polymers as the temporary scaffolds either to grow cells/tissues *in vitro* for tissue engineering applications or to regenerate tissues *in vivo* has very recently become a highly important aspect of research and development that broadens this class of biodegradable polymers beyond their traditional use in wound closure and drug control/release biomaterials. The scaffolds used in either tissue engineering or regeneration provide support for cellular attachment and subsequent controlled proliferation into a predefined shape or form. Obviously, a biodegradable scaffold would be preferred because of the elimination of chronic foreign body reaction and the generation of additional volume for regenerated tissues.

Although many other biodegradable polymers of natural origin like alginate [Atala et al., 1994], hyaluronate [Benedetti et al., 1993; Larsen et al., 1993], collagen [Hirai et al., 1995], and laminin [Dixit, 1994] have been studied for such a purpose, synthetic biodegradable polymers of linear aliphatic polyesters like PGA, PLA, and their copolymers [Bowald et al., 1979, 1980; Freed et al., 1993; Greisler, 1982, 1988, 1991; Greisler et al., 1985, 1987a and b, 1988a and b; Kim et al., 1998; Mikos et al., 1993; Mooney et al., 1994, 1995, 1996a, b, and c; Yu et al., 1993, 1994] have received more attention because of their consistent sources, reproducible properties, means to tailor their properties, and versatility in manufacturing processes.

Biodegradable polymers must be fabricated into stable textile structures before they can be used as the scaffold for tissue engineering or regeneration. The stability of the scaffold structure is important during tissue engineering and regeneration in order to maintain its proper size, shape, or form upon the shear force imposed by the circulating culture media in a bioreactor, the contractile force imposed by the growing cells on the scaffold surface, and other forces like the compression from surrounding tissues.

Kim et al. reported that, although ordinary non-woven PGA matrices have very good porosity (to facilitate diffusion of nutrients) with a high surface to volume ratio (to promote cell attachment and proliferation) and have been used to engineer dental pulp and smooth muscle tissues having comparable biological contents as the native tissues [Kim et al., 1998; Mooney et al., 1996c], these non-woven PGA matrices could not maintain their original structure during tissue engineering due to the relatively weak non-woven textile structure and stronger contractile force exerted by the attached and proliferated cells/tissues [Kim and Mooney, 1998a]. This led to deformed engineered tissues that may have undesirable properties; for example, the smooth muscle engineered on collagen gels exhibited significant contraction over time [Hirai et al., 1995; Zeigler et al., 1994].

Because of this shortcoming of the existing non-woven PGA matrices, Kim et al. very recently reported the use of PLLA to stabilize the PGA matrices [Kim et al., 1998]. A 5% w/v PLLA solution in chloroform was sprayed onto PGA non-woven matrices (made of 12-μm-diameter PGA fibers) of 97% porosity and either 3- or 0.5-mm thickness. The PLLA-impregnated PGA non-wovens could be subjected to additional heat treatment at 195°C to enhance their structural stability further. Figure 5.3 shows the morphology of such a heat-annealed PLLA-impregnated PGA non-woven matrix [Kim et al., 1998]. The PLLA was deposited mainly on the crosspoints of PGA fibers and hence interlocked the possible sliding of PGA fibers upon external force. Depending on the amount of PLLA used and subsequent heat treatment, the resulting PLLA-impregnated PGA non-woven matrices had an increase in compressive modulus of 10- to 35-fold when compared with the original PGA non-woven. The PLLA-impregnated PGA non-woven matrices also retained their initial volume (101 ± 4%) and about same shape as the original during the 7 weeks in culture, while the untreated PGA non-woven exhibited severe distortion in shape and contracted about 5% of its original volume. Since PLLA is well known to degrade at a much slower rate than PGA, its presence on the PGA fibers surface would be expected to make the treated PGA non-woven matrices degrade at a much slower rate than the untreated PGA non-woven. For example, the PLLA treated PGA non-woven retained about 80% of its initial mass, while the untreated PGA control had only 10% at the end of the 7-week culture.

Linear aliphatic polyesters like PGA, its lactide copolymer, and poly-*p*-dioxanone have also been fabricated into both woven and knitted forms for the *in vivo* regeneration of blood vessels in animals [Bowald et al., 1979, 1980; Greisler, 1982; Greisler et al., 1985, 1987a, 1988b, 1991; Yu et al., 1993, 1994]. The published results from a variety of animals like dogs and rabbits indicate that full-wall healing with pseudo-endothelial lining was observed. This class of synthetic biodegradable polymers are promising candidates for the regeneration of vascular tissue.

FIGURE 5.3 Scanning electron micrograph of the exterior of PLLA-impregnated and annealed PGA matrix. (*Source:* Kim, B.S. and Mooney, D.J., 1998. *J. Biomed. Mater. Res.*, 41(2):322–332. With permission.)

These encouraging findings were believed to be associated with the intense macrophage/biomaterial interactions. [Greisler, 1988; Greisler et al., 1989]. This interaction leads to a differential activation of the macrophage which, in turn, yields different macrophage products being released into the micro-environment [Greisler et al., 1991]. Greisler et al. have documented active stimulatory or inhibitory effects of various bioresorbable and non-resorbable materials on myofibroblast, vascular smooth muscle cell, and endothelial cell regeneration and has shown a transinterstitial migration to be their source when lactide/glycolide copolymeric prostheses are used [Greisler et al., 1988]. The rate of tissue ingrowth parallels the kinetics of macrophage-mediated prosthetic resorption in all lactide/glycolides studied [Gresler, 1982; Greisler et al., 1985, 1987a, 1988a]. Macrophage phagocytosis of the prosthetic material is observed histologically as early as 1 week following implantation of a rapidly resorbed material, such as PGA or polyglactin 910 (PG910), and is followed by an extensive increase in the myofibroblast population and neovascularization of the inner capsules [Greisler, 1982; Greisler et al., 1985, 1986]. Autoradiographic analyses using tritiated thymidine demonstrated a significantly increased mitotic index within these inner capsular cells, that mitotic index paralleling the course of prosthetic resorption [Greisler, 1991]. Polyglactin 910, for example, resulted in a mitotic index of 20.1 ± 16.6% 3 weeks following implantation, progressively decreasing to 1.2 ± 1.3% after 12 weeks. The more slowly resorbed polydioxanone prostheses demonstrated a persistently elevated mitotic index, 7.1 ± 3.8%, 12 weeks after implantation, a time in which the prosthetic material was still being resorbed. By contrast Dacron never yielded greater than a 1.2 ± 1.3% mitotic index [Greisler, 1991]. These mitotic indices correlated closely with the slopes of the inner capsule thickening curves suggesting that myofibroblast proliferation contributed heavily to this tissue deposition.

Therefore, the degradation property of synthetic biodegradable polymers somehow relates to macrophage activation which subsequently leads to the macrophage production of the required growth factors that initiate tissue regeneration. Different degradation properties of synthetic biodegradable polymers would thus be expected to result in different levels of macrophage activation, i.e., different degrees of tissue regeneration.

Defining Terms

Biodegradation: Materials that could be broken down by nature through hydrolytic mechanisms without the help of enzymes and/or enzymatic mechanism. It is loosely associated with absorbable, erodable, resorbable.

Tissue engineering: The ability to regenerate tissue through the help of artifical materials and devices.

References

Ali, S.A.M., Zhong, S.P., Doherty, P.J., and Williams, D.F., 1993. Mechanisms of polymer degradation in implantable devices. I. Poly(caprolactone). *Biomaterials*, 14:648.

Atala, A., Kim, W., Paige, K.T., Vancanti, C.A., and Retil, A., 1994. Endoscopic treatment of vesicoureterall reflux with a chondrocye-alginate suspension. *J. Urol.*, 152:641–643.

Babior, B.M., Kipnes R.S., and Cumutte, J.T., 1973. Biological defense mechanisms. The production by leukocytes of superoxide, a potential bactercidal agent. *J. Clin. Invest.*, 52: 741.

Badwey, J.A. and Kamovsky, M.L., 1980. Active oxygen species and the functions of phagocytic leucocytes. *Ann. Rev. Biochem.*, 49:695.

Barrows, T.H., 1986. Degradable implant materials: a review of synthetic absorbable polymers and their applications. *Clin. Mater.*, 1:233–257.

Barrows, T.H., 1994. *Bioabsorbable Poly(ester-amides)*. In: *Biomedical Polymers: Designed-to-Degrade Systems*, S.W. Shalaby, Ed., Hanser, New York, chap. 4.

Benedetti, L., Cortivo, R., Berti, T., Berti, A., and Pea, F., 1993. Biocompatibility and biodegradation of different hyaluronan derivatives (Hyaff) implanted in rats. *Biomaterials*, 14:1154–1160.

Bezwada, R.S., Jamiolkowski, D.D., Lee, I.Y., Agarwal, V., Persivale, J., Trenka-Benthin, S., Erneta, M., Suryadevara, J., Yang, A., and Liu, S., 1995. Monocryl suture: a new ultra-pliable absorbable monofilament suture, *Biomaterials*, 16: 1141–1148.

Bezwada, R.S., Shalaby, S.W., Newman, H.D. Jr., and Kafrawy, A., 1990. Bioabsorbable copolymers of p-dioxanone and lactide for surgical devices. *Trans. Soc. Biomater.*, 13:194.

Bostman, O., Hirvensalo, E., Vainionpaa, S. et al., 1990. Degradable polyglycolide rods for the internal fixation of displaced bimalleolar fractures. *Intern. Orthop. (Germany)*, 14(1):1–8.

Bowald, S., Busch, C., and Eriksson, I., 1979. Arterial regeneration following polyglactin 910 suture mesh grafting, *Surgery*, 86(5):722–729.

Bowald, S., Busch, C., and Eriksson, I., 1980. Absorbable material in vascular prosthesis. *Acta Chir. Scand.*, 146: 391–395.

Brandrup, J. and Immergut, E.H., 1975. *Polymer Handbook*, 2nd ed., Wiley, New York.

Campbell, N.D. and Chu, C.C., 1981. The effect of γ-irradiation on the biodegradation of polyglycolic acid synthetic sutures, the Tensile Strength Study. *27th International Symposium on Macromolecules*, Abstracts of Communications, Vol. II, pp. 1348–1352, Strasbourg, France, July 6–9.

Casey, D.J. and Roby, M.S., 1984. Synthetic copolymer surgical articles and method of manufacturing the same. U.S. Patent 4,429,080, American Cyanamid.

Chatani, Y., Suehiro, K., Okita, Y., Tadokoro, H., and Chujo, K., 1968. Structural studies of polyesters, I. Crystal structure of polyglycolide. *Makromol. Chemie*, 113:215–229.

Chu, C.C., 1981. The *in-vitro* degradation of poly(glycolic acid) sutures: effect of pH. *J. Biomed. Mater. Res.*, 15: 795–804.

Chu, C.C., 1982. The effect of pH on the *in vitro* degradation of poly(glycolide lactide) copolymer absorbable sutures. *J. Biomed. Mater. Res.*, 16:117–124.

Chu, C.C., 1985a. Strain-accelerated hydrolytic degradation of synthetic absorbable sutures. In: *Surgical Research Recent Development*, C.W. Hall, Ed., Pergamon Press, San Antonio, TX.

Chu, C.C., 1985b. The degradation and biocompatibility of suture materials. In: *CRC Critical Reviews in Biocompatibility*, D.F. Williams, Ed., Vol. 1(3), CRC Press, Boca Raton, FL, pp. 261–322.

Chu, C.C., 1991. Recent advancements in suture fibers for wound closure. In: *High-Tech Fibrous Materials: Composites, Biomedical Materials, Protective Clothing, and Geotextiles*, T.L. Vigo and A.F. Turbak, Eds., ACS Symposium Series No. 457, American Chemical Society, Washington, D.C., pp. 167–213.

Chu, C.C., 1995a. Biodegradable suture materials: intrinsic and extrinsic factors affecting biodegradation phenomena. In: *Handbook of Biomaterials and Applications*, D.L. Wise, D.E. Altobelli, E.R. Schwartz, M. Yszemski, J. D. Gresser, and D.J. Trantolo, Eds., Marcel Dekker, New York.

Chu, C.C. 1995b. Biodegradable suture materials: intrinsic and extrinsic factors affecting biodegradation. In: *Encyclopedic Handbook of Biomaterials and Applications*, Part A: *Materials*, Vol. 1, D.L. Wise, Ed., Marcel Dekker, chap. 17, pp. 543–688.

Chu, C.C. and Browning, A., 1988. The study of thermal and gross morphologic properties of polyglycolic acid upon annealing and degradation treatments. *J. Biomed. Mater. Res.*, 22(8):699–712.

Chu, C.C. and Campbell, N.D., 1982. Scanning electron microscope study of the hydrolytic degradation of poly(glycolic acid) suture. *J. Biomed. Mater. Res.*, 16(4):417–430.

Chu, C.C. and Kizil, Z., 1989. The effect of polymer morphology on the hydrolytic degradation of synthetic absorbable sutures. *3rd International ITV Conference on Biomaterials—Medical Textiles*, Stuttgart, Germany, June 14–16.

Chu, C.C. and Louie, M., 1985. A chemical means to study the degradation phenomena of polyglycolic acid absorbable polymer. *J. Appl. Polym. Sci.*, 30:3133–3141.

Chu, C.C. and Williams, D.F., 1983. The effect of γ-irradiation on the enzymatic degradation of polyglycolic acid absorbable sutures. *J. Biomed. Mater. Res.*, 17(6):1029.

Chu, C.C., Hsu, A., Appel, M., and Beth, M. 1992. The effect of macrophage cell media on the *in vitro* hydrolytic degradation of synthetic absorbable sutures. *4th World Biomaterials Congress*, April 27–May 1, Berlin, Germany.

Chu, C.C., von Fraunhofer, J.A., and Greisler, H.P., 1996. *Wound Closure Biomaterials and Devices*. CRC Press, Boca Raton, FL.

Chu, C.C., Zhang, L., and Coyne, L., 1995. Effect of irradiation temperature on hydrolytic degradation properties of synthetic absorbable sutures and polymers. *J. Appl. Polym. Sci.*, 56:1275–1294.

Chujo, K., Kobayashi, H., Suzuki, J., Tokuhara, S., and Tanabe, M., 1967a. Ring-opening polymerization of glycolide. *Die Makromol. Chemie*, 100:262–266.

Chujo, K., Kobayashi, H., Suzuki, J., and Tokuhara, S., 1967b. Physical and chemical characteristics of polyglycolide. *Die Makromol. Chemie*, 100:267–270.

Daniels, A.U., Taylor, M.S., Andriano, K.P., and Heller, J., 1992. Toxicity of absorbable polymers proposed for fracture fixation devices. *Trans. 38th Ann. Mtg. Orthop. Res. Soc.*, 17:88.

Devereux, D.F., O'Connell, S.M., Liesch, J.B., Weinstein, M., and Robertson, F.M., 1991. Induction of leukocyte activation by meshes surgically implanted in the peritoneal cavity. *Am. J. Surg.*, 162:243.

Dixit, V., 1994. Development of a bioartificial liver using isolated hepatocytes. *Artif. Organs*, 18:371–384.

Eitenmüller, K.L., Schmickal, G.T., and Muhr, G., 1989. Die Versorgung von Sprunggelenksfrakturen unter Verwendung von Platten und Schrauben aus resorbierbarem polymer Material. Presented at Jahrestagung der Deutschen Gesellschaft für Unfallheilkunde, Berlin, November.

Forrester, A.R. and Purushotham, V., 1984. Mechanism of hydrolysis of esters by superoxide. *J. Chem. Soc., Chem. Commun.*, 1505.

Forrester, A.R. and Purushotham, V., 1987. Reactions of carboxylic acid derivatives with superoxide. *J. Chem. Soc. Perkin Trans.* 1,945.

Fredericks, R.J., Melveger, A.J., and Dolegiewitz, L.J., 1984. Morphological and structural changes in a copolymer of glycolide and lactide occurring as a result of hydrolysis. *J. Polym. Sci. Phy. Ed.*, 22:57–66.

Freed, L.E., Marquis, J.C. Nohia, A., Emmanual, J., Mikos, A.G., and Langer, R., 1993. Neocartilage formation *in vitro* and *in vivo* using cells cultured on synthetic biodegradable polymers. *J. Biomed. Mater. Res.*, 27:11–23.

Fukuzaki, H., Yoshida, M., Asano, M., Aiba, Y., and Kumakura, M., 1989. Direct copolymerization of glycolic acid with lactones in the absence of catalysts. *Eur. Polym. J.*, 26:457–461.

Fukuzaki, H., Yoshida, M., Asano, M., Kumakura, M., Mashimo, T., Yuasa, H., Imai, K., Yamandka, H., Kawaharada, U., and Suzuki, K., 1991. A new biodegradable copolymer of glycolic acid and lactones with relatively low molecular weight prepared by direct copolycondensation in the absence of catalysts. *J. Biomed. Mater. Res.*, 25:315–328.

Gogolewski, S. and Pennings, A.J., 1983. Resorbable materials of poly(L-lactide). II. Fibres spun from solutions of poly(L-lactide) in good solvents. *J. Appl. Polym. Sci.*, 28:1045–1061.

Greisler, H.P., 1982. Arterial regeneration over absorbable prostheses. *Arch. Surg.*, 117:1425-1431.

Greisler, H.P., 1988. Macrophage-biomaterial interactions with bioresorbable vascular prostheses. *Trans. ASAIO*, 34(4):1051–1059.

Greisler, H.P., 1991. Macrophage activation in bioresorbable vascular grafts. In: *Vascular Endothelium: Physiological Basis of Clinical Problems*. Catravas, J.D., Callow, A.D., Gillis, C.N., and Ryan, U., Eds., Plenum Press, New York, NATO Advanced Study Institute, pp. 253–254.

Greisler, H.P., Kim, D.U., Price, J.B., and Voorhees, A.B., 1985. Arterial regenerative activity after prosthetic implantation. *Arch. Surg.*, 120: 315–323.

Greisler, H.P., Schwarcz, T.H., Ellinger, J., and Kim, D.U., 1986. Dacron inhibition of arterial regenerative activity. *J. Vasc. Surg.*, 747–756.

Greisler, H.P., Ellinger, J., Schwarcz, T.H., Golan, J., Raymond, R.M., and Kim, D.U., 1987a. Arterial regeneration over polydioxanone prostheses in the rabbit. *Arch. Surg.*, 122:715–721.

Greisler, H.P., Kim, D.U., Dennis, J.W., Klosak, J.J., Widerborg, K.A., Endean, E.D., Raymond, R.M., and Ellinger, J., 1987b. Compound polyglactin 910/polypropylene small vessel prostheses. *J. Vasc. Surg.*, 5:572–583.

Greisler, H.P., Dennis, J.W., Endean, E.D., and Kim, D.U., 1988a. Derivation of neointima of vascular grafts. *Circ. Suppl. I*, 78:I6–I12.

Greisler, H.P., Endean, E.D., Klosak, J.J., Ellinger, J., Dennis, J.W., Buttle, K., and Kim, D.U., 1988b. Polyglactin 910/polydioxanone bicomponent totally resorbable vascular prostheses. *J. Vasc. Surg.*, 7:697–705.

Greisler, H.P., Dennis, J.W., Endean, E.D., Ellinger, J., Friesel, R., and Burgess, W., 1989. Macrophage/biomaterial interactions: the stimulation of endotherlialization. *J. Vasc. Surg.*, 9(4):588–593.

Greisler, H.P., Tattersall, C.W., Kloask, J.J. et al., 1991. Partially bioresorbable vascular grafts in dogs. *Surgery*, 110(4):645–655.

Gross, R.A., 1994. Bacterial polyesters: structural variability in microbial synthesis. In: *Biomedical Polymers: Designed-to-Degrade Systems*, S.W. Shalaby, Ed., Hanser, New York, chap. 7.

Haber, F. and Weiss, J., 1934. The catalytic decomposition of hydrogen peroxide by iron salts. *Proc. R. Soc. Lond. A*, 147:332.

Helder, J., Feijen, J., Lee, S.J., and Kim, W., 1986. Copolymers of DL-lactic acid and glycine. *Makromol. Chem., Rapid. Commun.* 7:193.

Hirai, J. and Matsuda, T., 1995. Self-organized, tubular hybrid vascular tissue composed of vascular cells and collagen for low pressure-loaded venous system, *Cell Transplant*, 4:597–608.

Hofmann, G.O., 1992. Biodegradable implants in orthopaedic surgery—a review of the state of the art. *Clin. Mater.*, 10(1 & 2):75.

Hollinger, J.O., 1995. *Biomedical Applications of Synthetic Biodegradable Polymers*, CRC Press, Boca Raton, FL.

Jamiokowski, D.D., and Shalaby, S.W., 1991. A polymeric radiostabilizer for absorbable polyesters. In: *Radiation Effect of Polymers*, R.L. Clough and S.W. Shalaby, Eds., chap. 18, pp. 300–309. ACS Symposium Series #475, American Chemical Society, Washington, D.C.

Johnson, R.A., 1976. *Tetrahedron Lett.*, 331.

Katsarava, R., Beridze, V., Arabuli, N. Kharadze, D., Chu, C.C., and Won, C.Y., 1999. Amino acid-based bioanalogous polymers. Synthesis, and study of regular poly(ester amide)s based on *bis*(α-amino acid) α, ω-alkylene diesters and aliphatic dicarboxylic acids. *J. Polym. Sci. Part A: Polym. Chem.*, 37(4):391–407.

Katz, A., Mukherjee, D.P., Kaganov, A.L., and Gordon, S., 1985. A new synthetic monofilament absorbable suture made from polytrimethylene carbonate. *Surg. Gynecol. Obstet.*, 161:213–222.

Kim, B.S. and Mooney, D.J., 1998. Engineering smooth muscle tissue with a predefined structure. *J. Biomed. Mater. Res.*, 41(2):322.

Kim, B.S., Putman, A.J., Kulik, T.J., and Mooney, D.J., 1998. Optimizing seeding and culture methods to engineer smooth muscle tissue on biodegradable polymer matrices. *Biotechnol. Bioeng.*, 57:64–54.

Kimura, Y., 1993. Biodegradable polymers. In: *Biomedical Applications of Polymeric Materials*, T. Tsuruta, T. Hayashi, K. Kataoka, K. Ishihara, and Y. Kimura, Eds., pp.164–190. CRC Press, Boca Raton, FL.

Koelmel, D.F., Jamiokowski, D.D., Shalaby, S.W., and Bezwada, R.S., 1991. Low modulus radiation sterilizable monofilament sutures. *Polym. Prepr.*, 32(2):235–236.

Larsen, N.E., Pollak, C.T., Reiner, K., Leshchiner, E., and Balazs, E.A., 1993. Hylan gel biomaterial: dermal and immunologic compatibility. *J. Biomed. Meter. Res.*, 27:1129–1134.

Lee, K.H. and Chu, C.C., 1996. The role of free radicals in hydrolytic degradation of absorable polymeric biomaterials. 5th World Biomaterials Congress, Toronto, Canada, May 29–June 2.

Lee, K.H. and Chu, C.C., 1998. Molecular design of biologically active biodegradable polymers for biomedical applications. *Macromol. Symp.*, 130:71.

Lee, K.H., Chu, C.C., and Fred, J., 1996a. Aminoxyl-containing radical spin in polymers and copolymers. *U.S. Patent* 5,516,881.

Lee, K.H., Won, C.Y., and Chu, C.C., 1996b. Hydrolysis of absorable polymeric biomaterials by superoxide. 5th World Biomaterials Congress, Toronto, Canada, May 29–June 2.

Leenslag, J.W. and Pennings, A.J., 1984. Synthesis of high-molecular-weight poly(L-lactide) initiated with tin 2-ethylhexanoate. *Makromol. Chem.*, 188(8):1809–1814.

Li, S., Anjard, S., Tashkov, I., and Vert, M., 1998a. Hydrolytic degradation of PLA/PEO/PLA triblock copolymers prepared in the presence of Zn metal or CaH$_2$. *Polymer*, 39(22):5421–5430.

Li, Y. and Kissel, T., 1998b. Synthesis, characteristics and *in vitro* degradation of star-block copolymers consisting of L-lactide, glycolide and branched multi-arm poly(ethylene oxide). *Polymer*, 39(18): 4421–4427.

Loh, I.H., Chu, C.C., and Lin, H.L., 1992. Plasma surface modification of synthetic absorbable fibers for wound closure. *J. Appl. Biomater.*, 3(2):131–146.

Magno, F. and Bontempelli, G., 1976. *J. Electroanal. Chem.*, 68: 337.

Matlaga, V.F. and Salthouse, T.N., 1980. Electron microscopic observations of polyglactin 910 suture sites, In *First World Biomaterials Congress Abstr.*, Baden, Austria, April 8–12, p. 2.

Mikos, A.G., Sarakinos, G., Leite, S.M., Vacanti, J.P., and Langer, R., 1993. Laminated three-dimensional biodegradable forms for use in tissue engineering. *Biomaterials*, 14:323–330.

Miller, N.D. and Williams, D.F., 1984. The *in vivo* and *in vitro* degradation of poly(glycolic acid) suture material as a function of applied strain. *Biomaterials*, 5:365–368.

Mooney, D.J., Organ, G., Vacanti, J.P., and Langer, R., 1994. Design and fabrication of biodegradable polymer devices to engineer tubular tissue. *Cell Transplant*, 3:203–210.

Mooney, D.J., Breuer, C., McNamara, K., Vacanti, J.P., and Langer, R., 1995. Fabricating tubular devices from polymers of lactic and glycolic acid for tissue engineering. *Tissue Eng.*, 1:107–118.

Mooney, D.J., Baldwin, D.F., Vacanti, J.P., and Langer, R., 1996a. Novel approach to fabricate porous sponges of poly(D,L-lactic-*co*-glycolic acid) without the use of organic solvents. *Biomaterials*, 17:1417–1422.

Mooney, D.J., Mazzoni, C.L., Breuer, K., McNamara, J.P., Vacanti, J.P., and Langer, R., 1996b. Stabilized polyglycolic acid fibre-based tubes for tissue engineering. *Biomaterials,* 17:115–124.

Mooney, D.J, Powell, C., Piana, J., and Rutherford, B., 1996c. Engineering dental pulp-like tissue *in vitro. Biotechnol. Prog.,* 12:865–868.

Nathan, A. and Kohn, J., 1994. Amino acid derived polymers. In: *Biomedical Polymers: Designed-to-Degrade Systems,* S.W. Shalaby, Ed., chap. 5. Hanser Publishers, New York.

Park, K., Shalaby, W.S.W., and Park. H., 1993. *Biodegradable Hydrogels for Drug Delivery,* Technomic, Lancaster, PA.

Pratt, L. and Chu, C.C., 1993. Hydrolytic degradation of α-substituted polyglycolic acid: a semi-empirical computational study. *J. Comp. Chem.,* 14(7):809–817.

Pratt, L. and Chu, C.C., 1994a. The effect of electron donating and electron withdrawing substituents on the degradation rate of bioabsorbable polymers: a semi-empirical computational study. *J. Molec. Structure,* 304:213–226.

Pratt, L. and Chu, C.C., 1994b. A computational study of the hydrolysis of degradable polysaccharide biomaterials: substituent effects on the hydrolytic mechanism. *J. Comp. Chem.,* 15:241–248.

Pratt, L., Chu, A., Kim, J., Hsu, A. and Chu, C.C., 1993. The effect of electrolytes on the *in vitro* hydrolytic degradation of synthetic biodegradable polymers: mechanical properties, thermodynamics and molecular modeling. *J. Polym. Sci. Chem Ed.,* 31:1759–1769.

Puelacher, W.C., Mooney, D., Langer, R., Upton, J., Vacanti, J.P., and Vananti, C.A., 1994. Design of nasoseptal cartilage replacements sunthesized from biodegradable polymers and chondrocytes. *Biomaterials,* 15:774–778.

San Fillipo, Jr, J., Romano, L.J., Chem, C.I., and Valentine, J.S., 1976. Cleavage of esters by superoxide. *J. Org. Chem.,* 4:586.

Shalaby, S.W., Ed., 1994. *Biomedical Polymers: Designed-to-Degrade Systems,* Hanser Publishers, New York.

Shieh, S.J., Zimmerman, M.C., and Parsons, J.R., 1990. Preliminary characterization of bioresorbable and nonresorbable synthetic fibers for the repair of soft tissue injuries. *J. Biomed. Mater. Res.,* 24:789–808.

Sugnuma, J., Alexander, H., Traub, J., and Ricci, J.L., 1992. Biological response of intramedullary bone to poly-L-lactic acid. In: *Tissue-Inducing Biomater,* L.G. Cima and E.S. Ron, Eds., *Mater. Res. Soc. Sump. Proc.,* 252:339–343.

Tunc, D.C., 1983. A high strength absorbable polymer for internal bone fixation. *Trans. Soc. Biomater.,* 6:47.

Vert, M., Feijen, J., Albertsson, A., Scott, G., and Chiellini, E., 1992. *Biodegradable Polymers and Plastics,* Royal Society of Chemistry, Cambridge, England.

Williams, D.F., 1979. Some observations on the role of cellular enzymes in the *in vivo* degradation of polymers. *ASTM Spec. Tech. Publ.,* 684:61–75.

Williams, D.F., 1990. Biodegradation of medical polymers. In: *Concise Encyclopedia of Medical and Dental Materials,* D.F. Williams, Ed., pp. 69–74. Pergamon Press, New York.

Williams, D.F., and Chu, C.C., 1984. The effects of enzymes and gamma irradiation on the tensile strength and morphology of poly(*p*-dioxanone) fibers. *J. Appl. Polym. Sci.,* 29:1865–1877.

Williams, D.F., and Mort, E., 1977. Enzyme-accelerated hydrolysis of polyglycolic acid. *J. Bioeng.* 1:231–238.

Williams, D.F. and Zhong, S.P., 1991. Are free radicals involved in the biodegradation of implanted polymers. *Adv. Mater.,* 3:623.

Winet, H. and Hollinger, J.O., 1993. Incorporation of polylactide-polyglycolide in a cortical defect: neoosteogenesis in a bone chamber. *J. Biomed. Mater. Res.,* 27:667–676.

Wise, D.L., Fellmann, T.D., Sanderson, J.E., and Wentworth, R.L., 1979. Lactic/glycolic acid polymers. In: *Drug Carriers in Biology and Medicine,* G. Gregoriadis, Ed., pp. 237–270. Academic Press, New York.

Yu, T.J. and Chu, C.C., 1993. Bicomponent vascular grafts consisting of synthetic biodegradable fibers. Part I. *In vitro* study. *J. Biomed. Mater. Res.,* 27:1329–1339.

Yu, T.J., Ho, D.M., and Chu, C.C., 1994. Bicomponent vascular grafts consisting of synthetic biodegradable fibers. Part II. *In vivo* healing response. *J. Inv. Surg.* 7:195–211.

Zhang, L., Loh, I.H., and Chu, C.C., 1993. A combined γ-irradiation and plasma deposition treatment to achieve the ideal degradation properties of synthetic absorbable polymers. *J. Biomed. Mater. Res.*, 27:1425–1441.

Zhong, S.P., Doherty, P.J., and Williams, D.F., 1994. A preliminary study on the free radical degradation of glycolic acid/lactic acid copolymer. *Elastics, Rubber and Composites Processing and Application*, 21:89.

Ziegler, T. and Nerem, R.M., 1994. Tissue engineering a blood vessel: regulation of vascular biology by mechanical stress, *J. Cell. Biochem.*, 56:204–209.

Further Information

Several publications provide very comprehensive descriptions of a variety of biodegradable polymeric biomaterials, their synthesis, and physical, chemical, mechanical, biodegradable, and biological properties.

Barrows, T.H., 1986, Degradable implant materials: a review of synthetic absorbable polymers and their applications, *Clin. Mater.*, 1:233–257.

Chu, C.C., 1995. Biodegradable suture materials: intrinsic and extrinsic factors affecting biodegradation phenomena. In: *Handbook of Biomaterials and Applications*, D.L. Wise, D.E. Altobelli, E.R. Schwartz, M. Yszemski, J.D. Gresser, and D.J. Trantolo, Eds., Marcel Dekker, New York.

Chu, C.C., von Fraunhofer, J.A., and Greisler, H.P., 1996. *Wound Closure Biomaterials and Devices*, CRC Press, Boca Raton, FL.

Hollinger, J.O., Ed., 1995. *Biomedical Applications of Synthetic Biodegradable Polymers*, CRC Press, Boca Raton, FL.

Kimura, Y., 1993, Biodegradable polymers. In: *Biomedical Applications of Polymeric Materials*, T. Tsuruta, T. Hayashi, K. Kataoka, K. Ishihara, and Y. Kimura, Eds., pp. 164–190. CRC Press, Boca Raton, FL.

Park, K., Shalaby, W.S.W., and Park. H., 1993. *Biodegradable Hydrogels for Drug Delivery*, Technomic, Lancaster, PA.

Shalaby, S.W., 1994. *Biomedical Polymers: Designed-to-Degrade Systems*, Hanser Publishers, New York.

Vert, M., Feijen, J., Albertsson, A., Scott, G., and Chiellini, E., 1992. *Biodegradable Polymers and Plastics*, Royal Society of Chemistry, Cambridge, England.

The review by Barrows is brief with an emphasis on their applications and an extensive lists of patents. The book and chapter by Chu et al. focus on the most successful use of biodegradable polymers in medicine, namely wound closure biomaterials like sutures, and provide the most comprehensive review of all aspects of biodegradable wound closure biomaterials with very detailed chemical, physical, mechanical, biodegradable, and biological information. The chapter by Kimura is an overview of the subject with some interesting new polymers. The chapter includes both enzymatically degradable natural polymers and non-enzymatically degradable synthetic polymers. The biodegradable hydrogel book by Park et al. is the only book available that focuses on hydrogel. Probably the most broad coverage of biodegradable polymeric biomaterials is the book edited by Shalaby. It has eight chapters and covers almost all commercially and experimentally available biodegradable polymers. The book edited by Vert et al. is based on the Proceedings of the 2nd International Scientific Workshop on Biodegradable Polymers and Plastics held in Montpellier, France in November 1991. The book covers both medical and non-medical applications of biodegradable polymers. It has broader coverage of biodegradable polymers with far more chapters than Shalaby's book, but its chapters are shorter and less comprehensive than Shalaby's book, which is far more focused on biomedical use.

Topics of biodegradable polymeric biomaterials can also be found in *Journal of Biomedical Materials Research, Journal of Applied Biomaterials, Biomaterials, Journal of Biomaterials Science: Polymer Ed., Journal of Applied Polymer Science, Journal of Materials Science,* and *Journal Polymer Science.*

6

Biologic Biomaterials: Tissue-Derived Biomaterials (Collagen)

Shu-Tung Li
Collagen Matrix, Inc.

6.1   Structure and Properties of Collagen and Collagen-Rich Tissues

Structure of Collagen

Collagen is a multifunctional family of proteins of unique structural characteristics. It is the most abundant and ubiquitous protein in the body, its functions ranging from serving crucial biomechanical functions in bone, skin, tendon, and ligament to controlling cellular gene expressions in development [Nimni and Harkness, 1988]. Collagen molecules like all proteins are formed *in vivo* by enzymatic-regulated step-wise polymerization reaction between amino and carboxyl groups of amino acids, where R is a side group of an amino acid residue:

$$(-\overset{\overset{O}{\|}}{C}-\overset{\overset{H}{|}}{N}-\overset{\overset{H}{|}}{\underset{\underset{R}{|}}{C}}-)_n \tag{6.1}$$

The simplest amino acid is *glycine* (Gly) (R = H), where a hypothetical flat sheet organization of polyglycine molecules can form and be stabilized by intermolecular hydrogen bonds (Fig. 6.1a). However, when R is a large group as in most other amino acids, the stereochemical constraints frequently force the *polypeptide* chain to adopt a less constraining conformation by rotating the bulky R groups away from the crowded interactions, forming a helix, where the large R groups are directed toward the surface of the helix (Fig. 6.1b). The hydrogen bonds are allowed to form within a helix between the hydrogen

FIGURE 6.1   (a) Hypothetical flat sheet structure of a protein. (b) Helical arrangement of a protein chain.

attached to nitrogen in one amino acid residue and the oxygen attached to a second amino acid residue. Thus, the final conformation of a protein, which is directly related to its function, is governed primarily by the amino acid sequence of the particular protein.

Collagen is a protein comprised of three polypeptides (α chains), each having a general amino acid sequence of $(-Gly-X-Y-)_n$, where X is any other amino acid and is frequently *proline* (Pro) and Y is any other amino acid and is frequently *hydroxyproline* (Hyp). A typical amino acid composition of collagen is shown in Table 6.1. The application of helical diffraction theory to high-angle collagen x-ray diffraction pattern [Rich and Crick, 1961] and the stereochemical constraints from the unusual amino acid composition [Eastoe, 1967] led to the initial triple-helical model and subsequent modified triple helix of the collagen molecule. Thus, collagen can be broadly defined as a protein which has a typical triple helix extending over the major part of the molecule. Within the triple helix, glycine must be present as every third amino acid, and proline and hydroxyproline are required to form and stabilize the triple helix.

To date, 19 proteins can be classified as collagen [Fukai et al., 1994]. Among the various collagens, type I collagen is the most abundant and is the major constituent of bone, skin, ligament, and tendon. Due to the abundance and ready accessibility of these tissues, they have been frequently used as a source for the preparation of collagen. This chapter will not review the details of the structure of the different collagens. The readers are referred to reviews for a more in-depth discussion of this subject [Nimni, 1988; van der Rest et al., 1990; Fukai et al., 1994; Brodsky and Ramshaw, 1997]. It is, however, of particular relevance to review some salient structural features of the type I collagen in order to facilitate the subsequent discussions of properties and its relation to biomedical applications.

TABLE 6.1   Amino Acid Content of Collagen

Amino Acid	Content (Residues/1000 residues[a])
Gly	334
Pro	122
Hyp	96
Acid polar (Asp, Glu, Asn)	124
Basic polar (Lys, Arg, His)	91
Other	233

[a] Reported values are average values of 10 different determinations for tendon tissue.

Source: Eastoe [1967].

FIGURE 6.2   Diagram depicting the formation of collagen, which can be visualized as taking place in several steps: (a) single-chain left-handed helix; (b) three single chains intertwined into a triple-stranded helix; (c) a collagen (tropocollagen) molecule; (d) collagen molecules aligned in *D* staggered fashion in a fibril producing overlap and hole regions.

A type I collagen molecule (also referred to as *tropocollagen*) isolated from various tissues has a molecular weight of about 283,000 daltons. It is comprised of three left-handed helical polypeptide chains (Figure 6.2a) which are intertwined forming a right-handed helix around a central molecular axis (Figure 6.2b). Two of the polypeptide chains are identical (α_1), having 1056 amino acid residues, and the third polypeptide chain (α_2) has 1029 amino acid residues [Miller, 1984]. The triple-helical structure has a rise per residue of 0.286 nm and a unit twist of 108°, with 10 residues in three turns and a helical pitch (repeating distance within a single chain) of 30 residues or 8.68 nm [Fraser et al., 1983]. Over 95% of the amino acids have the sequence of Gly–*X*–*Y*. The remaining 5% of the molecule does not have the sequence of Gly–*X*–*Y* and is therefore not triple helical. These nonhelical portions of the molecule are located at the N- and C-terminal ends and are referred to as *telopeptides* (9~26 residues) [Miller, 1984]. The whole molecule has a length of about 280 nm and a diameter of about 1.5 nm and has a conformation similar to a rigid rod (Fig. 6.2c).

The triple-helical structure of a collagen molecule is stabilized by several factors (Fig. 6.3): (1) a tight fit of the amino acids within the triple-helix—this geometrical stabilization factor can be appreciated from a space-filling model constructed from a triple helix with (Gly–Pro–Hyp) sequence (Fig. 6.3); (2) the interchain hydrogen bond formation between the backbone carbonyl and amino hydrogen interactions; and (3) the contribution of water molecules to the interchain hydrogen bond formation.

The telopeptides are regions where *intermolecular crosslinks* are formed *in vivo*. A common intermolecular crosslink is formed between an *allysine* (the ε-amino group of lysine or hydroxy-lysine has been converted to an aldehyde) of one telopeptide of one molecule and an ε-amino group of a lysine or hydroxylysine in the triple helix or a second molecule (Fig. 6.2). Thus the method commonly used to solubilize the collagen molecules from crosslinked fibrils with *proteolytic enzymes* such as *pepsin* removes the telopeptides (cleaves the intermolecular crosslinks) from the collagen molecule. The pepsin solubilized collagen is occasionally referred to as *atelocollagen* [Stenzl, 1974].

FIGURE 6.3   A space-filling model of the collagen triple helix, showing all the atoms in a ten-residue segment of repeating triplet sequence $(Gly–Pro–Hyp)_n$. The arrow shows an interchain hydrogen bond. The arrow heads identify the hydroxy groups of hydroxyproline in one chain. The circle shows a hydrogen-bonded water molecule. The short white lines identify the ridge of amino acid chains. The short black lines indicate the supercoil of one chain [Piez, 1984].

$$Pr–CH_2–CH_2–CH_2–CHO \quad + \quad H_2N–CH_2–\overset{\overset{\textstyle OH}{\textstyle |}}{CH}–CH_2–CH_2–Pr$$

$$\text{Allysine} \qquad\qquad\qquad \text{Hydroxylysine} \tag{6.2}$$

$$\rightarrow Pr–CH_2–CH_2–CH_2–CH{=}N–CH_2–\overset{\overset{\textstyle OH}{\textstyle |}}{CH}–CH_2–CH_2–Pr$$

$$\text{Dehydrohydroxylysinonorleucine}$$

Since the presence of hydroxyproline is unique in collagen (*elastin* contains a small amount), the determination of collagen content in a collagen-rich tissue is readily done by assaying the hydroxyproline content.

Collagen does not appear to exist as isolated molecules in the extracellular space in the body. Instead, collagen molecules aggregate into *fibrils*. Depending on the tissue and age, a collagen fibril varies from about 50 nm to about 300 nm in diameter with indeterminate length and can be easily seen under electron microscopy (Fig. 6.4). The fibrils are important structural building units for large *fibers* (Fig. 6.5). Collagen molecules are arranged in specific orders both longitudinally and in cross-section, and the organization of collagen molecules in a fibril is tissue specific [Katz and Li, 1972; 1973b]. The two-dimensional structure (the projection of a three-dimensional structure onto a two-dimensional plane) of a type I collagen fibril has been unequivocally defined both by an analysis of small-angle x-ray diffraction pattern along the meridian of a collagenous tissue [Bear, 1944] and by examination of the transmission electron micrographs of tissues stained with negative or positive stains [Hodge and Petruska, 1963]. In this structure (Fig. 6.2d), the collagen molecules are staggered with respect to one another by a distance of D (64 nm to 67 nm) or multiple of D, where D is the fundamental repeat distance seen in the small-angle x-ray diffraction pattern, or the repeating distance seen in the electron micrographs. Since a collagen molecule has a length of about 4.4 D, this staggering of collagen molecules creates overlap regions of about 0.4 D and hole or defect regions of about 0.6 D.

(a)

(b)   (c)

FIGURE 6.4 (a) Scanning electron micrograph of the surface of an adult rabbit bone matrix, showing how the collagen fibrils branch and interconnect in an intricate, woven pattern (4800×) [Tiffit, 1980]. (b) Transmission electron micrographs (24,000×) of parallel collagen fibrils in tendon [Fung, 1992]. (c) Transmission electron micrographs (24,000×) of mesh work of fibrils in skin [Fung, 1993].

UNIT FIBRILS
800Å-1000Å

1-4μ

FIGURE 6.5 Diagram showing the collagen fibers of the connective tissue in general, which are composed of unit collagen fibrils.

One interesting and important structural aspect of collagen is its approximate equal number of acidic (*aspartic* and *glutamic* acids) and basic (lysines and *arginines*) side groups. Since these groups are charged under physiological conditions, the collagen is essentially electrically neutral [Li and Katz, 1976]. The packing of collagen molecules with a D staggering results in clusters of regions where the charged groups are located [Hofmann and Kuhn, 1981]. These groups therefore are in close proximity to form intra- and intermolecular hydrogen-bonded *salt linkages* of the form (Pr–COO⁻ ⁺H₃N–Pr) [Li et al., 1975]. In addition, the side groups of many amino acids are nonpolar [*alanine* (Ala), *valine* (Val), *leucine* (Leu), *isoleucine* (Ile), *proline* (Pro), and *phenolalanine* (Phe)] in character and hence *hydrophobic;* therefore, chains with these amino acids avoid contact with water molecules and seek interactions with the nonpolar chains of amino acids. In fact, the result of molecular packing of collagen in a fibril is such that the nonpolar groups are also clustered, forming hydrophobic regions within collagen fibrils [Hofmann and Kuhn, 1981]. Indeed, the packing of the collagen molecules in various tissues is believed to be a result of intermolecular interactions involving both the electrostatic and hydrophobic interactions [Hofmann and Kuhn, 1981; Katz and Li, 1981; Li et al., 1975].

The three-dimensional organization of type I collagen molecules within a fibril has been the subject of extensive research over the past 40 years [Fraser et al., 1983; Katz and Li, 1972, 1973a, 1973b, 1981; Miller, 1976; Ramachandran, 1967; Yamuchi et al., 1986]. Many structural models have been proposed based on an analysis of equatorial and off-equatorial x-ray diffraction patterns of rat-tail-tendon collagen [Miller, 1976; North et al., 1954], *intrafibrillar volume* determination of various collagenous tissues [Katz and Li, 1972, 1973a, 1973b], intermolecular side chain interactions [Hofmann and Kuhn, 1981; Katz and Li, 1981; Li et al., 1981], and intermolecular crosslinking patterns studies [Yamuchi et al., 1986]. The general understanding of the three-dimensional molecular packing in type I collagen fibrils is that the collagen molecules are arranged in hexagonal or near hexagonal arrays [Katz and Li, 1972, 1981; Miller, 1976]. Depending on the tissue, the intermolecular distance varies from about 0.15 nm in rat tail tendon to as large as 0.18 nm in bone and dentin [Katz and Li, 1973b]. The axial staggering of the molecules by 1~4 D with respect to one another is tissue specific and has not yet been fully elucidated.

TABLE 6.2   Composition of Collagen-Rich Soft Tissues

Component	Composition (%)
Collagen	75 (dry), 30 (wet)
Proteoglycans and polysaccharides	20 (dry)
Elastin and glycoproteins	<5 (dry)
Water	60–70

Source: Park and Lakes [1992].

There are very few interspecies differences in the structure of type I collagen molecule. The extensive homology of the structure of type I collagen may explain why this collagen obtained from animal species is acceptable as a material for human implantation.

Properties of Collagen-Rich Tissue

The function of collagenous tissue is related to its structure and properties. This section reviews some important properties of collagen-rich tissues.

Physical and Biomechanical Properties

The physical properties of tissues vary according to the amount and structural variations of the collagen fibers. In general, a collagen-rich tissue contains about 75–90% of collagen on a dry weight basis. Table 6.2 is a typical composition of a collagen-rich soft tissue such as skin. Collagen fibers (bundles of collagen fibrils) are arranged in different configurations in different tissues for their respective functions at specific anatomic sites. For example, collagen fibers are arranged in parallel in tendon [Fig. 6.4b] and ligament for their high-tensile strength requirements, whereas collagen fibers in skin are arranged in random arrays [Fig. 6.4c] to provide the resiliency of the tissue under stress. Other structure-supporting functions of collagen such as transparency for the lens of the eye and shaping of the ear or tip of the nose can also be provided by the collagen fiber. Thus, an important physical property of collagen is the three-dimensional organization of the collagen fibers.

The collagen-rich tissues can be thought of as a composite polymeric material in which the highly oriented crystalline collagen fibrils are embedded in the amorphous ground substance of noncollagenous *polysaccharides, glycoproteins,* and elastin. When the tissue is heated, its specific volume increases, exhibiting a glass transition at about 40°C and a melting of the crystalline collagen fibrils at about 56°C. The melting temperature of crystalline collagen fibrils is referred to as the *denaturation temperature* of collagenous tissues.

The stress–strain curves of a collagenous tissue such as tendon exhibit nonlinear behavior (Fig. 6.6). This nonlinear behavior of stress–strain of tendon collagen is similar to that observed in synthetic fibers. The initial toe region represents alignment of fibers in the direction of stress. The steep rise in slope represents the majority of fibers stretched along their long axes. The decrease in slope following the steep rise may represent the breaking of individual fibers prior to the final catastrophic failure. Table 6.3 summarizes some mechanical properties of collagen and elastic fibers. The difference in biomechanical properties between collagen and elastin is a good example of the requirements for these proteins to serve their specific functions in the body.

Unlike tendon or ligament, skin consists of collagen fibers randomly arranged in layers or lamellae. Thus, skin tissues show mechanics anisotropy (Fig. 6.7). Another feature of the stress–strain curve of the skin is its extensibility under small load as compared to tendon. At small load the fibers are straightened and aligned rather than stretched. Upon further stretching the fibrous lamellae align with respect to each other and resist further extension. When the skin is highly stretched the modulus of elasticity approaches that of tendon as expected of the aligned collagen fibers.

Cartilage is another collagen-rich tissue which has two main physiological functions. One is the maintenance of shape (ear, tip of nose, and rings around the trachea), and the other is to provide bearing surfaces at joints. It contains very large and diffuse proteoglycan (protein-polysaccharide)

FIGURE 6.6   A typical stress–strain curve for tendon [Rigby et al., 1959].

TABLE 6.3   Elastic Properties of Collagen and
Elastic Fibers

Fibers	Modulus of Elasticity (MPa)	Tensile Strength (MPa)	Ultimate Elongation (%)
Collagen	1000	50–100	10
Elastin	0.6	1	100

Source: Park and Lakes [1992].

FIGURE 6.7   Stress–strain curves of human abdominal skin [Daly, 1966].

molecules which form a gel in which the collagen-rich molecules are entangled. They can affect the mechanical properties of the collagen by hindering the movements through the interstices of the collagenous matrix network.

TABLE 6.4 Mechanical Properties of Some Nonmineralized Human Tissues

Tissue	Tensile Strength (MPa)	Ultimate Elongation (%)
Skin	7.6	78.0
Tendon	53.0	9.4
Elastic cartilage	3.0	30.0
Heart valves (aortic)		
Radial	0.45	15.3
Circumferential	2.6	10.0
Aorta		
Transverse	1.1	77.0
Longitudinal	0.07	81.0

Source: Park and Lakes [1992].

The joint cartilage has a very low coefficient of friction (<0.01). This is largely attributed to the squeeze-film effect between cartilage and synovial fluid. The synovial fluid can be squeezed out through highly fenestrated cartilage upon compressive loading, and the reverse action will take place in tension. The lubricating function is carried out in conjunction with *glycosaminoglycans* (GAG), especially *chondroitin sulfates*. The modulus of elasticity (10.3~20.7 MPa) and tensile strength (3.4 MPa) are quite low. However, wherever high stress is required the cartilage is replaced by purely collagenous tissue. Mechanical properties of some collagen-rich tissues are given in Table 6.4 as a reference.

Physiochemical Properties

Electrostatic Properties. A collagen molecule has a total of approximately 240 ε-amino and guanidino groups of lysines, hydroxylysines, and arginines and 230 carboxyl groups of aspartic and glutamic acids. These groups are charged under physiological conditions. In a native fibril, most of these groups interact either intra- or intermolecularly forming salt-linkages providing significant stabilization energy to the collagen fibril [Li et al., 1975]. Only a small number of charged groups are free. However, the electrostatic state within a collagen fibril can be altered by changing the pH of the environment. Since the pK for an amino group is about 10 and about 4 for a carboxyl group, the electrostatic interactions are significantly perturbed at a pH below 4 and above 10. The net result of the pH change is a weakening of the intra- and intermolecular electrostatic interactions, resulting in a swelling of the fibrils. The fibril swelling can be prevented by chemically introducing covalent intermolecular crosslinks. Any bifunctional reagent which reacts with amino, carboxyl, and hydroxyl groups can serve as a crosslinking agent. The introduction of covalent intermolecular crosslinks fixes the physical state of the fibrillar structure and balances the swelling pressures obtained from any pH changes.

Another way of altering the electrostatic state of a collagen fibril is by chemically modifying the electrostatic side groups. For example, the positively charged ε-amino groups of lysine and hydroxylysine can be chemically modified with acetic anhydride, which converts the ε-amino groups to a neutral acetyl group [Green et al., 1954]. The result of this modification increases the number of the net negative charges of the fibril. Conversely, the negatively charged carboxyl groups of aspartic and glutamic acid can be chemically modified to a neutral group by methylation [Fraenkel-Conrat, 1944]. Thus, by adjusting the pH of the solution and applying chemical modification methods, a range of electrostatic properties of collagen can be obtained.

Ion and Macromolecular Binding Properties. In the native state and under physiological conditions, a collagen molecule has only about 60 free carboxyl groups [Li et al., 1975]. These groups have the capability of binding cations such as calcium with a free energy of formation for the protein $-COO-Ca^{++}$ of about 1.2 Kcal/mol. This energy is not large enough to compete for the hydrogen-bonded salt-linkage interactions, which have a free energy of formation of about -1.6 Kcal/mol. The extent of ion binding, however, can be enhanced in the presence of lyotropic salts such as KCNS, which breaks the salt linkages, or by shifting the pH away from the *isoelectric point* of collagen. Macromolecules can bind to collagen via covalent bonding, cooperative ionic binding, entrapment, entanglement, and a combination of the above. In addition, binding of charged ions and macromolecules can be significantly increased by modifying the charge profile of collagen as described previously. For example, a complete N-acetylation of collagen will eliminate all the positively charged ε-amino groups and, thus, will increase the free negatively charged groups. The resulting acetylated collagen enhances the binding of positively charged ions and macromolecules. On the other hand, the methylation of collagen will eliminate the negatively charged carboxyl groups and, thus, will increase the free positively charge moieties. The methylated collagen, therefore, enhances the binding of negatively charged ions and macromolecules [Li and Katz, 1976].

Fiber-Forming Properties.   Native collagen molecules are organized in tissues in specific orders. *Polymorphic* forms of collagen can be reconstituted from the collagen molecules, obtained either from enzymatic digestion of collagenous tissues or by extracting the tissues with salt solutions. The formation of polymorphic aggregates of collagen depends on the environment for reconstitution [Piez, 1984]. Native arrangement of the collagen molecules is formed under physiological conditions. Various polymorphic molecular aggregates may be formed by changing the state of intermolecular interactions. For example, when collagen molecules are aggregated under high concentrations of a neutral salt or under nonaqueous conditions, the collagen molecules associate into random arrays having no specific regularities detectable by electron microscopy. The collagen molecules can be induced to aggregate into other polymorphic forms such as the *segment-long-spacing* (SLS) form where all heads are aligned in parallel and the *fibrous-long-spacing* (FLS) form where the molecules are randomly aligned in either a head-to-tail, tail-to-tail, or head-to-head orientation.

Biologic Properties

Hemostatic Properties.   Native collagen aggregates are intrinsically hemostatic. The mechanism of collagen-induced hemostasis has been the subject of numerous investigations [Jaffe and Deykin, 1974; Wang et al., 1978; Wilner et al., 1968]. The general conclusion from these studies is that *platelets* first adhere to a collagen surface. This induces the release of platelet contents, followed by platelet aggregation, leading to the eventual hemostatic plug. The hemostatic activity of collagen is dependent on the size of the collagen aggregate and the native organization of the molecules [Wang et al., 1978]. Denatured collagen (*gelatin*) is not effective in inducing hemostasis [Jonas et al., 1988].

Cell Interaction Properties.   Collagen forms the essential framework of the tissues and organs. Many cells, such as epithelial and endothelial cells, are found resting on the collagenous surfaces or within a collagenous matrix such as that of many connective tissue cells. Collagen-cell interactions are essential features during the development stage and during wound healing and tissue remodeling in adults [Kleinman et al., 1981; Linbold and Kormos, 1991]. Studying collagen–cell interactions is useful in developing simulated tissue and organ structures and in investigating cell behavior in the *in vivo* simulated systems. Numerous studies have aimed at developing viable tissues and organs *in vitro* for transplantation applications [Bell et al., 1981; Montesano et al., 1983; Silbermann, 1990; Bellamkonda and Aebischer, 1994; Hubbel, 1995; Moghe et al., 1996; Sittinger et al., 1996].

Immunologic Properties.   Soluble collagen has long been known to be a poor immunogen [Timpl, 1982]. A significant level of antibodies cannot be raised without the use of Freund's complete adjuvant (a mixture of mineral oil and heat-killed *mycobacteria*) which augments antibody response. It is known that insoluble collagen is even less immunogenic [Stenzel et al., 1974]. Thus, xenogeneic collagenous tissue devices such as porcine and bovine pericardial heart valves are acceptable for long-term implantation in humans. The reasons for the low antibody response against collagen are not known. It may be related to the homology of the collagen structure from different species (low level of foreignness) or to certain structural features associated with collagen [Timpl, 1982].

6.2 Biotechnology of Collagen

Isolation and Purification of Collagen

There are two distinct ways of isolating and purifying collagen material. One is the molecular technology and the other is the fibrillar technology. These two technologies are briefly reviewed here.

Isolation and Purification of Soluble Collagen Molecules

The isolation and purification of soluble collagen molecules from a collagenous tissue is achieved by using a proteolytic enzyme such as pepsin to cleave the telopeptides [Miller and Rhodes, 1982]. Since telopeptides are the natural crosslinking sites of collagen, the removal of telopeptides renders the collagen molecules and small collagen aggregates soluble in an aqueous solution. The pepsin-solubilized collagen can be purified by repetitive precipitation with a neutral salt. Pepsin-solubilized collagen in monomeric form is generally soluble in a buffer solution at low temperature. The collagen molecules may be reconstituted into fibrils of various polymorphisms. However, the reconstitution of the pepsin-solubilized collagen into fibrils of native molecular packing is not as efficient as the intact molecules, since the telopeptides facilitate fibril formation [Comper and Veis, 1977].

Isolation and Purification of Fibrillar Collagen

The isolation and purification of collagen fibers relies on the removal of noncollagenous materials from the collagenous tissue. Salt extraction removes the newly synthesized collagen molecules that have not been covalently incorporated into the collagen fibrils. Salt also removes the noncollagenous materials that are soluble in aqueous conditions and are bound to collagen fibrils by nonspecific interactions. *Lipids* are removed by low-molecular-weight organic solvents such as low-molecular-weight ethers and alcohols. Acid extraction facilities the removal of acidic proteins and glycosaminoglycans due to weakening of the interactions between the acidic proteins and collagen fibrils. Alkaline extraction weakens the interaction between the basic proteins and collagen fibrils and thus facilitates the removal of basic proteins. In addition, various enzymes other than collagenase can be used to facilitate the removal of the small amounts of glycoproteins, proteoglycans, and elastins from the tissue. Purified collagen fibers can be obtained through these sequential extractions and enzymatic digestions from the collagen-rich tissues.

Matrix Fabrication Technology

The purified collagen materials obtained from either the molecular technology or from the fibrillar technology are subjected to additional processing to fabricate the materials into useful devices for specific medical applications. The different matrices and their medical applications are summarized in Table 6.5. The technologies used in fabricating these matrices are briefly outlined below.

TABLE 6.5 Summary of Different Collagen Matrices and Their Medical Applications

Matrix Form	Medical Application
Membrane (film, sheet)	Oral tissue repair; wound dressings; dura repair; patches
Porous (sponge, felt, fibers)	Hemostats; wound dressings; cartilage repair; soft-tissue augmentation
Gel	Drug and biologically active macromolecule delivery; soft- and hard-tissue augmentation
Solution	Soft-tissue augmentation; drug delivery
Filament	Tendon and ligament repair; sutures
Tubular (membrane, sponge)	Nerve repair; vascular repair
Composite	
Collagen/synthetic polymer	Vascular repair; skin repair; wound dressings
Collagen/biological polymer	Soft-tissue augmentation; skin repair
Collagen/ceramic	Hard-tissue repair

Membranous Matrix

Collagen membranes can be produced by drying a collagen solution or a fibrillar collagen dispersion cast on a nonadhesive surface. The thickness of the membrane is governed by the concentration and the initial thickness of the cast solution or dispersion. In general, membrane thickness of up to 0.5 mm can be easily obtained by air drying a cast collagen material. Additional chemical crosslinking is required to stabilize the membrane from dissolution or dissociation. The membrane produced by casting and air drying does not permit manipulation of the pore structure. Generally, the structure of a cast membrane is dense and amorphous with minimal *permeability* to macromolecules [Li et al., 1991]. Porous membranes may be obtained by freeze-drying a cast solution or dispersion of a predetermined density or by partially compressing a preformed porous matrix to a predetermined density and pore structure.

Porous Matrix

Porous collagen matrices are generally obtained by freeze-drying an aqueous volume of collagen solution or dispersion. The freeze-dried porous matrix requires chemical crosslinking to stabilize the structure. A convenient way to stabilize the porous matrix is to crosslink the matrix by vapor using a volatile crosslinking agent such as formaldehyde or glutaraldehyde. The pore structure of the matrix depends, to a large extent, on the concentration of the collagen in the solution or dispersion. Other factors that contribute to the pore structure include the rate of freezing, the size of fibers in the dispersion, and the presence and absence of other macromolecules. *Apparent densities* from 0.05 to 0.3 gram matrix per cubic centimeter matrix volume can be obtained. These porous matrices generally have pores from about 50 μm to as large as 1500 μm.

Gel Matrix

A *gel matrix* may be defined as a homogeneous phase between a liquid and a solid. As such, a gel may vary from a simple viscous fluid to a highly concentrated puttylike material. Collagen gels may be formed by shifting the pH of a dispersion away from its isoelectric point. Alternatively, the collagen material may be subjected to a chemical modification procedure to change its charge profile to a net positively charged or a net negatively charged protein before hydrating the material to form a gel matrix. For example, native fibers dispersed in water at pH 7 will be in the form of two phases. The dispersed fibers become gel when the pH changes from 7 to 3. Succinylating the primary amino groups of collagen, which converts the positively charged amino groups to negatively charged carboxyl groups, changes the isoelectric point of collagen from about 7 to about 4.5. Such a collagen material swells to a gel at a pH of 7.

Solution Matrix

A collagen solution is obtained by dissolving the collagen molecules in an aqueous solution. Collagen molecules are obtained by digesting the insoluble tissue with pepsin to cleave the crosslinking sites of collagen (telopeptides) as previously described. The solubility of collagen depends on the pH, the temperature, the ionic strength of the solution, and the molecular weight. Generally, collagen is more soluble in the cold. Collagen molecules aggregate into fibrils when the temperature of the solution increases to the body temperature. pH plays an important role in solubilizing collagen. Collagen is more soluble at a pH away from the isoelectric point of the protein. Collagen is less soluble at higher ionic strength of a solution. The solubility of collagen decreases with increasing the size of molecular aggregates. Thus, collagen becomes increasingly less soluble with increasing the extent of crosslinking [Bailey et al., 1970].

Filamentous Matrix

Collagen filaments can be produced by extrusion techniques [Kemp et al., 1995; Li and Stone, 1993; Schimpf and Rodriquez, 1976]. A collagen solution or dispersion having a concentration in the range of 0.5–1.5% (w/v) is first prepared. Collagen is extruded into a coacervation bath containing a high concentration of a salt or into an aqueous solution at a pH of the isoelectric point of the collagen. Tensile strength of 30 MPa has been obtained for the reconstituted filaments.

Tubular Matrix

Tubular matrices may be formed by extrusion through a coaxial cylinder [Stenzl et al., 1974], or by coating collagen onto a mandrel [Li, 1990]. Different properties of the tubular membranes can be obtained by controlling the drying properties.

Composite Matrix

Collagen can form a variety of homogeneous composites with other water-soluble materials. Ions, peptides, proteins, and polysaccharides can all be uniformly incorporated into a collagen matrix. The methods of homogeneous composite formation include ionic and covalent bonding, entrapment, entanglement, and coprecipitation. A heterogeneous composite can be formed between collagen, ceramics, and synthetic polymers that have distinct properties for medical applications [Li, 1988].

6.3 Design of a Resorbable Collagen-Based Medical Implant

Designing a medical implant for tissue or organ repair requires a thorough understanding of the structure and function of the tissue and organ to be repaired, the structure and properties of the materials used for repair, and the design requirements. There are at present two schools of thought regarding the design of an implant, namely the permanent implant and the *resorbable implant*. The permanent implants intended to permanently replace the damaged tissues or organs are fabricated from various materials including metals and natural or synthetic polymers. For example, most of the weight-bearing orthopedic and oral implants are made of metals or alloys. Non-weight-bearing tissues and organs are generally replaced with implants that are fabricated either from synthetic or natural materials. Implants for blood vessel, heart valve, and most soft tissue repair fall into this class. Permanent implants, particularly those made of synthetic and biological materials, frequently suffer from the long-term effects of material degradation. Material degradation can result from biological processes such as enzymatic degradation or environmentally induced degradation from mechanical, metal-catalyzed oxidation, and from the permeation of body fluids into the polymeric devices [Bruck, 1991]. The material degradation is particularly manifested in applications where there is repetitive stress–strain on the implant, such as artificial blood vessels and heart valves.

As a result of the lack of suitable materials for long-term implantation, the concept of using a resorbable template to guide host tissue regeneration (guided tissue regeneration) has received vigorous attention in recent years. This area of research can be categorized into synthetic and biological templates. *Polyglycolic acid* (PGA), *polylactic acid* (PLA), polyglycolic-polylactic acid copolymers, and *polydioxanone* are among the polymers most selected for resorbable medical implant development. Among the biological materials used for resorbable medical implant development, *collagen* has been one of the most popular materials in this category. Collagen-based templates have been developed for skin [Yannas and Burke, 1981], peripheral nerve [Li et al., 1990; Yannas et al., 1985], oral tissue [Altman and Li, 1990; Blumenthal, 1988], and meniscal regeneration [Li et al., 1994; Stone et al., 1997]. A variety of other collagen-based templates are being developed for tissue repair and regeneration applications [Goldstein et al., 1989; Ma et al., 1990; Li et al., 1997].

The following discussion is useful in designing a template for tissue repair and regeneration applications. By way of an example, the design parameters listed below are specifically applied to the development of a resorbable collagen based template for guiding meniscal tissue repair and regeneration in the knee joint.

Menisci are semilunar fibrocartilages that are anatomically located between the femoral condyles and tibial plateau, providing stability, weight bearing, and shock absorption, and assisting in lubrication of the knee joint. A major portion of the meniscal tissue is avascular except the peripheral rim, which comprises about 10–30% of the total width of the structure and which is nourished by the peripheral vasculature [Arnoczky and Warren, 1982]. Collagen is the major matrix material of the meniscus, and the fibers are oriented primarily in the circumferential direction in the line of stress for mechanical function. Repair of damaged meniscal tissue in the peripheral vascular rim can be accomplished with sutures. However, in cases where the injured site is in the avascular region, partial or total removal of the meniscal tissue is often indicated. This is primarily due to the inadequacy of the *fibrochondrocytes* alone to self-repair the damaged meniscal tissue. Studies in animals and humans have shown that removal of the meniscus is a prelude to degenerative knees manifested by the development of *osteoarthritis* [Hede and Sarberg, 1992; Shapiro and Glimcher, 1980]. At present there is no suitable permanent substitute for meniscal tissue.

Biocompatibility

Biocompatibility of the materials and their degraded products is a prerequisite for resorbable implant development. Purified collagen materials have been used either as implants or have been extensively tested in clinical studies as implants without adverse effects. The meniscus template can be fabricated from purified type I collagen fibers that are further crosslinked chemically to increase the stability and reduce the immunogenicity *in vivo*. In addition, small amounts of noncollagenous materials such as glycosaminoglycans and growth factors can be incorporated into the collagen matrix to improve the osmotic properties as well as the rate of tissue ingrowth.

Since the primary structure of a collagen molecule from bovine is homologous to human collagen [Miller, 1984], the *in vivo* degradation of bovine collagen implant should be similar to the normal host tissue remodeling process during wound healing. For a resorbable collagen template, the matrix is slowly degraded by the host over time. It is known that a number of cell types such as *polymorphonuclear leukocytes, fibroblasts,* and *macrophages,* during the wound healing period, are capable of secreting enzyme collagenases which cleave a collagen molecule at 1/4 position from the C-terminal end of the molecule [Woolley, 1984]. The enzyme first reduces a collagen molecule to two smaller triple helices which are not stable at body temperature and are subsequently denatured to random coiled polypeptides. These polypeptides are further degraded by proteases into amino acids and short peptides that are metabolized through normal metabolic pathways [Nimni and Harkness, 1988].

Despite the safety record of collagen materials for implantation, during the process of preparing the collagen template, small amounts of unwanted noncollagenous materials could be incorporated into the device such as salts and crosslinking agents. Therefore, a series of biocompatibility testing must be conducted to ensure the residuals of these materials do not cause any safety issues. The FDA has published a new guideline for biocompatibility testing of implantable devices [Biological Evaluation of Medical Devices, 1995].

Physical Dimension

The physical dimension of a template defines the boundary of regeneration. Thus, the size of the collagen template should match the tissue defect to be repaired. A properly sized meniscal substitute has been found to function better than a substitute which mismatches the physical dimension of the host meniscus [Rodkey et al., 1999a; Sommerlath et al., 1991]. For a porous, elastic matrix such as the one designed from collagen for meniscal tissue repair, the shape of the meniscus is further defined *in vivo* by the space available between the femoral condyles and tibial plateau within the synovial joint.

Apparent Density

The apparent density is defined as the weight of the dry matrix in a unit volume of matrix. Thus, the apparent density is a direct measure of the empty space which is not occupied by the matrix material per se in the dry state. For example, for a collagen matrix of an apparent density 0.2 g/cm^3, the empty space would be 0.86 cm^3 for a 1 cm^3 total space occupied by the matrix, taking the density of collagen to be 1.41 g/cm^3 [Noda, 1992]. The apparent density is also directly related to the mechanical strength of a matrix. In weight-bearing applications, the apparent density has to be optimized such that the mechanical properties are not compromised for the intended function of the resorbable implant as described in the mechanical properties section.

Pore Structure

The dimension of a mammalian fibrogenic cell body is on the order of 10–50 μm, depending on the substrate to which the cell adheres [Folkman et al., 1978]. In order for cells to infiltrate into the interstitial space of a matrix, the majority of the pores must be significantly larger than the dimension of a cell such that both the cell and its cellular processes can easily enter the interstitial space. In a number of studies using collagen-based matrices for tissue regeneration, it has been found that pore size plays an important role in the effectiveness of the collagen matrix to induce host tissue regeneration [Chvapil, 1982; Dagalailis et al., 1980; Yannas, 1996]. It was suggested that pore size in the range of 100–400 μm is optimal for tissue regeneration. Similar observations were also found to be true for porous metal implants in total hip replacement [Cook et al., 1991]. The question of interconnecting pores may not be a critical issue in a collagen template as collagenases are synthesized by most *inflammatory cells* during wound healing and remodeling processes. The interporous membranes which exist in the noninterconnecting pores should be digested as part of resorption and wound healing processes.

Mechanical Property

In designing a resorbable collagen implant for weight-bearing applications, not only is the initial mechanical strength important, but the gradual strength reduction of the partially resorbed template has to be compensated by the strength increase from the regenerated tissue such that at any given time point, the total mechanical properties of the template are maintained. In order to accomplish this goal, one must first be certain that the initial mechanical properties are adequate for supporting the weight-bearing application. For example, compressing the implant with multiple body weights should not cause fraying of the collagen matrix material. It is also of particular importance to design an implant having an adequate and consistent suture pullout strength in order to reduce the incidence of detachment of the implant from the host tissue. The suture pullout strength is also important during surgical procedures as the lack of suture pull strength may result in retrieval and reimplantation of the template. In meniscal tissue repair the suture pullout strength of 1 kg has been found to be adequate for arthroscopically assisted surgery in simulated placement procedures in human cadaver knees, and this suture pullout strength should be maintained as the minimal strength required for this particular application.

Hydrophilicity

Hydration of an implant facilitates nutrient diffusion. The extent of hydration would also provide information on the space available for tissue ingrowth. The porous collagen matrix is highly hydrophilic and therefore facilitates cellular ingrowth. The biomechanical properties of the hydrophilic collagen matrix such as fluid outflow under stress, fluid inflow in the absence of stress, and the resiliency for shock absorption are the properties also found in the weight-bearing cartilagenous tissues.

Permeability

The permeability of ions and macromolecules is of primary importance in tissues that do not rely on vascular transport of nutrients to the end organs. The diffusion of nutrients into the interstitial space ensures the survival of the cells and their continued ability of growth and synthesis of tissue specific extracellular matrix. Generally, the permeability of a macromolecule the size of the bovine serum albumin (MW 67,000) can be used as a guideline for probing accessibility of the interstitial space of a collagen template [Li et al., 1994].

In Vivo Stability

As stated above, the rate of template resorption and the rate of new tissue regeneration have to be balanced so that the adequate mechanical properties are maintained at all times. The rate of in vivo resorption of a collagen-based implant can be controlled by controlling the density of the implant and the extent of intermolecular crosslinking. The lower the density, the greater the interstitial space and generally the larger the pores for cell infiltration, leading to a higher rate of matrix degradation. The control of the extent of intermolecular crosslinking can be accomplished by using bifunctional crosslinking agents under conditions that do not denature the collagen. Glutaraldehyde, formaldehyde, adipyl chloride, hexamethylene diisocyanate, and carbodiimides are among the many agents used in crosslinking the collagen-based implants. Crosslinking can also be achieved through vapor phase of a crosslinking agent. The vapor phase crosslinking is effective using crosslinking agents of high vapor pressures such as formaldehyde and glutaraldehyde. The vapor crosslinking is particularly useful for thick implants of vapor permeable dense fibers where crosslinking in solution produces nonuniform crosslinking. In addition, intermolecular crosslinking can be achieved by heat treatment under high vacuum. This treatment causes the formation of an amide bond between an amino group of one molecule and the carboxyl group of an adjacent molecule and has often been referred to in the literature as dehydrothermal crosslinking.

The shrinkage temperature of the crosslinked matrix has been used as a guide for *in vivo* stability of a collagen implant [Li, 1988]. The temperature of shrinkage of collagen fibers measures the transition of the collagen molecules from the triple helix to a random coil conformation. This temperature depends on the number of intermolecular crosslinks formed by chemical means. Generally, the higher the number of intermolecular crosslinks, the higher the thermal shrinkage temperature and more stable the material *in vivo*.

A second method of assessing the *in vivo* stability is to determine the crosslinking density by applying the theory of rubber elasticity to denatured collagen [Wiederhorn and Beardon, 1952]. Thus, the *in vivo* stability can be directly correlated with the number of intermolecular crosslinks introduced by a given crosslinking agent.

Another method that has been frequently used in assessing the *in vivo* stability of a collagen-based implant is to conduct an *in vitro* collagenase digestion of a collagen implant. Bacterial collagenase is generally used in this application. The action of bacterial collagenase on collagen is different from that of mammalian collagenase [Woolley, 1984]. In addition, the enzymatic activity used in *in vitro* studies is arbitrarily defined. Thus, the data generated from the bacterial collagenase should be viewed with caution. The bacterial collagenase digestion studies, however, are useful in comparing a prototype with a collagen material of known rate of *in vivo* resorption.

Each of the above parameters should be considered in designing a resorbable implant. The interdependency of the parameters must also be balanced for maximal efficacy of the implant.

6.4   Tissue Engineering for Tissue and Organ Regeneration

Biomedical applications of collagen have entered a new era in the past decade. The potential use of collagen materials in medicine has increasingly been appreciated as the science and technology advances.

One major emerging field of biomedical research which has received rigorous attention in recent years is tissue engineering. Tissue engineering is an interdisciplinary science of biochemistry, cell and molecular biology, genetics, materials science, biomedical engineering, and medicine to produce innovative three-dimensional composites having structure/function properties that can be used either to replace or correct poorly functioning components in humans and animals or to introduce better functional components into these living systems. Thus, the field of tissue engineering requires a close collaboration among various disciplines for success.

Tissue engineering consists primarily of three components: (1) extracellular matrix, (2) cells, and (3) regulatory signals (e.g., tissue specific growth factors). One of the key elements in tissue engineering is the extracellular matrix which either provides a scaffolding for cells or acts as a delivery vehicle for regulatory signals such as growth factors.

Type I collagen is the major component of the extracellular matrix and is intimately associated with development, wound healing, and regeneration. The development of the type I collagen based matrices described in this review article will greatly facilitate the future development of tissue engineering products for tissue and organ repair and regeneration applications.

TABLE 6.6 Survey of Collagen-Based Medical Products, and Research and Development Activities

Application	Comments
Hemostasis	*Commercial products*: Sponge, fiber, and felt forms are used in cardiovascular [Abbott and Austin, 1975]; neurosurgical [Rybock and Long, 1977]; dermatological [Larson, 1988]; ob/gyn [Cornell et al., 1985]; orthopedic [Blanche and Chaux, 1988]; oral surgical applications [Stein et al., 1985]
Dermatology	*Commercial products*: Injectable collagen for soft tissue augmentation [Webster et al., 1984]; collagen-based artificial skins [Bell et al., 1981; Yannas and Burke, 1981]. *Research and development*: Collagen-based wound dressings [Armstrong et al., 1986]
Cardiovascular surgery and cardiology	*Commercial products*: Collagen-coated and gelatin-coated vascular grafts [Jonas et al., 1988, Li, 1988]; chemically processed human vein graft [Dardik et al., 1974]; bovine arterial grafts [Sawyer et al., 1977]; porcine heart valves [Angell et al., 1982]; bovine pericardial heart valves [Walker et al., 1983]; vascular puncture hole seal device [Merino et al., 1992]
Neurosurgery	*Research and development*: Guiding peripheral nerve regeneration [Archibald et al., 1991; Yannas et al., 1985]; dura replacement material [Collins et al., 1991]
Periodontal and oral surgery	*Research and development*: Collagen membranes for periodontal ligament regeneration [Blumenthal, 1988]; resorbable oral tissue wound dressings [Ceravalo and Li, 1988]; collagen/hydroxyapatite for augmentation of alveolar ridge [Gongloff and Montgomery, 1985]
Ophthalmology	*Commercial products*: Collagen corneal shield to facilitate epithelial healing [Ruffini et al., 1989]. *Research and development*: Collagen shield for drug delivery to the eye [Reidy et al., 1990]
Orthopedic surgery	*Commercial products*: Collagen with hydroxyapatite and autogenous bone marrow for bone repair [Hollinger et al., 1989]. *Research and development*: Collagen matrix for meniscus regeneration [Li et al., 1994]; collagenous material for replacement and regeneration of Achilles tendon [Kato et al., 1991]; reconstituted collagen template for ACL reconstruction [Li et al., 1997]
Other applications	*Research and development*: Drug delivery support [Sorensen et al., 1990]; delivery vehicles for growth factors and bioactive macromolecules [Deatherage and Miller, 1987; Li et al., 1996]; collagenous matrix for delivery of cells for tissue and organ regeneration [Bell et al., 1981]

To date, collagen-based implants have been attempted for many tissue and organ repair and regeneration applications. A complete historical survey of all potential medical applications of collagen is a formidable task but a selected survey of collagen-based medical products and the research and development activities are summarized in Table 6.6 as a reference.

Defining Terms

Alanine (Ala): One of the amino acids in collagen molecules.

Allysine: The ε-amino group of lysine has been enzymatically modified to an aldehyde group.

Apparent density: Calculated as the weight of the dry collagen matrix per unit volume of matrix.

Arginine (Arg): One of the amino acids in collagen molecules.

Aspartic acid (Asp): One of the amino acids in collagen molecules.

Atelocollagen: A collagen molecule without the telopeptides.

Chondroitin sulfate: Sulfated polysaccharide commonly found in cartilages, bone, corea, tendon, and skin.

Collagen: A family fibrous insoluble proteins having a triple helical conformation extending over a major part of the molecule. Glycine is present at every third amino acid in the triple helix and proline and hydroxyproline are required in the triple helix.

Collagenase: A proteolytic enzyme that specifically catalyzes the degradation of collagen molecules.

Dehydrohydroxylysinonorleucine (deH-HLNL): A covalently crosslinked product between an allysine and a hydroxylysine residues in collagen fibrils.

D spacing: The repeat distance observed in collagen fibrils by electron microscopic and x-ray diffraction methods.

Elastin: One of the proteins in connective tissue. It is highly stable at high temperatures and in chemicals. It also has rubberlike properties.

Fiber: A bundled group of collagen fibrils.

Fibril: A self-assembled group of collagen molecules.

Fibroblast: Any cell from which connective tissue is developed.

Fibrochondrocyte: Type of cells that are associated with special types of cartilage tissues such as meniscus of the knee and intervertebral disc of the spine.

Fibrous long spacing (FLS):   One of the polymorphic forms of collagen where the collagen molecules are randomly aligned in either head-to-tail, tail-to-tail, or head-to-head orientation.

Gelatin: A random coiled form (denatured form) of collagen molecules.

Glutamic acid (Glu):   One of the amino acids in collagen molecules.

Glycine (Gly):   One of the amino acids in collagen molecules having the simplest structure.

Glycoprotein: A compound consisting of a carbohydrate protein. The carbohydrate is generally hexosamine, an amino sugar.

Glycosaminoglycan (GAG):   A polymerized sugar (see polysaccharide) commonly found in various connective tissues.

Helical pitch: Repeating distance within a single polypeptide chain in a collagen molecule.

Hemostat: Device or medicine which arrests the flow of blood.

Hydrophilicity: The tendency to attract and hold water.

Hydrophobicity: The tendency to repel or avoid contact with water. Substances generally are nonpolar in character, such as lipids and nonpolar amino acids.

Hydroxylysine (Hyl):   One of the amino acids in collagen molecules.

Hydroxyproline (Hyp):   One of the amino acids uniquely present in collagen molecules.

Inflammatory cell: Cells associated with the succession of changes which occur in living tissue when it is injured. These include macrophages, polymorphonuclear leukocytes, and lymphocytes.

Intermolecular crosslink: Covalent bonds formed *in vivo* between a side group of one molecule and a side group of another molecule; covalent bonds formed between a side group of one molecule and one end of a bifunctional agent and between a side group of a second molecule and the other end of a bifunctional agent.

Intrafibrillar volume: The volume of a fibril excluding the volume occupied by the collagen molecule.

In vitro: In glass, as in a test tube. An *in vitro* test is one done in the laboratory, usually involving isolated tissues, organs, or cells.

In vivo: In the living body or organism. A test performed on a living organism.

Isoelectric point: Generally used to refer to a particular pH of a protein solution. At this pH, there is no net electric charge on the molecule.

Isoleucine (Ile):   One of the amino acids in collagen molecules.

Leucine (Leu):   One of the amino acids in collagen molecules.

Lipid: Any one of a group of fats or fat-like substances, characterized by their insolubility in water and solubility in fat solvents such as alcohol, ether, and chloroform.

Lysine (Lys):   One of the amino acids in collagen molecules.

Macrophage: Cells of the reticuloendothelial system having the ability to phagocytose particulate substances and to store vital dyes and other colloidal substances. They are found in loose connective tissues and various organs of the body.

Meniscus: A C-shaped fibrocartilage anatomically located between the femoral condyles and tibial plateau providing stability and shock absorption and assisting in lubrication of the knee joint.

Mycobacterium: A genus of acid-fast organisms belonging to the Mycobacteriaceae which includes the causative organisms of tuberculosis and leprosy. They are slender, nonmotile, gram-positive rods and do not produce spores or capsules.

Osteoarthritis: A chronic disease involving the joint, especially those bearing the weight, characterized by destruction of articular cartilage, overgrown of bone with impaired function.

Permeability: The space within a collagen matrix, excluding the space occupied by collagen molecules, which is accessible to a given size of molecule.

Pepsin: A proteolytic enzyme commonly found in the gastric juice. It is formed by the chief cells of gastric glands and produces maximum activity at a pH of 1.5–2.0.

Phenolalanine (Phe):   One of the amino acids in collagen molecules.

Platelet: A round or oval disk, 2 to 4 μm in diameter, found in the blood of vertebrates. Platelets contain no hemoglobin.

Polydioxanone: A synthetic polymer formed from dioxanone monomers which degrades by hydrolysis.

Polyglycolic acid (PGA):   A synthetic polymer formed from glycolic acid monomers which degrades by hydrolysis.

Polylactic acid (PLA):   A synthetic polymer formed from lactic acid monomers which degrades by hydrolysis.

Polymorphism: Different types of aggregated states of the collagen molecules.

Polymorphonuclear leukocyte: A white blood cell which possesses a nucleus composed of two or more lobes or parts; a granulocyte (neutrophil, eosinophil, basophil).

Polypeptide: Polymerized amino acid molecules formed by enzymatically regulated stepwise polymerization *in vivo* between the carboxyl group of one amino acid and the amino group of a second amino acid.

Polysaccharide: Polymerized sugar molecules found in tissues as lubricant (synovial fluid) or cement (between osteons, tooth root attachment) or complexed with proteins such as glycoproteins or proteoglycans.

Proline (Pro):   One of the amino acids commonly occurring in collagen molecules.

Proteolytic enzyme: Enzymes which catalyze the breakdown of native proteins.

Resorbable collagen: Collagen which can be biodegraded *in vivo*.

Salt-linkage: An electrostatic bond formed between a negative charge group and a positive charge group in collagen molecules and fibrils.

Segment-long-spacing (SLS):   One of the polymorphic forms of collagen where all heads of collagen molecules are aligned in parallel.

Soluble collagen: Collagen molecules that can be extracted with salts and dilute acids. Soluble collagen molecules contain the telopeptides.

Telopeptide: The two short nontriple helical peptide segments located at the ends of collagen molecules.

Valine (Val):   One of the amino acids in collagen molecules.

References

Abbott WM, Austin WG. 1975. The effectiveness of mechanism of collagen-induced topical hemostasis. *Surgery* 78:723–729.

Altman R, Li ST. 1990. Collagen matrix for oral surgical applications. *Int J Oral Implantol* 7:75.

Angell WW, Angell JD, Kosek JC. 1982. Twelve year experience with gluteraldehyde preserved porcine xenografts. *J Thorac Cardiovasc Surg* 83:493–502.

Archibald SJ, Krarup C, Shefner J, Li ST, Madison R. 1991. Collagen-based nerve conduits are as effective as nerve grafts to repair transected peripheral nerves in rodents and non-human primates. *J Comp Neurol* 306:685–696.

Armstrong RB, Nichols J, Pachance J. 1986. Punch biopsy wounds treated with Monsel's solution or a collagen matrix. *Arch Dermatol* 122:546–549.

Arnoczky SP, Warren RF. 1982. Microvasculature of the human meniscus. *Am J Sport Med* 10:90–95.

Baily AJ, Rhodes DN. 1964. Irradiation-induced crosslinking of collagen. *Radiation Res* 22:606–621.

Bear RS. 1952. The structure of collagen fibrils. *Adv Prot Chem* 7:69–160.

Bell E, Ehrlich HP, Buttle DJ, Nakatsuji T. 1981. Living tissue formed *in vitro* and accepted as skin equivalent tissue of full thickness. *Science* 211:1042–1054.

Bellamkonda R, Aebischer P. 1994. Review: Tissue engineering in the nerve system. *Biotechnol Bioeng* 43:543–554.

Biological Evaluation and Medical Devices. Use of International Standard ISO-10993. Blue Book Memorandon G95-1, Rockville, MD, FDA, CDRH, Office of Device Evaluation, May 1, 1995.

Blanche C, Chaux A. 1988. The use of absorbable microfibrillation collagen to control sternal bone marrow bleeding. *Joint Surg* 73:42–43.

Blumenthal NM. 1988. The use of collagen membranes to guide regeneration of new connective tissue attachment in dogs. *J Periodontol* 59(12):830–836.

Brodsky B, Ramshaw JA. 1997. The collagen triple-helix structure. *Matrix Biol* 15:545–554.

Bruck SD. 1991. Biostability of materials and implants. *J Long-Term Effects Med Implants* 1(1):89–106.

Ceravolo F, Li ST. 1988. Alveolar ridge augmentation utilizing collagen wound dressing. *Int J Oral Implantol* 4:15–18.

Chvapil M. 1982. Considerations on manufacturing principles of a synthetic burn dressing: a review. *J Biomed Mater Res* 16:245–263.

Collins RL, Christiansen D, Zazanis GA, Silver FH. 1991. Use of collagen film as a dural substitute: preliminary animal studies. *J Biomed Mater Res* 25:267–276.

Comper WD, Veis A. 1977. Characterization of nuclei *in vitro* collagen fibril formation. *Biopolymers* 16:2133–2142.

Cook SD, Thomas KA, Dalton JE, Volkman T, Kay JF. 1991. Enhancement of bone ingrowth and fixation strength by hydroxyapatite coating porous implants. *Trans Orthop Res Soc* 16:550.

Correll JT, Prentice HR, Wise RC. 1985. Biological investigations of a new absorbable sponge. *Surg Gynecol Obstet* 81:585–589.

Dagalailis N, Flink J, Stasikalis P, Burke JF, Yannas IV. 1980. Design of an artificial skin. III. Control of pore structure. *J Biomed Mater Res* 14:511–528.

Daly CH. 1966. The biomechanical characteristics of human skin. Ph.D. thesis, University of Strathclyde, Scotland.

Dardik H, Veith FJ, Spreyregen S, Dardik I. 1974. Arterial reconstruction with a modified collagen tube. *Ann Surg* 180:144–146.

Deatherage JR, Miller EJ. 1987. Packaging and delivery of bone induction factors in a collagen implant. *Collagen Rel Res* 7:225–231.

Eastoe JE. 1967. Composition of collagen and allied proteins. In *Treatise on Collagen*, GN Ramachandran, Ed., pp. 1–72, Academic Press, New York.

Ellis DL, Yannas IV. 1996. Recent advances in tissue synthesis *in vivo* by use of collagen-glycosamino-glycans copolymers. *Biomaterials* 17:291–299.

Folkman J, Moscona A. 1978. Role of cell shape in growth control. *Nature* 273:345–349.

Fraenkel-Conrat H, Olcott HS. 1945. Esterification of proteins with alcohols of low molecular weight. *J Biol Chem* 161:259–268.

Fraser RDB, MacRae TP, Miller A, Suzuki E. 1983. Molecular conformation and packing in collagen fibrils. *J Mol Biol* 167:497–510.

Fukai N, Apte SS, Olsen BR. 1994. Nonfibrillar collagens. *Meth Enzymol* 245:3–28.

Fung, YC. 1993. Bioviscoelastic solids. In *Biomechanics, Mechanical Properties of Living Tissues*, 2nd ed., p. 255, Springer-Verlag, New York.

Goldstein JD, Tria AJ, Zawadsky JP, Kato YP, Christiansen D, Silver FH. 1989. Development of a reconstituted collagen tendon prosthesis. A preliminary implantation study. *J Bone Joint Surg* 71-A:1183–1191.

Gongloff RK, Whitlow W, Montgomery CK. 1985. Use of collagen tubes for implantation of hydroxyl-apatite. *J Oral Maxillofac Surg* 43(8):570–573.

Green RW, Ang KP, Lam LC. 1953. Acetylation of collagen. *Biochem J* 54:181–187.

Guidon R, Marcean D, Rao TJ, Merhi Y, Roy P, Martin L, Duval M. 1987. *In vitro* and *in vivo* character-ization of an impervious polyester arterial prosthesis: The Gelseal Triaxial graft. *Biomaterials* 8:433–441.

Hede A, Larson E, Sanberg H. 1992. The long term outcome of open total and partial meniscectomy related to the quantity and site of the meniscus removed. *Int Orthop* 16:122–125.

Hodge AJ, Petruska JA. 1963. Recent studies with the electron microscope on the ordered aggregates of the tropocollagen molecule. In *Aspects of Proteins Structure,* GN Ramachandran, Ed., pp. 289–300, Academic Press, New York.

Hofmann H, Kuhn K. 1981. Statistical analysis of collagen sequences with regard to fibril assembly and evolution. In *Structural Aspects of Recognition and Assembly in Biological Macromolecules,* M. Balaban, JL Sussman, W. Traub, A. Yonath, Eds., pp. 403–425, Balabann ISS, Rehovot.

Hollinger J, Mark DE, Bach DE, Reddi AH, Seyfer AE. 1989. Calvarial bone regeneration using osteogenin. *J Oral Maxillofac Surg* 47:1182–1186.

Hubbell JA. 1995. Biomaterials in tissue engineering. *Bio/technology* 13:565–576.

Jaffe R, Deykin DJ. 1974. Evidence for a structural requirement for the aggregation of platelet by collagen. *Clin Invest* 53:875–883.

Kato YP, Dunn MG, Zawadsky JP, Tria AJ, Silver FH. 1991. Regeneration of Achilles tendon with a collagen tendon prosthesis. *J Bone Joint Surg* 73-A:561–574.

Katz EP, Li ST. 1972. The molecular organization of collagen in mineralized and nonmineralized tissues. *Biochem Biophys Res Commun* 3:1368–1373.

Katz EP, Li ST. 1973a. The intermolecular space of reconstituted collagen fibrils. *J Mol Biol* 73:351–369.

Katz EP, Li ST. 1973b. Structure and function of bone collagen fibrils. *J Mol Biol* 80:1–15.

Katz EP, Li ST. 1981. The molecular packing of type I collagen fibrils. In *The Chemistry and Biology of Mineralized Connective Tissues,* A Veis, Ed., pp. 101–105, Elsevier, Amsterdam.

Kemp PD, Cavallaro JF, Hastings DN. 1995. Effects of carbodiimide crosslinking and load environment on the remodeling of collagen scaffolds. *Tissue Eng* 1:71–79.

Kleinman HK, Klebe RJ, Martin GR. 1981. Role of collagenous matrices in the adhesion and growth of cells. *J Cell Biol* 88:473–485.

Larson PO. 1988. Topical hemostatic agents for dermatologic surgery. *J Dermatol Surg Oncol* 14(6):623–632.

Li ST. 1988. Collagen and vascular prosthesis. In *Collagen,* Vol. III, ME Nimni, Ed., pp. 253–271, CRC Press, Boca Raton, FL.

Li ST. 1990. A multi-layered, semipermeable conduit for nerve regeneration comprised of type I collagen, its method of manufacture and a method of nerve regeneration using said conduit. U.S. Patent No. 4,963,146.

Li ST, Katz EP. 1976. An electrostatic model for collagen fibrils: the interaction of reconstituted collagen with Ca^{++}, Na$^+$, and Cl$^-$. *Biopolymers* 15:1439–1460.

Li ST, Stone KR. 1993. Prosthetic ligament. U.S. Patent No. 5,263,984.

Li ST, Golub E, Katz EP. 1975. On electrostatic side chain complimentarity in collagen fibrils. *J Mol Biol* 98:835–839.

Li ST, Sullman S, Katz EP. 1981. Hydrogen bonded salt linkages in collagen. In *The Chemistry and Biology of Mineralized Tissues,* A Veis, Ed., pp. 123–127, Elsevier, Amsterdam.

Li ST, Archibald SJ, Krarup C, Madison R. 1990. Semipermeable collagen nerve conduits for peripheral nerve regeneration. *Poly Mater Sci Eng* 62:575–582.

Li ST, Archibald SJ, Krarup C, Madison RD. 1991. The development of collagen nerve guiding conduits that promote peripheral nerve regeneration. In *Biotechnology and Polymers,* CG Gebelein, Ed., pp. 282–293, Plenum Press, New York.

Li ST, Yuen D, Li PC, Rodkey WG, Stone KR. 1994. Collagen as a biomaterial: an application in knee meniscal fibrocartilage regeneration. *Mater Res Soc Symp Proc* 331:25–32.

Li ST, Bolton W, Helm G, Gillies G, Frenkel S. 1996. Collagen as a delivery vehicle for bone morphogenetic protein (BMP). *Trans Orthop Res Soc,* p. 647.

Li ST, Yuen D, Charoenkul W, Ulreich JB, Speer DP. 1997. A type I collagen ligament for ACL reconstruction. *Trans Soc Biomater,* p. 407.

Lindblad WJ, Kormos AI. 1991. Collagen: a multifunctional family of proteins. *J Reconstructive Microsurg* 7:37–43.

Ma S, Chen G, Reddi AH. 1990. Collaboration between collagenous matrix and osteoginin is required for bone induction. *Ann NY Acad Sci* 580:524–525.

Merino A, Faulkner C, Corvalan A, Sanborn TA. 1992. Percutaneous vascular hemostasis device for interventional procedures. *Catheterization Cardiovas Diag* 26:319–322.

Miller A. 1976. Molecular packing in collagen fibrils. In *Biochemistry of Collagen*, GN Ramachandran, H Reddi, Eds., pp. 85–136, Plenum Press, New York.

Miller EJ. 1984. Chemistry of the collagens and their distribution. In *Extracellular Matrix Biochemistry*, KA Piez, AH Reddi, Eds., pp. 41–82, Elsevier, New York.

Miller EJ, Rhodes RK. 1982. Preparation and characterization of the different types of collagen. *Meth Enzymol* 82:33–63.

Moghe PV, Berthiaume F, Ezzell RM, Toner M, Tompkins RC, Yarmush ML. 1996. Culture matrix configuration and composition in the maintenance of hepatocyte polarity and function. *Biomaterials* 17:373–385.

Montesano R, Mouron P, Amherdt M, Orci L. 1983. Collagen matrix promotes reorganization of pancreatic endocrine cell monolayers into islet-like organoids. *J Cell Biol* 97:935–939.

Nimni ME, Ed. 1988. *Collagen*, Vols. I, II, and III, CRC Press, Boca Raton, FL.

Nimni ME, Harkness RD. 1988. Molecular structures and functions of collagen. In *Collagen*, Vol. I, ME Nimni, Ed., pp. 1–78, CRC Press, Boca Raton, FL.

Noda H. 1972. Partial specific volume of collagen. *J Biochem* 71:699–703.

Park JB, Lakes RS. 1992. Structure-property relationships of biological materials. In *Biomaterials: An Introduction*, 2nd ed., pp. 185–222, Plenum Press, New York.

Piez KA. 1984. Molecular and aggregate structures of the collagens. In *Extracellular Matrix Biochemistry*, KA Piez, AH Reddi, Eds., p. 5, Elsevier, New York

Ramachandran GN. 1967. Structure of collagen at the molecular level. In *Treatise on Collagen*, Vol. I, GN Ramachandran, Ed., pp. 103–183, Academic Press, New York.

Reidy JJ, Limberg M, Kaufman HE. 1990. Delivery of fluorescein to the anterior chamber using the corneal collagen shield. *Ophthalmology* 97(9):1201–1203.

Rich A, Crick FHC. 1961. The molecular structure of collagen. *J Mol Biol* 3:483–505.

Rigby BJ, Hiraci N, Spikes JD, Eyring H. 1959. The mechanical properties of rat tail tendon. *J Gen Physiol* 43:265–283.

Rodkey WG, Steadman JR, Li ST. 1999a. A clinical study of collagen meniscus implants to restore the injured meniscus. *Clin Orthop Rel Res* 367S:S281–S292.

Rodney WG, Steadman JR, Li ST. 1999b. Collagen scaffolds: a new method to preserve and restore the severely injured meniscus. *Sports Med Arthroscopy Rev* 7:63–73.

Ruffini JJ, Aquavella JV, LoCascio JA. 1989. Effect of collagen shields on corneal epithelialization following penetrating keratoplasty. *Ophthal Surg* 20:21–25.

Rybock JD, Long DM. 1977. Use of microfibrillar collagen as a topical hemostatic agent in brain tissue. *J Neurosurg* 46:501–505.

Sawyer PN, Stanczewski B, Kirschenbaum D. 1977. The development of polymeric cardiovascular collagen prosthesis. *Artif Organs* 1:83–91.

Schimpf WC, Rodriquez F. 1976. Fibers from regenerated collagen. *Ind Eng Chem Prod Res Rev* 16:90–92.

Shapiro F, Glimcher MJ. 1980. Induction of osteoarthrosis in the rabbit knee joint: histologic changes following meniscectomy and meniscal lesions. *Clin Orthop* 147:287–295.

Silbermann M. 1990. *In vitro* systems for inducers of cartilage and bone development. *Biomaterials* 11:47–49.

Sittinger JB, Bugia J, Rotter N, Reitzel D, Minuth WW, Burmester GR. 1996. Tissue engineering and autologous transplant formation: prectical approaches with resorbable biomaterials and new cell culture techniques. *Biomaterials* 17:237–242.

Sommerlath K, Gallino M, Gillquist J. 1991. Biomechanical characteristics of different artificial substitutes for the rabbit medial meniscus and the effect of prosthesis size on cartilage. *Trans Orthop Res Soc* 16:375.

Sorensen TS, Sorensen AI, Merser S. 1990. Rapid release of gentamicin from collagen sponge. *Acta Orthop Scand* 61(4):353–356.

Steadman JR, Rodkey WG, Li S. 2000. The collagen meniscus implant: development and clinical trials of a device to treat meniscus injuries of the knee. *Sport Orthop Traumatol* 16:173–177.

Stein MD, Salkin LM, Freedman AL, Glushko V. 1985. Collagen sponge as a topical hemostatic agent in mucogingival surgery. *J Periodontol* 56:35–38.

Stenzl KH, Miyata T, Rubin AL. 1974. Collagen as a biomaterial. *Annu Rev Biophys Bioeng* 3:231–253.

Stone KR, Steadman JR, Rodkey WR, Li ST. 1997. Regeneration of meniscal cartilage with the use of a collagen scaffold. *J Bone Joint Surg* 79-A:1770–1777.

Tiffit JT. 1980. The organic matrix of bone tissue. In *Fundamental and Clinical Bone Physiology*, MR Urist, Ed., p. 51, J.B. Lippincott, Philadelphia, PA.

Timpl R. 1982. Antibodies to collagen and procollagen. *Meth Enzymol* 82:472–498.

van der Rest M, Dublet B, Champliaud MF. 1990. Fibril-associated collagens. *Biomaterials* 11:28–31.

Walker WE, Duncan JM, Frazier OH, Liversay JJ, Ott DA, Reul GJ, Cooly DA. 1983. Early experience with the Ionescu-Shiley pericardial xenograft valve. *J Thorac Cardiovasc Surg* 86:570–575.

Wang C-L, Miyata T, Weksler B, Rubin A, Stenzel KH. 1978. Collagen-induced platelet aggregation and release: critical size and structural requirements of collagen. *Biochim Biophys Acta* 544:568–577.

Webster RC, Kattner MD, Smith RC. 1984. Injectable collagen for augmentation of facial areas. *Arch Otolaryngol* 110:652–656.

Wiederhorn N, Beardon GV. 1952. Studies concerned with the structure of collagen: II. Stress–strain behavior of thermally controlled collagen. *J Polymer Sci* 9:315–325.

Wilner GD, Nossel HL, Leroy EC. 1968. Activation of Hageman factor by collagen. *J Clin Invest* 47:2608–2615.

Woolley DE. 1984. Mammalian collagenases. In *Extracellular Matrix Biochemistry*, KA Piez, AH Reddi, Eds., pp. 119–151, Elsevier, New York.

Yamuchi M, Katz EP, Mechanic GL. 1986. Intermolecular cross-linking and stereospecific molecular packing in type I collagen fibrils of the periodontal ligament. *Biochemistry* 25:4907–4913.

Yannas IV, Burke JF. 1981. Design of an artificial skin. I. Basic design principles. *J Biomed Mater Res* 14:65–80.

Yannas IV, Orgill DP, Silver J, Norregaad T, Ervas NN, Schoene WC. 1985. Polymeric template facilitates regeneration of sciatic nerve across a 15 mm gap. *Poly Mater Sci Eng* 53:216–218.

7

Soft Tissue Replacements

K. B. Chandran
University of Iowa

Karen J. L. Burg
Carolinas Medical Center

S. W. Shalaby
Poly-Med, Inc.

7.1 Blood-Interfacing Implants

K. B. Chandran

Introduction

Blood comes in contact with foreign materials for a short term in extracorporeal devices such as *dialyzers*, *blood oxygenators*, ventricular assist devices, and *catheters*. Long-term vascular implants include heart valve prostheses, *vascular grafts*, and *cardiac pacemakers*, among others. In this section, we will be concerned with development of biomaterials for long-term implants, specifically for heart valve prostheses, total artificial heart (*TAH*), and vascular grafts. The primary requirements for biomaterials for long-term implants are biocompatibility, nontoxicity, and durability. Furthermore, the material should be nonirritating to the tissue, resistant to *platelet* and *thrombus* deposition, nondegradable in the physiological environment, and neither absorb blood constituents nor release foreign substances into the blood stream [Shim and Lenker, 1988]. In addition, design considerations include that the implant should mimic the function of the organ that it replaces without interfering with the surrounding anatomical structures and must be of suitable size and weight. The biomaterials chosen must be easily available, inexpensive, easily machinable, and sterilizable and have a long storage life. The selection of material will also be dictated by the strength requirement for the implant being made. As an example, an artificial heart valve prosthesis is required to open and close on an average once every second. The biomaterial chosen must be such that the valve is durable and will not fail under *fatigue stress* after implantation in a patient. As sophisticated measurement techniques and detailed computational analyses become available with the advent of super computers, our knowledge of the complex dynamics of the functioning of the implants is increasing. Improvements in design based on such knowledge and improvements in selection and manufacture of biomaterials will minimize problems associated with blood-interfacing implants and significantly improve the quality of life for patients with implants. We will discuss the

TABLE 7.1   Heart Valve Prostheses Developed and Currently Available in the U.S.

Type	Name	Manufacturer
Caged ball	Starr–Edwards	Baxter Health Care, Irvine, CA
Tilting disc	Medtronic–Hall	Medtronic Blood Systems, Minneapolis, MN
	Lillehei–Kaster	Medical Inc., Inner Grove Heights, MN
	Omni–Science	
Bileaflet	St. Jude Medical	St. Jude Medical, Inc., St. Paul, MN
	Carbomedics	CarboMedics, Austin, TX
	ATS valve[a]	ATS Medical, St. Paul, MN
	On-X valve[a]	Medical Carbon Research Inst., Austin, TX
Porcine bioprostheses	Carpentier–Edwards Standard	Baxter Health Care, Irvine, CA
	Hancock Standard	Medtronic Blood Systems, Santa Ana, CA
	Hancock modified orifice	
	Hancock II	
Pericardial bioprostheses	Carpentier–Edwards	Edwards Laboratories, Santa Ana, CA

[a] FDA approval pending

development of biomaterials for the blood-interfacing implants, problems associated with the same, and future directions in the development of such implants.

Heart Valve Prostheses

Attempts at replacing diseased natural human valves with prostheses began about four decades ago. The details of the development of heart valve prostheses, design considerations, *in vitro* functional testing, and durability testing of valve prototypes can be found in several monographs [Shim and Lenker, 1988; Chandran, 1992]. The heart valve prostheses can be broadly classified into *mechanical prostheses* (made of non-biological material) and *bioprostheses* (made of biological tissue). Currently available mechanical and tissue heart valve prostheses in the U.S. are listed in Table 7.1.

Mechanical Heart Valves

Lefrak and Starr [1970] describe the early history of mechanical valve development. The initial designs of mechanical valves were of centrally occluding caged ball or caged disc type. The Starr–Edwards caged ball prostheses, commercially available at the present time, was successfully implanted in the mitral position in 1961. The caged ball prosthesis is made of a polished Co–Cr alloy (Stellite 21®) cage and a silicone rubber ball (Silastic®) which contains 2% by weight barium sulfate for *radiopacity* (Fig. 7.1). The valve *sewing rings* use a silicone rubber insert under a knitted composite polytetrafluorethylene (PTFE-Teflon®) and *polypropylene* cloth. Even though these valves have proven to be durable, the centrally occluding design of the valve results in a larger pressure drop in flow across the valve and higher *turbulent stresses* distal to the valve compared to other designs of mechanical valve prostheses [Yoganathan et al., 1979a,b; 1986; Chandran et al., 1983]. The relatively large profile design of caged ball or disc construction also increases the possibility of interference with anatomical structures after implantation. The *tilting disc valves*, with improved hemodynamic characteristics, were introduced in the late 1960s. The initial design consisted of a polyacetal (Delrin®) disc with a Teflon® sewing ring. Delrin acetal resins are thermoplastic polymers manufactured by the polymerization of *formaldehyde* [Shim and Lenker, 1988]. Even though Delrin exhibited excellent wear resistance and mechanical strength with satisfactory performance after more than 20 years of implantation, it was also found to swell when exposed to humid environments such as *autoclaving* and blood contact. To avoid design and manufacturing difficulties due to the swelling phenomenon, the Delrin disc was soon replaced by the *pyrolytic carbon* disc, which has become the preferred material for mechanical valve prostheses occluders to date. Pyrolytic carbons are formed in a fluidized bed by pyrolysis of a gaseous hydrocarbon in the range of 1000 to 2400°C. For biomedical applications, carbon is deposited onto a preformed polycrystalline graphite substrate at

FIGURE 7.1 A caged-ball heart valve prosthesis. (Courtesy of Baxter Health Care, Irvine, CA.)

temperatures below 1500°C (low temperature isotropic pyrolytic carbon, LTI Pyrolite®). Increase in strength and wear resistance is obtained by codepositing silicone (up to 10% by weight) with carbon in applications for heart valve prostheses. The pyrolytic carbon discs exhibit excellent blood compatibility, as well as wear and fatigue resistance. The guiding *struts* of tilting disc valves are made of *titanium* or Co–Cr alloys (Haynes 25® and Stellite 21®). The Co–Cr based alloys, along with pure titanium and its alloy (Ti6A14V) exhibit excellent mechanical properties as well as resistance to corrosion and thrombus deposition. A typical commercially available tilting disc valve with a pyrolytic carbon disk is shown in Fig. 7.2a. A tilting disc valve with the leaflet made of *ultra-high-molecular-weight polyethylene* (Chitra valve—Fig. 7.2b) is currently marketed in India. The advantages of *leaflets* with relatively more flexibility compared to pyrolytic carbon leaflets are discussed in Chandran et al. [1994a]. Another new concept in a tilting disc valve design introduced by Reul et al. [1995] has an S-shaped leaflet with leading and trailing edges being parallel to the direction of blood flow. The housing for the valve is nozzle shaped to minimize

FIGURE 7.2a Photograph of a typical tilting disc valve prosthesis. (Courtesy of Medtronic Heart Valves, Minneapolis, MN.)

FIGURE 7.2b Chitra tilting disc valve prosthesis with the occluder made of ultra-high-molecular-weight poly-ethylene. (Courtesy of Sree Chitra Tirunal Institute for Medical Sciences and Technology, India).

flow separation at the inlet and energy loss in flow across the valve. Results from *in vitro* evaluation and animal implantation have been encouraging.

In the late 1970s, a bileaflet design was introduced for mechanical valve prostheses and several different bileaflet models are being introduced into the market today. The leaflets as well as the housing of the bileaflet valves are made of pyrolytic carbon and the bileaflet valves show improved hemodynamic characteristics, especially in smaller sizes, compared to tilting disc valves. A typical bileaflet valve is shown in Fig. 7.3. Design features to improve the hydrodynamic characteristics of the mechanical valves include the opening angle of the leaflets [Baldwin et al., 1997] as well as having an open-pivot design in which the pivot area protrudes into the orifice and is exposed to the washing action of flowing blood [Drogue and Villafana, 1997]. Other design modifications to improve the mechanical valve function include: the use of double polyester (Dacron®) velour material for the suture ring to encourage rapid and controlled tissue ingrowth,

FIGURE 7.3 A CarboMedics bileaflet valve with pyrolytic carbon leaflets and housing (Courtesy of Sulzer-Carbo-Medics, Austin, TX.)

FIGURE 7.4   Two views of a tri-leaflet heart valve prosthesis under development. (Courtesy of Triflo Medical, Inc., Costa Mesa, CA.)

and mounting the cuff on a rotation ring which surrounds the orifice ring to protect the cuff mounting mechanism from deeply placed annulus sutures. A PTFE (Teflon®) insert in the cuff provides pliability without excessive drag on the sutures. Tungsten (20% by weight) is incorporated into the leaflet substrate in order to visualize the leaflet motion *in vivo*.

Another attempt to design a mechanical valve that mimics the geometry and function of the tri-leaflet aortic valve is that of Lapeyre et al. [1994; Fig. 7.4]. The geometry of the valve affords true central flow characteristics with reduced backflow. Accelerated fatigue tests have also shown good wear characteristics for this design and the valve is undergoing further evaluation including animal studies. Other improvements in the mechanical valves which augment performance include: machining of the valve housing to fit a disk so as to produce optimal washing and minimal regurgitation [McKenna, 1997]; a supra-annular design so that a larger-sized valve can be inserted in the aortic position in the case of patients with small aortic annulus [Bell, 1997]; and coating of a titanium alloy ring with a thin, uniform, and strongly adherent film of high-density turbostratic carbon (Carbofilm™) [Bona et al., 1997] in order to integrate the structural stability of the metal alloy to the non-thrombogenecity of pyrolytic carbon.

Details of contemporary design efforts in mechanical valve design and potential future biomaterials such as Boralyn® (boron carbide) are discussed in Wieting [1997].

In spite of the desirable characteristics of the biomaterials used in the heart valve prostheses, problems with *thrombo-embolic* complications are significant with implanted valves, and patients with mechanical valves are under long-term anticoagulant therapy. The mechanical stresses induced by the flow of blood across the valve prostheses have been linked to the lysis and activation of *formed elements of blood* (red blood cells, white blood cells, and platelets) resulting in the deposition of thrombi in regions with relative stasis in the vicinity of the prostheses. Numerous *in vitro* studies with mechanical valves in pulse duplicators simulating physiological flow have been reported in the literature and have been reviewed by Chandran [1988] and Dellsperger and Chandran [1991]. Such studies have included measurement of velocity profiles and turbulent stresses distal to the valve due to flow across the valve. The aim of these studies has been the correlation of regions prone to thrombus deposition and tissue overgrowth with explanted valves and the experimentally measured bulk turbulent shear stresses as well as regions of relative stasis. In spite of improvements in design of the prostheses to afford a centralized flow with minimal flow disturbances and fluid mechanical stresses, the problems with thrombus deposition remain significant.

Reports of strut failure, material *erosion* and leaflet escapes, as well as *pitting* and erosion of valve leaflets and housing, have resulted in numerous investigations of the *closing dynamics* of mechanical valves. The dynamics of the leaflet motion and its impact with the valve housing or seat stop are very complex and a number of experimental and numerical studies have appeared recently in the literature. As the leaflet impacts against the seat stop and comes to rest instantaneously, high positive and negative pressure transients are present on the outflow and inflow side of the occluder, respectively, at the instant when the leaflet impacts against the seat stop or the guiding strut [Leuer, 1986; Chandran et al., 1994a]. The *negative pressure transients* have been shown to reach magnitudes below the *liquid vapor pressure* and have been demonstrated to be a function of the loading rate on the leaflet inducing the valve closure. As the magnitudes of negative pressure transients go below the liquid vapor pressure, *cavitation bubbles* are initiated and the subsequent collapse of the cavitation bubbles may also be a factor in the lysis of red blood cells, platelets, and *valvular structures* [Chandran et al., 1994a; Lee et al., 1994]. Typical cavitation bubbles visualized in an *in vitro* study with tilting disc and bileaflet valves are shown in Fig. 7.5. A correlation is also observed between the region where cavitation bubbles are present, even though for a period of time less than a millisecond after valve closure, and sites of pitting and erosion reported in the pyrolytic carbon material in the valve housing and on the leaflets with explanted valves [Kafesjian, 1994] as well as those used in total artificial hearts [Leuer, 1987]. An electron micrograph of pitting and erosion observed in the pyrolytic carbon valve housing of an explanted bileaflet mechanical valve is shown in Fig. 7.6. The pressure transients at valve closure are substantially smaller in mechanical valves with a flexible occluder and leaflets made of ultra-high-molecular-weight polyethylene (Fig. 7.2b) may prove to be advantageous based on the closing dynamic analysis [Chandran et al., 1994a]. A correlation between the average velocity of the leaflet edge and the negative pressure transients in the same region at the instant of valve closure, as well as the presence of cavitation bubbles, has been reported recently [Chandran et al., 1997]. This study demonstrated that for the valves of the same geometry (e.g., tilting disk) and size, the leaflet edge velocity as well as the negative pressure transients were similar. However, the presence of cavitation bubbles depended on the local interaction between the leaflet and the seat stop. Hence, it was pointed out that magnitudes of leaflet velocity or presence of pressure transients below the liquid vapor pressure might not necessarily indicate cavitation inception with mechanical valve closure. Chandran et al. [1998] have also demonstrated the presence of negative pressure transients in the atrial chamber with implanted mechanical valves in the mitral position in animals, demonstrating that the *potential* for cavitation exists with implanted mechanical valves. Similar to the *in vitro* results, the transients were of smaller magnitudes with the Chitra valve made of flexible leaflets, and no pressure transients were observed with tissue valve implanted in the mitral position *in vivo*. The demonstration of the negative pressure transients with mechanical valve closure also shows that this phenomenon is

FIGURE 7.5 Cavitation bubbles visualized on the inflow side of the valves *in vitro* [Chandran et al., 1994a]: (a) Medtronic–Hall tilting disc valve; (b) Edwards–Duromedics bileaflet valve.

localized and the flow chamber or valve holder rigidity with the *in vitro* experiments will not affect the valve closing dynamics.

The pressure distribution on the leaflets and impact forces between the leaflets and guiding struts have also been experimentally measured in order to understand the causes for strut failure [Chandran et al., 1994b]. The flow through the clearance between the leaflet and the housing at the instant of valve closure [Lee and Chandran, 1994a,b] and in the fully closed position [Reif, 1991] and the resulting wall shear stresses within the clearance are also being suggested as responsible for clinically significant hemolysis and thrombus initiation. Detailed analysis of the complex closing dynamics of the leaflets may also be exploited in improving the design of the mechanical valves to minimize problems with structural failure [Cheon and Chandran, 1994]. Further improvements in the design of the valves based on the closing dynamics as well as improvements in material may result in minimizing thrombo-embolic complications with implanted mechanical valves.

(c)

FIGURE 7.5 (continued) Cavitation bubbles visualized on the inflow side of the valves *in vitro* [Chandran et al., 1994a]: (c) CarboMedics bileaflet valve.

FIGURE 7.6 Photographs showing pitting on pyrolytic carbon surface of a mechanical heart valve. (Courtesy of Baxter Health Care, Irvine, CA.)

Biological Heart Valves

The first biological valves implanted were *homografts* with valves explanted from cadavers within 48 hours after death. Preservation of the valves included various techniques of sterilization, freeze drying, and immersing in antibiotic solution. The use of homografts is not popular due to problems with long-term durability and due to limited availability except in a few centers [Shim and Lenker, 1988; Lee and Boughner, 1991]. Attempts were also made in the early 1960s in the use of *xenografts* (valves made from animal tissue) and porcine bioprostheses became commercially available after the introduction of the gluteraldehyde (rather than formaldehyde, which was initially used) fixation technique. Gluteraldehyde reacts with tissue proteins to form crosslinks and results in improved durability [Carpentier et al., 1969]. The valves are harvested from 7- to 12-month-old pigs and attached to supporting *stents* and preserved.

FIGURE 7.7 Typical bioprostheses: (a) Hancock porcine bioprosthesis (courtesy of Medtronic Heart Valves, Minneapolis, MN); (b) PhotoFix™ α pericardial prosthesis (courtesy of Sulzer–CarboMedics, Inc., Austin, TX.)

The stent provided support to preserve the valve in the natural shape and to achieve normal opening and closing. Initial supports were made of metal and subsequently flexible polypropylene stents were introduced. The flexible stents provided the advantage of ease of assembling the valve and finite element analyses have demonstrated reduction in stresses at the juncture between the stent and tissue leaflets resulting in increased durability and increased leaflet coaptation area [Reis et al., 1971; Hamid et al., 1985]. A typical porcine bioprosthesis is included in Fig. 7.7a.

Fixed bovine pericardial tissue is also used to construct heart valves in which design characteristics such as orifice area, valve height, and degree of coaptation can be specified and controlled. Thus, the geometry and flow dynamics past *pericardial prostheses* mimic those of the natural human aortic valves more closely. Due to the low profile design of pericardial prostheses and increased orifice area, these valves are less stenotic compared to porcine bioprostheses, especially in smaller sizes [Chandran et al., 1984]. In the currently available bioprostheses, the stents are constructed from polypropylene, *Acetol®* homopolymer, or copolymer, Elgiloy wire, or titanium. A stainless steel radiopaque marker is also introduced to visualize the valve *in vivo*. Other biomaterials which have been employed in making the bioprostheses

TABLE 7.2   Biomaterial Used in Heart Valve Prostheses

Prosthesis Type	Component	Biomaterial
Caged ball	Ball/occluder	Silastic
	Cage	Stellite 21®/Titanium
	Suture ring	Silicone rubber insert under knitted composite Teflon®/polypropylene cloth
Tilting disc	Leaflet	Delrin®; pyrolytic carbon (carbon deposited on graphite substrate); ultra high molecular polyethylene (UHMPE)
	Housing/strut	Haynes 25®/Titanium
	Suture ring	Teflon®/Dacron®
Bileaflet	Leaflets	Pyrolytic carbon
	Housing	Pyrolytic carbon
	Suture ring	Double velour Dacron® tricot knit polyester
Porcine bioprostheses	Leaflets	Porcine aortic valve fixed by stabilized gluteraldehyde
	Stents	Polypropylene stent covered with Dacron®; lightweight Elgiloy wire covered with porous knitted Teflon® cloth
	Suture ring	Dacron®; soft silicone rubber insert covered with porous, seamless Teflon® cloth
Pericardial bioprostheses	Leaflets	Porcine pericardial tissue fixed by stabilized gluteraldehyde before leaflets are sewn to the valve stents
	Stents	Polypropylene stent covered with Dacron®; Elgiloy wire and nylon support band covered with polyester and Teflon® cloth
	Suture ring	PTFE fabric over silicone rubber filter

Source: Shim and Lenker [1988]; Dellsperger and Chandran [1988].

include *fascia lata* tissue as well as human *duramater* tissue. The former was prone to deterioration and hence unsuitable for bioprosthetic application, while the latter lacked commercial availability.

The advantage with bioprostheses is the freedom from thrombo-embolism and hence not requiring long-term anticoagulant therapy in general. These prostheses are preferable in patients who do not tolerate anticoagulants. On the other hand, bioprosthetic valves are prone to *calcification* and leaflet tear with an average lifetime of about 10 years before replacement is necessary, generally attributed to the tissue fixation process. Numerous attempts are being made to improve the design as well as fixation in bioprostheses in order to minimize problems with calcification and increase duration of the function of the implant. As an example, a bovine pericardial trileaflet valve (Fig. 7.7b) treated with a non-aldehyde fixation resulting in collagen crosslink formation without a new "foreign" chemical process [Phillips and Printz, 1997] has been introduced in the European market. A non-aldehyde iodine-based sterilization process also sterilizes the valve.

Numerous studies linking the mechanical stresses on the leaflets with calcification, focal thinning, and leaflet failure [Thubrikar et al., 1982a; Sabbah et al., 1985] and design improvements to minimize the stresses on the leaflets [Thubrikar et al., 1982b] have been reported in the literature. Further details on the effects of tissue fixation and mechanical effects of fixation on the leaflets are reported elsewhere [Lee and Boughner, 1991]. Improvements in fixation techniques as well as in design of the bioprostheses are continually being made in order to minimize problems with calcification of the leaflets and improve the durability and functional characteristics of bioprosthetic heart valves [Piwnica and Westaby, 1998]. The biomaterials used in commercially available mechanical and bioprosthetic heart valves are included in Table 7.2. Table 7.3 includes a summary of the problems associated with implanted artificial heart valves.

Synthetic Heart Valves

Concurrently, efforts have also been made in the development of valve prostheses made of synthetic material. Several attempts to make bileaflet [Braunwald et al., 1960] and trileaflet valves [Roe et al., 1958; Hufnagel, 1977; Gerring et al., 1974; Ghista and Reul, 1977] made of polyurethanes, polyester fabrics, and silicone rubber were not successful due to problems with durability of relatively thin leaflets made of synthetic material. With the advent of the total artificial hearts (TAHs) and *left ventricular assist devices* (LVADs) in the 1980s, an additional impetus on the development of synthetic valves is present. Due to

TABLE 7.3 Common Problems with Implanted
Prosthetic Heart Valves

I. *Mechanical Valves:*
    a) Thrombo-embolism
    b) Structural failure
    c) Red blood cell and platelet destruction
    d) Tissue overgrowth
    e) Damage to endothelial lining
    f) Paravalvular/perivalvular leakage
    g) Tearing of sutures
    h) Infection

II. *Bioprosthetic Valves:*
    a) Tissue calcification
    b) Leaflet rupture
    c) Paravalvular/perivalvular leakage
    d) Infection

Source: Yoganathan et al. [1979a]; Shim and Lenker
[1988]; Chandran [1992].

problems with thrombus deposition in the vicinity of the mechanical valves used in the TAH and subsequent stroke episodes in patients with permanent implants, the use of the device is currently restricted as a bridge to transplantation. In such temporary use before a donor heart becomes available (on an average of several weeks), the four mechanical prostheses used in the TAH result in substantial cost. Hence, efforts are being made to replace the mechanical valves with those made with synthetic material. With *vacuum forming* or *solution casting* techniques, synthetic valves can be made at a fraction of the cost of mechanical valves, provided their function in a TAH environment for several weeks will be satisfactory. Implantation of synthetic trileaflet valves [Russel et al., 1980; Harold et al., 1987], even more recently, has resulted in limited success due to leaflet failure and calcification. Hemodynamic comparison of vacuum formed and solution cast trileaflet valves to currently available bioprostheses have produced satisfactory results [Chandran et al., 1989a,b]. *Finite element analysis* of synthetic valves can be exploited in design improvements similar to those reported for bioprostheses [Chandran et al., 1991a].

Total Artificial Hearts (TAHs) or Ventricular Assist Devices (VADs)

Artificial circulatory support can be broadly classified into two categories. The first category is for those patients who undergo open heart surgery to correct *valvular disorders*, ventricular *aneurysm*, or coronary *artery* disease. In several cases, the heart may not recover sufficiently after surgery to take over the pumping action. In such patients ventricular assist devices are used as extracorporeal devices to maintain circulation until the heart recovers. Other ventricular assist devices include *intra-aortic balloon pumps* as well as *cardiopulmonary* bypass. Within several days or weeks, when the natural heart has recovered, these devices are removed. In the second category are patients who have advanced stages of cardiomyopathy and are subjects for heart transplantation. Due to problems in the availability of suitable donor hearts, not all patients with a failed heart are candidates for heart transplantation. For those patients not selected for transplantation, the concept of replacing the natural heart with a total artificial heart has gained considerable attention [Akutsu and Kolff, 1958; Jarvick, 1981; DeVries and Joyce, 1983; Unger, 1989; Kambic and Nose, 1991]. A number of attempts in the permanent implantation of TAHs with pneumatically powered units were made in the 1980s. However, due to neurological complications as a result of thrombo-embolism, infection, and hematological and renal complications, permanent implantations are currently suspended. If a suitable donor heart is not readily available, TAHs can be used as bridges to transplantation for several weeks until a donor heart becomes available. Until recently, most of the circulatory assist devices were pneumatically driven; a typical pneumatic heart is shown in Fig. 7.8a. It has two chambers for the left and right ventricle with inlet and outlet valves for each of the chambers. A line coming from the external pneumatic driver passes through the skin and is attached to the

(a)

(b)

FIGURE 7.8 Typical prototype designs of total artificial hearts: (a) pneumatically powered TAH. The right and left ventricular chambers, inflow and outflow valves, as well as the connector for the pneumatic line are visible in the photograph; (b) electrically powered TAH. Shown are the external battery pack, transcutaneous energy transmission system (TETS) primary and secondary coils, implanted electronics, energy converter and the blood pumps, compliance chamber, and the subcutaneous access port. (Courtesy of G. Rosenberg, Pennsylvania State University.)

diaphragm housing through the connector shown in the photograph. Thus, the patient is tethered to an external pneumatic drive. He can move around for a short period of time by attaching the pneumatic line to a portable driver that he can carry.

Electrically driven blood pumps, which can afford tether-free operation within the body, unlike those of the pneumatically powered pumps, are currently at various stages of development for long-term use (of more than two years). The components of such devices include the blood pump in direct contact with blood, energy converter (from electrical to mechanical energy), variable column compensator, implantable batteries, transcutaneous energy transmission system, and external batteries. The blood pump configuration in these devices includes sac, diaphragm, and *pusher plate devices*. Materials used in blood-contacting surfaces in these devices are synthetic polymers (polyurethanes, segmented polyurethanes, Biomer®, and others). Segmented polyurethane elastomer used in prosthetic ventricles with a thromboresistant additive modifying the polymeric surface have resulted in improved blood compatibility and reduced thrombo-embolic risk in animal trials [Farrar et al., 1988]. Design considerations include reduction of regions of stagnation of blood within the blood chamber and minimizing the mechanical stresses induced on the formed elements in blood. Apart from the characteristics of these materials to withstand repetitive high mechanical stresses and minimize failure due to fatigue, surface interaction with blood is also another crucial factor. An electrically powered total artificial heart intended for long-term implantation is shown in Fig. 7.8b. The details of the design considerations for the circulatory assist devices are included in Rosenberg [1995] and details of the evaluation of the electrically powered heart are included in Rosenberg et al. [1995].

Due to significant problems with thrombo-embolic complications and subsequent neurological problems with long-term implantation of TAHs in humans, attention has been focused on minimizing factors responsible for thrombus deposition. In order to eliminate crevices formed with the quick connect system, valves sutured in place at the inflow and outflow orifices were offered as an alternative in the Philadelphia Heart [Wurzel et al., 1988]. An alternative, quick-connect system using precision machined components has been demonstrated to reduce valve- and connector-associated thrombus formation substantially [Holfert et al., 1987]. Several *in vitro* studies have been reported in the literature in order to assess the effect of fluid dynamic stresses on thrombus deposition [Phillips et al., 1979; Tarbell et al., 1986; Baldwin et al., 1990; Jarvis et al., 1991]. These have included flow visualization and laser Doppler anemometry velocity and turbulence measurements within the ventricular chamber as well as in the vicinity of the inflow and outflow orifices. The results of such studies indicate that the flow within the chamber generally has a smooth washout of blood in each pulsatile flow cycle with relatively large turbulent stresses and regions of stasis found near the valves. The thrombus deposition found with implanted TAHs in the vicinity of the inflow valves also indicates that the major problem with the working of these devices are still with the flow dynamics across the mechanical valves. Computational flow dynamic analysis within the ventricular chamber may also be exploited to improve the design of the valve chambers and the mechanical valves in order to reduce the turbulent stresses near the vicinity of the inflow and outflow orifices [Kim et al., 1992]. Structural failure of the mechanical valves initially reported with the TAH may have been the result of increased load on the valves during closure due to the relatively large dp/dt (p is pressure, t is time) at which the TAH was operated. Attempts at reducing the dp/dt during closure of the inflow valves have also been reported with modified designs of the artificial heart driver [Wurzel et al., 1988]. Due to the relatively large dp/dt at which TAHs are operated, there is increased possibility of cavitation bubble initiation, and subsequent collapse of the bubbles may also be another important reason for thrombus deposition near the mechanical valve at the inflow orifice. Introducing synthetic valves to replace the mechanical valves [Chandran et al., 1991b] may prove to be advantageous with respect to cavitation initiation and may minimize thrombus formation.

Vascular Prostheses

In advanced stages of vascular diseases such as obstructive *atherosclerosis* and aneurysmal dilatation, when other treatment modalities fail, replacement of diseased segments with vascular prostheses is a common practice. Vascular prostheses can be classified as given in Table 7.4.

TABLE 7.4   Classification of Vascular Prostheses

Prosthesis	Comments
Surgically Implanted Biological Grafts	
Autograft	Graft transplanted from part of a patient's body to another. *Example:* saphenous vein graft for peripheral bypass.
Allograft	Homograft. Transplanted vascular graft tissues derived from the same species as recipient. *Example:* glutaraldehyde treated umbilical cord vein graft.
Xenograft	Heterograft. Surgical graft of vascular tissues derived from one species to a recipient of another species. *Example:* modified bovine heterograft.
Surgically Implanted Synthetic Grafts	
Dacron (polyethylene terephthalate)	Woven, knitted
PTFE (polytetrafluoroethylene)	Expanded, knitted
Other	Nylon, polyurethane

Surgically Implanted Biological Grafts

Arterial homografts, even though initially used in large scale, resulted in aneurysm formation especially in the proximal suture line [Strandness and Sumner, 1975]. Still, a viable alternative is to use the saphenous vein graft from the same patient. Vein grafts have a failure rate of about 20% in one year and up to 30% in five years after implantation. Vein grafts from the same patients are also unavailable or unsuitable in about 10 to 30% of the patients [Abbott and Bouchier-Hayes, 1978]. Modified *bovine heterografts* and gluteraldehyde-treated *umbilical cord vein grafts* have also been employed as vascular prostheses with less success compared to autologous vein grafts.

Surgically Implanted Synthetic Grafts

Prostheses made of synthetic material for vascular replacement have been used for over 40 years. Poly-meric material currently used as implants include *nylon*, polyester, *polytetrafluoroethylene* (PTFE), polypropylene, polyacrylonitrile, and silicone rubber [Park and Lakes, 1992]. However, Dacron® (poly-ethylene terephthalate) and PTFE are the more common vascular prostheses materials currently available. These materials exhibit the essential qualities for implants—they are biocompatible, resilient, flexible, durable, and resistant to sterilization and biodegradation. Detailed discussion on the properties, manu-facturing techniques, and testing of Dacron® prostheses is included in Guidoin and Couture [1992]. Figure 7.9a depicts a Dacron vascular graft having a bifurcated configuration. Figure 7.9b shows expanded PTFE vascular grafts having a variety of configurations and sizes: straight, straight with external rein-forcement rings (to resist external compression), and bifurcated.

Synthetic vascular grafts implanted as large-vessel replacements have resulted in reasonable degrees of success. However, in medium- and small-diameter prostheses (less than 6 mm in diameter), loss of *patency* within several months after implantation is more acute. Graft failure due to thrombosis or intimal hyperplasia with thrombosis is primarily responsible in failures within 30 days after implantation, and intimal hyperplasia formation is the reason for failure within 6 months after surgery. Soon after implan-tation, layers of *fibrin* and fibrous tissue cover the intimal and outer surface of the prosthesis, respectively. A layer of *fibroblasts* replaces the fibrin and is referred to as *neointima*. In the later stages, *neointimal hyperplasia* formation occurs and ultimately results in the occlusion of the vessels in small-diameter vascular grafts. Attempts are being made to suitably modify the surface characteristics of the prostheses in order to reduce the problems with loss of patency. Studies are also being performed in order to understand the mechanical stresses induced at the anastomotic region, which may result in deposits on the intimal surface and occlusion of the vessels [Chandran and Kim, 1994]. The alterations in mechanical stresses with the implantation of vascular prostheses in the arterial circulation may include changes in the deformation and stress concentrations at the anastomotic site. Altered fluid shear stresses at the

FIGURE 7.9a Photograph of a Dacron vascular graft having a bifurcated configuration. (Courtesy of W. L. Gore and Associates, Inc., Flagstaff, AZ.)

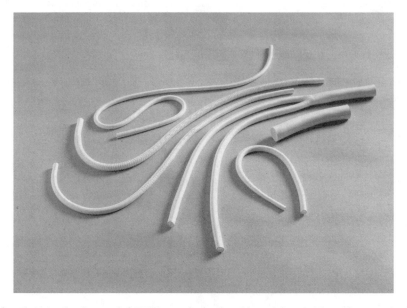

FIGURE 7.9b Photograph of expanded PTFE vascular grafts with straight, straight with external reinforcement rings to resist compression, and bifurcated configurations. (Courtesy of W. L. Gore and Associates, Inc., Flagstaff, AZ.)

intimal surface in the vicinity of the anastomosis has also been suggested as important particularly since the loss of patency is present more often at the distal anastomosis. The vascular prosthesis should have the same dynamic response after implantation as the host artery in order to reduce the effect of abnormal mechanical stresses at the junction. For a replacement graft of the same size as the host artery, mismatch in *compliance* may be the most important factor resulting in graft failure [Abbott and Bouchier-Hayes, 1978]. In implanting the prostheses, end-to-end configuration is common in the reconstruction of peripheral arteries. *End-to-side configuration* is common in coronary artery bypass where blood will flow from the host artery (aorta) to the prosthesis branching out at the anastomotic site. At the other end, the graft is attached distal to the occlusion in the host (coronary) vessel to enable perfusion of the vascular bed downstream from the occlusion. Numerous studies analyzing the abnormal flow dynamics within the anastomotic geometry and stress distribution within the vascular material at the junction to the prostheses have been reported in delineating the causes for intimal hyperplasia formation and loss of patency [Kim and Chandran, 1993; Kim et al., 1993; Ojha et al., 1990; Keynton et al., 1991: Chandran et al., 1992; Rodgers et al., 1987; Rhee and Tarbell, 1994] and a detailed discussion on the mechanical aspects of vascular prostheses can be found in Chandran and Kim [1994]. Improvements in the blood–surface interactions are also being attempted in order to improve the functioning capability of vascular grafts. Attempts at seeding the grafts with *endothelial cells* [Hunter et al., 1983], and modifying the graft material properties by removing the *crimping* and heat fusing a coil of bendable and dimensionally stable polypropylene at the outer surface to make it kink resistant [Guidoin et al., 1983], and employing a compliant and biodegradable graft which will promote regeneration of arterial wall in small caliber vessels [Van der Lei et al., 1985, 1986] are a few examples of such improvements.

Transluminally Placed Endovascular Prostheses (Stent-Grafts)

Endoluminal approaches to treating vascular disease involve the insertion of a prosthetic device into the vasculature through a small, often percutaneous, access site created in a remote vessel, followed by the intraluminal delivery and deployment of a prosthesis via transcatheter techniques [Veith et al., 1995]. In contrast to conventional surgical therapies for vascular disease, transluminally placed endovascular prostheses are distinguished by their "minimally invasive" nature. Because these techniques do not require extensive surgical intervention, they have the potential to simplify the delivery of vascular therapy, improve procedural outcomes, decrease procedural costs, reduce morbidity, and broaden the patient population that may benefit from treatment. Not surprisingly, endoluminal therapies have generated intense interest within the vascular surgery, interventional radiology, and cardiology communities over recent years.

The feasibility of using transluminally placed endovascular prostheses, or stent-grafts, for the treatment of traumatic vascular injury [Marin et al., 1994], atherosclerotic obstructions [Cragg and Dake, 1993], and aneurysmal vascular disease [Parodi et al., 1991; Yusuf et al., 1994; Dake et al., 1994] has been demonstrated in human beings. Endoluminal stent-grafts continue to evolve to address a number of cardiovascular pathologies at all levels of the arterial tree. Figure 7.10a depicts endoluminal stent-grafts having a variety of configurations (straight, bifurcated) and functional diameters (peripheral, aortic) that are currently under clinical investigation.

Endoluminal stent-grafts are catheter-deliverable endoluminal prostheses comprised of an intravascular stent component and a biocompatible graft component. The function of these devices is to provide an intraluminal conduit that enables blood flow through pathologic vascular segments without the need for open surgery. The stent component functions as an arterial attachment mechanism and provides structural support to both the graft and the treated vascular segment. By design, stents are delivered to the vasculature in a low profile, small diameter delivery configuration, and can be elastically or plastically expanded to a secondary, large diameter configuration upon deployment. Vascular attachment is achieved by the interference fit created when a stent is deployed within the lumen of a vessel having a diameter smaller than that of the stent. The graft component, on the other hand, is generally constructed from a biocompatible material such as expanded polytetrafluoroethylene (ePTFE), woven polyester (Dacron), or polyurethane. The graft component has a number of real and theoretical functions, including: segregating potential thromboemboli or atheroemboli from the bloodstream, presenting a physical barrier to mass transport between the bloodstream and arterial wall, and mitigating cellular infiltration and the host inflammatory response. Figure 7.10b shows a stent-graft implant consisting of an ePTFE graft that is externally supported along its entire length by a self-expanding nitinol stent. The implant is radially constrained and attached to the leading end of a dual lumen polyethylene delivery catheter that allows transluminal delivery and deployment. Following introduction into the vascular system, the implant is positioned fluoroscopically within the diseased segment and released from the delivery system.

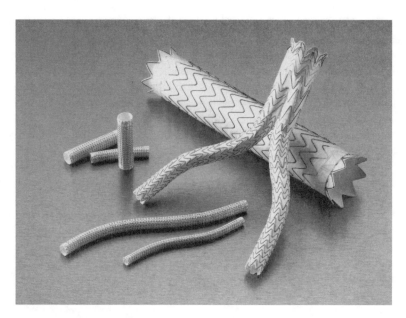

FIGURE 7.10a Endoluminal stent-grafts of straight and bifurcated configurations and sizes currently under clinical investigation. (Courtesy of W. L. Gore and Associates, Inc., Flagstaff, AZ.)

FIGURE 7.10b A stent-graft implant consisting of an expanded PTFE graft that is externally supported by a self-expanding nitinol stent. (Courtesy of W. L. Gore and Associates, Inc., Flagstaff, AZ.)

Mechanical properties play an important role in determining the *in vivo* performance of an endoluminal stent-graft. Since the graft component typically lacks significant structural integrity, the mechanical behavior of the stent-graft predominantly depends upon the mechanical properties of its stent component. The type of mechanism required to induce dilatation from the delivery (small diameter) configuration to the deployed (large diameter) configuration typically classifies stents. Self-expanding stents are designed to spontaneously dilate (i.e., elastically recover) from the delivery diameter up to a maximal, pre-determined deployed diameter, whereas balloon-expandable stents are designed to be plastically enlarged over a range of values with the use of appropriately sized and pressurized dilatation balloons. Consequently, self-expanding stents exert a continuous, radially outward directed force on periluminal tissues, while balloon-expandable stents assume a fixed diameter that resists recoil of the surrounding periluminal tissues. Both types of stents exhibit utilitarian features. For example, in comparison to balloon-expandable devices, self-expanding stents can be rapidly deployed without the use of dilatation balloons, are elastic and therefore less prone to external compression, can radially adapt to post-deployment vascular remodeling, and retain some of the natural compliance of the vascular tissues. In contrast, balloon-expandable stents are much more versatile when it comes to conforming to irregular vascular morphologies because their diameter can be radially adjusted via balloon dilatation. Since the luminal diameter of self-expanding stents cannot be adjusted (i.e., enlarged) to any appreciable degree, accurate sizing of the host vessel is critical. A sizing mismatch resulting in oversizing can cause overcompression of the self-expanding stent and obstructive invagination of the stent into the lumen. Undersizing, in turn, can result in a poor interference fit, inadequate anchoring, device migration, and/or leakage of blood into the abluminal compartment. In either case, the stent provides a scaffold that structurally supports the graft material. Ongoing work in the field of biomedical engineering is directed at optimizing the biomechanical and biological performance of these devices.

Conclusions

In the last four decades, we have observed significant advances in the development of biocompatible materials to be used in blood-interfacing implants. In the case of mechanical heart valve prostheses, pyrolytic carbon has become the material of choice for the occluder and the housing. The pyrolytic carbon is chemically inert and exhibits very little wear even after more than 20 years of use. However, thrombo-embolic complications still remain significant with mechanical valve implantation. The complex dynamics of valve function and the resulting mechanical stresses on the formed elements of blood appear to be the main cause for initiation of thrombus. More recent reports of structural failure with implanted mechanical valves and pitting and erosion observed on the pyrolytic carbon surfaces have resulted in investigations on cavitation bubble formation during valve closure. Along with further improvements in biomaterials for heart valves, detailed analysis of the closing dynamics and design improvements to minimize the adverse effects of mechanical stresses may be the key to reducing thrombus deposition. Improvements on mechanical heart valves or further developments in durable synthetic leaflet valves may also be vital for the development of TAHs for long-term implantation without neurologic complications.

In the case of vascular grafts, the mismatch of material properties (compliance) between the host artery and the graft, as well as geometric considerations in end-to-side anastomoses, appear to be important for the loss of patency within several months after implantation particularly with medium and small diameter arterial replacement. Most of the vascular grafts are stiffer compared to the host artery and it has been suggested that the mechanical stresses resulting from the discontinuity at the junction is the major cause for neointimal hyperplasia formation and subsequent occlusion of the conduit. Developments with more compliant grafts and in modifying the surface interaction of the graft with blood (endothelialization or other treatment of the graft material) may result in reducing the problems with loss of patency. Recent advances in the use of minimally invasive stent-grafts also show promise in improving the quality of life of patients with vascular disease.

Defining Terms

Acetol: Product of the addition of two moles of alcohol to one of an aldehyde.
Aneurysms: Abnormal bulging or dilatation of a segment of a blood vessel or myocardium.
Artery: Blood vessel transporting blood in a direction away from the heart.
Atherosclerosis: Lipid deposits in the intima of arteries.
ATS valve: A bileaflet mechanical valve made by ATS (Advancing The Standard) Inc.
Autoclaving: Sterilizing by steam under pressure.

Biomer®:   Segmented polyurethane elastomer.

Bioprostheses: Prosthetic heart valves made of biological tissue.

Blood oxygenators: Extracorporeal devices to oxygenate blood during heart bypass surgery.

Bovine heterograft: Graft material (arterial) transplanted from bovine species.

Calcification: Deposition of insoluble salts of calcium.

Cardiac pacemakers: Prosthesis implanted to stimulate cardiac muscles to contract.

Cardiopulmonary bypass: Connectors bypassing circulation to the heart and the lungs.

Catheters: Hollow cylindrical tubing to be passed through the blood vessels or other canals.

Cavitation bubbles (vapor cavitation):   Formation of vapor bubbles due to transient reduction in pressure to below the liquid vapor pressure.

Closing dynamics: Dynamics during the closing phase of heart valves.

Compliance: A measure of ease with which a structure can be deformed; ratio of volumetric strain to increase in unit pressure.

Crimping: Creasing of the synthetic vascular grafts in the longitudinal direction to accommodate the large intermittent flow of blood.

Delrin®:   Polyacetal made by Union Carbide.

Dialysers: Devices to filter the blood of waste products taking over the function of the kidney.

dp/dt: Slope of the pressure vs. time curve of the ventricles.

Duramater: A tough fibrous membrane forming the outer cover of the brain and the spinal cord.

Electrohydraulic blood pump: Blood pumps energized by the conversion of electrical to hydraulic energy.

End-to-end configuration: End of the vascular graft anastamosed to the end of the host artery.

End-to-side configuration: End of the vascular graft anastamosed to the side of the host.

Endothelial cells: A layer of flat cells lining the intimal surface of blood vessels.

Erosion: A state of being worn away.

Fascia lata: A sheet of fibrous tissue enveloping the muscles of the thigh.

Fatigue stress: Level of stress below which the material would not undergo fatigue failure (10^7 cycles is used as the normal limit).

Fibrin: An elastic filamentous protein derived from fibrinogen in coagulation of the blood.

Fibroblasts: An elongated cell with cytoplasmic processes present in connective tissue capable of forming collagen fibers.

Finite element analysis: Structural analysis with the aid of a computer which divides the structure into finite elements and applies the laws of mechanics on each element.

Formaldehyde: Formic aldehyde, methyl aldehyde, a pungent gas used as antiseptic.

Formed elements in blood: Red blood cells, white blood cells, platelets, and other cells in whole blood.

Haynes 25®:   Co–Cr alloy.

Homografts: Transplants (heart valves, arterial segments, etc.) from the same species.

Intra-aortic balloon pumps: A balloon catheter inserted in the descending aorta and alternately inflated and deflated timed to the EKG in order to assist the ventricular pumping.

Laser Doppler anemometry: A velocity measurement device using the principle of Doppler shifted frequency of laser light by particles moving with the fluid.

Leaflets: Occluders on valves which open and close to aid blood flow in one direction.

Left ventricular assist devices: Prosthetic devices to assist the left ventricle in pumping blood.

Liquid vapor pressure: Pressure at which liquid vaporizes.

LTI: Low temperature (below 1500°C) isotropic pyrolytic carbon.

Mechanical prostheses: Prostheses made of non-biological material.

Negative pressure transients: Reduction in pressure for a short duration.

Neointima: Newly formed intimal surface.

Neointimal hyperplasia: Growth of new intimal surface formed by fibroblasts.

Nylon: Synthetic polymer with condensation polymerization.

Patency: State of being freely open.

Pericardial prostheses: Heart valve prosthesis made with fixed bovine pericardial tissue.

Pitting: Depression or indent on a surface.

Platelet: One of the formed elements of blood responsible for blood coagulation.

Polypropylene: One of the vinyl polymers with good flex life and good environmental stress crack resistance.

Polytetrafluoroethylene (PTFE): A fluorocarbon polymer known as Teflon®.

Pusher plate devices: Artificial heart devices working with pusher plates moving the blood.

Pyrolytic carbon: Carbon deposited onto preformed polycrystalline graphite substrate.

Radiopacity: Being opaque to x-ray.

Sewing rings: Rings surrounding the housing of artificial heart valves used to sew the valve to the tissue orifice with suture.

Solution casting: Casting by pouring molten material on dyes to form a structure.

Stellite 21®: Co–Cr alloy.

Stent: A device used to maintain the bodily orifice or cavity.

Strut: A projection in the structure such as guiding struts in heart valves used to guide the leaflets during opening and closing.

TAH: Total artificial heart replacing a failed natural heart.

Teflon®: See PTFE.

Thrombo-embolic complications: Complications due to breaking away (emboli) of thrombus blocking the distal blood vessels.

Thrombus: A clot in the blood vessels or in the cavities of the heart formed from the constituents of blood.

Tilting disc valves: Valves with a single leaflet tilting open and shut.

Titanium: Highly reactive metal having low density, good mechanical properties, and biocompatibility due to tenacious oxide layer formation.

Turbulent stresses: Stresses generated in the fluid due to agitated random motion of particles.

Ultra-high-molecular-weight polyethylene: Linear thermoplastics with very high molecular weight ($>2 \times 10^6$ g/mol) used for orthopedic devices such as acetabular cup for hip joint replacement.

Umbilical cord vein grafts: Vascular graft made from umbilical cord veins.

Vacuum forming: A manufacturing technique for thermoplastic polymer in which a sheet is heated and formed over a mold while a vacuum is present under the sheet.

Valvular disorders: Diseased states of valves such as stenosis.

Valvular structures: Components of valves such as leaflets, struts, etc.

Vascular grafts: Grafts to replace segments of diseased vessels.

Xenografts: Grafts obtained from species other than that of the recipient.

References

Abbott, W.M. and Bouchier-Hayes, D.J. 1978. The role of mechanical properties in graft design. In *Graft Materials in Vascular Surgery*, Dardick, H., Ed., Year Book Medical Publishers, Chicago, IL, 59–78.

Akutsu, T. and Kolff, W.J. 1958. Permanent substitutes for valves and hearts. *Trans. Amer. Soc. Art. Intern. Organs (ASAIO)* 4:230–235.

Baldwin, J.T., Tarbell, J.M., Deutsch, S., Geselowitz, D.B., and Rosenberg, G. 1988. Hot-film wall shear probe measurements inside a ventricular assist device. *Am. Soc. Mech. Eng. (ASME) J. Biomech. Eng.* 110:326–333.

Baldwin, J.T., Campbell, A., Luck, C., Ogilvie, W., and Sauter, J. 1997. Hydrodynamics of the Carbo-Medics® aortic kinetic™ prosthetic heart valve. In *Surgery for Acquired Aortic Valve Disease*. Piwnica, A. and Westaby, S., Eds., ISIS Medical Media, Oxford, 365–370.

Bell, R.S. 1997. CarboMedics® supra-annular Top Hat™ aortic valve. In *Surgery for Acquired Aortic Valve Disease*. Piwnica, A. and Westaby, S., Eds., ISIS Medical Media, Oxford, 371–375.

Bona, G., Rinaldi, S., and Vallana, F. 1997. Design characteristics of the BICARBON™ bileaflet heart valve prosthesis. In *Surgery for Acquired Aortic Valve Disease*. Piwnica, A. and Westaby, S. Eds., ISIS Medical Media, Oxford, 392–396.

Braunwald, N.S., Cooper, T., and Morrow, A.G. 1960. Complete replacement of the mitral valve: successful application of a flexible polyurethane prosthesis. *J. Thorac. Cardiovasc. Surg.*, 40:1–11.

Carpentier, A., Lamaigre, C.G., Robert, L., Carpentier, S., and Dubost, C. 1969. Biological factors affecting long-term results of valvular heterografts. *J. Thorac. Cardiovasc. Surg.* 58:467–483.

Chandran, K.B. 1988. Heart valve prostheses: *In vitro* flow dynamics. In *Encyclopedia of Medical Devices and Instrumentation*, Vol. 3, Webster, J.G., Ed., Wiley Interscience, New York, 1475–1483.

Chandran, K.B. 1992. *Cardiovascular Biomechanics*. New York University Press, New York.

Chandran, K.B. and Aluri, S. 1997. Mechanical valve closing dynamics. Relationship between velocity of closing, pressure transients, and cavitation initiation. *Ann. Biomed. Eng.* 25: 926–938.

Chandran, K.B. and Kim, Y.H. 1994. Mechanical aspects of vascular graft-host artery anastomoses. *Inst. Elec. Electr. Engrs. (IEEE) Eng. Med. Bio. Mag.* 13: 517–524.

Chandran, K.B., Cabell, G.N., Khalighi, B., and Chen, C.J. 1983. Laser anemometry measurements of pulsatile flow past aortic valve prostheses. *J. Biomech.* 16:865–873.

Chandran, K.B., Cabell, G.N., Khalighi, B., and Chen, C.J. 1984. Pulsatile flow past aortic valve bioprostheses in a model human aorta. *J. Biomech.* 17:609–619.

Chandran, K.B., Fatemi, R., Schoephoerster, R., Wurzel, D., Hansen, G., Pantalos, G., Yu, L-S., and Kolff, W.J. 1989a. *In vitro* comparison of velocity profiles and turbulent shear distal to polyurethane trileaflet and pericardial prosthetic valves. *Art. Org.* 13:148–154.

Chandran, K.B., Schoephoerster, R.T., Wurzel, D., Hansen, G., Yu, L.-S., Pantalos, G., and Kolff, W.J. 1989b. Hemodynamic comparison of polyurethane trileaflet and bioprosthetic heart valves. *Trans. Amer. Soc. Art. Intern. Organs (ASAIO)* 35:132–138.

Chandran, K.B., Kim, S-H., and Han, G. 1991a. Stress distribution on the cusps of a polyurethane trileaflet heart valve prosthesis in the closed position. *J. Biomech.* 24:385–395.

Chandran, K.B., Lee, C.S., Shipkowitz, T., Chen, L.D., Yu, L.S. and Wurzel, D. 1991b. *In vitro* hemodynamic analysis of flexible artificial ventricle. *Art. Org.* 15:420–426.

Chandran, K.B., Gao, D., Han, G., Baraniewski, H., and Corson, J.D. 1992. Finite element analysis of arterial anastomosis with vein, Dacron® and PTFE grafts. *Med. Biol. Eng. Comp.* 30:413–418.

Chandran, K.B., Lee, C.S., and Chen, L.D. 1994a. Pressure field in the vicinity of mechanical valve occluders at the instant of valve closure: correlation with cavitation initiation. *J. Heart Valve Dis.* 3 (Suppl. 1):S 65—S 76.

Chandran, K.B., Lee, C.S., Aluri, S., Dellsperger, K.C., Schreck, S., and Wieting, D.W. 1994b. Pressure distribution near the occluders and impact forces on the outlet struts of Björk-Shiley convexo-concave valves during closing. *J. Heart Valve Dis.* 5: 199–206.

Chandran, K.B., Dexter, E.U., Aluri, S., and Richenbacher, W.E. 1998. Negative pressure transients with mechanical heart-valve closure: correlation between *in vitro* and *in vivo* results. *Ann. Biomed. Eng.* 26: 546–556.

Cheon, G.J. and Chandran, K.B. 1994. Transient behavior analysis of a mechanical monoleaflet heart valve prosthesis in the closing phase. *Amer. Soc. Mech. Eng. J. Biomech. Eng.* 116: 452–459.

Cragg A.H. and Dake M.D. 1993. Percutaneous femoropoliteal graft placement. *Radiology* 187:643–648.

Dake M.D., Miller D.C., Semba C.P. et al. 1994. Transluminal placement of endovascular stent-grafts for the treatment of descending thoracic aortic aneurysms. *New Engl. J. Med.* 331:1729–1734.

Dellsperger, K.C. and Chandran, K.B. 1991. Prosthetic heart valves. In *Blood Compatible Materials and Devices. Perspectives towards the 21st Century*, Sharma, C.P. and Szycher, M., Eds., Technomic, Lancaster, PA, 153–165.

DeVries, W.C. and Joyce, L.D. 1983. The artificial heart. *CIBA Clinical Symposia*, 35(6).

Drogue, J. and Villafana, M. 1997. ATS Medical open pivot™ valve. In *Surgery for Acquired Aortic Valve Disease*. Piwnica, A. and Westaby, S., Eds., ISIS Medical Media, Oxford, 410–416.

Farrar, D.J., Litwak, P., Lawson, J.H., Ward, R.S., White, K.A., Robinson, A.J., Rodvein, R., and Hill, J.D. 1988. *In vivo* evaluations of a new thromboresistant polyurethane for artificial heart blood pumps. *J. Thorac. Cardiovasc. Surg.* 95:191–200.

Gerring, E.L., Bellhouse, B.J., Bellhouse, F.H., and Haworth, F.H. 1974. Long term animal trials of the Oxford aortic/pulmonary valve prosthesis without anticoagulants. *Trans. ASAIO* 20:703–708.

Ghista, D.N. and Reul, H. 1977. Optimal prosthetic aortic leaflet valve: design, parametric and longevity analysis: development of the Avcothane-51 leaflet valve based on the optimal design analysis. *J. Biomech.* 10:313–324.

Guidoin, R. and Couture, J. 1991. Polyester prostheses: the outlook for the future. In *Blood Compatible Materials and Devices. Perspectives towards the 21st Century,* Sharma, C.P. and Szycher, M., Eds., Technomic, Lancaster, PA, 153–165.

Guidoin, R., Gosselin, C., Martin, L., Marios, M., Laroche, F., King, M., Gunasekara, K., Domurado, D., and Sigot-Luizard, M.F. 1983. Polyester prostheses as substitutes in the thoracic aorta of dogs. I. Evaluation of commercial prostheses. *J. Biomed. Mat. Res.* 17:1049–1077.

Hamid, M.S., Sabbah, H.N., and Stein, P.D. 1985. Finite element evaluation of stresses on closed leaflets of bioprosthetic heart valves with flexible stents. *Finite Elem. Analysis Des.* 1:213–225.

Harold, M., Lo, H.B., Reul, H., Muchter, H., Taguchi, K., Gierspien, M., Birkle, G., Hollweg, G., Rau, G., and Messmer, B.J. 1987. The Helmholtz Institute tri-leaflet polyurethane heart valve prosthesis: design, manufacturing, and first *in vitro* and *in vivo* results. In *Polyurethanes in Biomedical Engineering II.* Planck, H., Syre, I., and Dauner, M. Eds., Elsevier, Amsterdam, 321–356.

Holfert, J.W., Reibman, J.B., Dew, P.A., De Paulis, R., Burns, G.L., and Olsen, D.B. 1987. A new connector system for total artificial hearts: preliminary results. *Trans. ASAIO* 10:151–156.

Hufnagel, C.A. 1977. Reflections on the development of valvular prostheses. *Med. Instrum.* 11:74–76.

Hunter, G.C., Schmidt, S.P., Sharp, W.V. and Malindzak, G.S. 1983. Controlled flow studies in 4 mm endothelialized Dacron® grafts. *Trans. ASAIO* 29:177–182.

Jarvick, R.K. 1981. The total artificial heart. *Sci. Amer.,* 244:66–72.

Jarvis, P., Tarbell, J.M., and Frangos, J.A. 1991. An *in vitro* evaluation of an artificial heart. *Trans. ASAIO,* 37:27–32.

Kafesjian, R., Howanec, M., Ward, G.D., Diep, L., Wagstaff, L.S., and Rhee, R. 1994. Cavitation damage of pyrolytic carbon in mechanical heart valves. *J. Heart Valve Dis.* 3 (Suppl. 1):S 2–S 7.

Kambic, H.E. and Nose, Y. 1991. Biomaterials for blood pumps. In *Blood Compatible Materials and Devices. Perspectives towards the 21st Century,* Sharma, C.P. and Szycher, M., Eds., Technomic, Lancaster, PA, 141–151.

Keynton, R.S., Rittgers, S.E., and Shu, M.C.S. 1991. The effect of angle and flow rate upon hemodynamics in distal vascular graft anastomoses: an *in vitro* model study. *ASME J. Biomech. Eng.* 113:458–463.

Kim, S.H., Chandran, K.B., and Chen, C.J. 1992. Numerical simulation of steady flow in a two-dimensional total artificial heart model. *ASME J. Biomech. Eng.,* 114:497–503.

Kim, Y.H. and Chandran, K.B. 1993. Steady flow analysis in the vicinity of an end-to-end anastomosis. *Biorheology* 30:117–130.

Kim, Y.H., Chandran, K.B., Bower, T.J., and Corson, J.D. 1993. Flow dynamics across end-to-end vascular bypass graft anastomoses. *Ann. Biomed. Eng.* 21:311–320.

Lapeyre, D.M., Frazier, O.H., and Conger, J.L. 1994. *In vivo* evaluation of a trileaflet mechanical heart valve. *ASAIO J.* 40:M707–M713.

Lee, C.S. and Chandran, K.B. 1994. Instantaneous backflow through peripheral clearance of Medtronic Hall valve at the moment of closure. *Ann. Biomed. Eng.* 22:371–380.

Lee, C.S. and Chandran, K.B. 1995. Numerical simulation of instantaneous backflow through central clearance of bileaflet mechanical heart valves at the moment of closure: shear stress and pressure fields within the clearance. *Med. Biol. Eng. Comp.* 33:257–263.

Lee, C.S., Chandran, K.B., and Chen, L.D. 1994. Cavitation dynamics of mechanical heart valve prostheses. *Art. Org.* 18:758–767.

Lee, J.M. and Boughner, D.R. 1991. Bioprosthetic heart valves: tissue mechanics and implications for design. In *Blood Compatible Materials and Devices. Perspectives towards the 21st Century*, Sharma, C.P. and Szycher, M., Eds., Technomic, Lancaster, PA, 167–188.

Lefrak, E.A. and Starr, A., Eds. 1970. *Cardiac Valve Prostheses*. Appleton-Century-Crofts, New York.

Leuer, L. 1987. Dynamics of mechanical valves in the artificial heart. *Proc. 40th Annu. Conf. Eng. Med. Biol. (ACEMB)*, p. 82.

Marin, M.L., Veith, F.J., Panetta, T.F. et al. 1994. Transluminally placed endovascular stented graft repair for arterial trauma. *J. Vasc. Surg.* 20:466–473.

McKenna, J. 1997. The Ultracor™ prosthetic heart valve. In *Surgery for Acquired Aortic Valve Disease*. Piwnica, A. and Westaby, S., Eds., ISIS Medical Media, Oxford, 337–340.

Ojha, M., Ethier, C.R., Johnston, K.W., and Cobbold, R.S.C. 1990. Steady and pulsatile flow fields in an end-to-side arterial anastomosis model. *J. Vasc. Surg.* 12:747–753.

Park, J.B. and Lakes, R.S. 1992. *Biomaterials: An Introduction*. 2nd ed., Plenum Press, New York.

Parodi, J.C., Palmaz, J.C., and Barone, H.D., 1991. Transfemoral intraluminal graft implantation for abdominal aortic aneurysms. *Ann. Vasc. Surg.* 1991; 5:491–499.

Phillips, W.M., Brighton, J.A., and Pierce, W.S. 1979. Laser Doppler anemometer studies in unsteady ventricular flows. *Trans. ASAIO* 25:56–60.

Phillips, R.E. and Printz, L.K. 1997. PhotoFix™ α: a pericardial aortic prosthesis. In *Surgery for Acquired Aortic Valve Disease*. Piwnica, A. and Westaby, S., Eds., ISIS Medical Media, Oxford, 376–381.

Piwnica, A. and Westaby, S., Eds. 1997. *Surgery for Acquired Aortic Valve Disease*, ISIS Medical Media, Oxford.

Reif, T.H. 1991. A numerical analysis of the back flow between the leaflets of a St. Jude Medical cardiac valve prosthesis. *J. Biomech.* 24:733–741.

Reis, R.L., Hancock, W.D., Yarbrough, J.W., Glancy, D.L., and Morrow, A.G. 1971. The flexible stent. *J. Thorac. Cardiovasc. Surg.* 62:683–691.

Reul, H., Steinseifer, U., Knoch, M., and Rau, G. 1995. Development, manufacturing and validation of a single leaflet mechanical heart valve prosthesis. *J. Heart Valve Dis.* 4:513–519.

Rhee, K. and Tarbell, J.M. 1994. A study of wall shear rate distribution near the end-to-end anastomosis of a rigid graft and a compliant artery. *J. Biomech.* 27:329–338.

Rodgers, V.G.J., Teodori, M.F., and Borovetz, H.S. 1987. Experimental determination of mechanical shear stress about an anastomotic junction. *J. Biomech.* 20:795–803.

Roe, B.B., Owsley, J.W., and Boudoures, P.C. 1958. Experimental results with a prosthetic aortic valve. *J. Thorac. Cardiovasc. Surg.* 36:563–570.

Rosenberg, G. 1995. Artificial heart and circulatory assist devices. In *The Biomedical Engineering Handbook*. Bronzino, J.D., Ed., CRC Press, Boca Raton, FL, 1839–1846.

Rosenberg, G., Snyder, A. J., Weiss, W.J., Sapirstein, J.S., and Pierce, W.S. 1995. *In vivo* testing of a clinical-size totally implantable artificial heart. In *Assisted Circulation 4*, F. Unger, Ed., Springer-Verlag, Berlin, 235–248.

Russel, F.B., Lederman, D.M., Singh, P.I., Cumming, R.D., Levine, F.H., Austen, W.G., and Buckley, M.J. 1980. Development of seamless trileaflet valves. *Trans. ASAIO* 26:66–70.

Sabbah, H.N., Hamid, M.S., and Stein, P.D. 1985. Estimation of mechanical stresses on closed cusps of porcine bioprosthetic valves: effect of stiffening, focal calcium and focal thinning. *Am. J. Cardiol.* 55:1091–1097.

Shim, H.S. and Lenker, J.A. 1988. Heart valve prostheses. In *Encyclopedia of Medical Devices and Instrumentation*, Vol. 3, Webster, J.G., Ed., Wiley Interscience, New York, 1457–1474.

Strandness, D.E. and Sumner, D.S. 1975. Grafts and grafting. In *Hemodynamics for Surgeons*, Grune and Stratton, New York, 342–395.

Tarbell, J.M., Gunishan, J.P., Geselowitz, D.B., Rosenberg, G., Shung, K.K., and Pierce, W.S. 1986. Pulsed ultrasonic Doppler velocity measurements inside a left ventricular assist device. *ASME J. Biomech. Eng.* 108:232–238.

Thubrikar, M.J., Skinner, J.R., and Nolan, S.P. 1982a. Design and stress analysis of bioprosthetic valves *in vivo*. In *Cardiac Bioprostheses*, Cohn, L.H. and Gallucci, V., Eds., Yorke Medical Books, New York, 445–455.

Thubrikar, M.J., Skinner, J.R., Eppink, T.R., and Nolan, S.P. 1982b. Stress analysis of porcine bioprosthetic heart valves *in vivo*. *J. Biomed. Mat. Res.*, 16:811–826.

Unger, F. 1989. *Assisted Circulation*, Vol. 3, Springer-Verlag, Berlin.

Van der Lei, B., Wildevuur, C.R.H., Niewenhuis, P., Blaauw, E.H., Dijk, F., Hulstaert, C.E., and Molenaar, I. 1985. Regeneration of the arterial wall in microporous, compliant, biodegradable vascular grafts after implantation into the rat abdominal aorta. *Cell Tissue Res.* 242:569–578.

Van der Lei, B., Wildevuur, C.R.H., and Nieuwenhuis, P. 1986. Compliance and biodegradation of vascular grafts stimulate the regeneration of elastic laminae in neoarterial tissue: an experimental study in rats. *Surgery* 99:45–51.

Veith, F.J., Abbott, W.M., Yao, J.S.T. et al. 1995. Guidelines for development and use of transluminally placed endovascular prosthetic grafts in the arterial system. *J. Vasc. Surg.* 21:670–685.

Wieting, D.W. 1997. Prosthetic heart valves in the future. In *Surgery for Acquired Aortic Valve Disease*. Piwnica, A. and Westaby, S., Eds., ISIS Medical Media, Oxford, 460–478.

Wurzel, D., Kolff, J., Missfeldt, W., Wildevuur, W., Hansen, G., Brownstein, L., Reibman, J., De Paulis, R., and Kolff, W.J. 1988. Development of the Philadelphia heart system. *Art. Org.* 12:410–422.

Yoganathan, A.P., Corcoran, W.H., and Harrison, E.C. 1979a. *In vitro* velocity measurements in the vicinity of aortic prostheses. *J. Biomech.* 12:135–152.

Yoganathan, A.P., Corcoran, W.H., and Harrison, E.C. 1979b. Pressure drops across prosthetic aortic heart valves under steady and pulsatile flow—*in vitro* measurements. *J. Biomech.* 12:153–164.

Yoganathan, A.P., Woo, Y.R., and Sung, H.W. 1986. Turbulent shear stress measurements in the vicinity of aortic heart valve prostheses. *J. Biomech.* 19:433–442.

Yusef, S.W., Baker, D.M., Chuter, T.A.M. et al. 1994. Transfemoral endoluminal repair of abdominal aortic aneurysm with bifurcated graft. *Lancet* 344:650–1.

7.2   Non-Blood-Interfacing Implants for Soft Tissues

Karen J.L. Burg and S.W. Shalaby

Most tissues other than bone and cartilage are of the soft category. Implants do not generally interface directly with blood; the exceptions are located primarily in the cardiovascular systems. Non-blood-interfacing soft tissue implants are used to augment or replace natural tissues or to redirect specific biological functions. The implants can be transient; that is, of short-term function and thus made of absorbable materials, or they can be long-term implants which are expected to have prolonged functions and are made of nonabsorbable materials.

Toward the successful development of a new biomedical device or implant, including those used for soft tissues, the following milestones must be achieved: (1) acquire certain biologic and biomechanic data about the implant site and its function to aid in the selection of materials and engineering design of such an implant, to meet carefully developed product requirements; (2) construct a prototype and evaluate its physical and biologic properties both *in vitro* and *in vivo*, using the appropriate animal model; and (3) conduct a clinical study following a successful battery of animal safety studies depending on intended application and availability of historical safety and clinical data on the material or design. Extent of the studies associated with any specific milestone can vary considerably. Although different applications require different materials with specific properties, minimum requirements for soft-tissue implants should be met. The implant must (1) exhibit physical properties (e.g., flexibility and texture) which are equivalent or comparable to those called for in the product profile; (2) maintain the expected physical properties after implantation for a specific period; (3) elicit no adverse tissue reaction; (4) display no carcinogenic, toxic, allergenic, and/or immunogenic effect; and (5) achieve assured sterility without compromising the physicochemical properties. In addition to these criteria, a product of potentially broad applications is expected to (1) be easily mass produced at a reasonable cost; (2) have acceptable aesthetic quality; (3) be enclosed in durable, properly labeled, easy-access packaging; and (4) have adequate shelf stability.

The most common types of soft-tissue implants are (1) sutures and allied augmentation devices; (2) percutaneous and cutaneous systems; (3) maxillofacial devices; (4) ear and eye prostheses; (5) space-filling articles; and (6) fluid transfer devices.

Sutures and Allied Augmentation Devices

Sutures and staples are the most common types of augmentation devices. In recent years, interest in using tapes and adhesives has increased and may continue to do so, should new efficacious systems be developed.

Sutures and Suture Anchors

Sutures are usually packaged as a thread attached to a metallic needle. Although most needles are made of stainless steel alloys, the thread component can be made of various materials, and the type used determines the class of the entire suture. In fact, it is common to refer to the thread as the suture. Presently, most needles are drilled (mechanically or by laser) at one end for thread insertion. Securing the thread in the needle hole can be achieved by crimping or adhesive attachment. Among the critical physical properties of sutures are their diameter, *in vitro* knot strength, needle-holding strength, needle penetration force, ease of knotting, knot security, and *in vitro* strength retention profile.

Two types of threads are used in suture manufacturing and are distinguished according to the retention of their properties in the biologic environment, namely, absorbable and nonabsorbable. These may also be classified according to their source of raw materials, that is, natural (catgut, silk, and cotton), synthetic (nylon, polypropylene, polyethylene terephthalate, and polyglycolide and its copolymers), or metallic (stainless steel and tantalum). Sutures may also be classified according to their physical form, that is, monofilament and twisted or braided multifilament (or simply braids).

The first known suture, the absorbable catgut, is made primarily of collagen derived from sheep intestinal submucosa. It is usually treated with a chromic salt to increase its *in vivo* strength retention and through imparted crosslinking that retards absorption. Such treatment extends the functional performance of catgut suture from 1 to 2 weeks up to about 3 weeks. The catgut sutures are packaged in a specially formulated fluid to prevent drying and maintain necessary compliance for surgical handling and knot formation.

The use of synthetic absorbable sutures exceeded that of catgut over the past two decades. This is attributed to many factors including (1) higher initial breaking strength and superior handling characteristics; (2) availability of sutures with a broad range of *in vivo* strength retention profiles; (3) considerably milder tissue reactions and no immunogenic response; and (4) reproducible properties and highly predictable *in vivo* performance. Polyglycolide (PG) was the first synthetic absorbable suture to be introduced, about three decades ago. Because of the high modulus of oriented fibers, PG is made mostly in the braided form. A typical PG suture braid absorbs in about 4 months and retains partial *in vivo* strength after 3 weeks. However, braids made of the 90/10 glycolide/l-lactide copolymer have a comparable or improved strength retention profile and faster absorption rate relative to PG. The copolymeric sutures absorb in about 3 months and have gained wide acceptance by the surgical community.

As with other types of braided sutures, an absorbable coating which improves suture handling and knot formation has been added to the absorbable braids. To minimize the risk of infection and tissue drag that are sometimes associated with braided sutures, four types of monofilament sutures have been commercialized. The absorbable monofilaments were designed specifically to approach the engineering compliance of braided sutures, by combining appropriate materials to achieve low moduli, e.g., polydioxanone and copolymers of glycolide with caprolactone or trimethylene carbonate.

Members of the nonabsorbable family of sutures include braided silk (a natural protein), nylon, and polyethylene terephthalate (PET). These braids are used as coated sutures. Although silk sutures have retained wide acceptance by surgeons, nylon and particularly PET sutures are used for critical procedures where high strength and predictable long-term performance are required. Meanwhile, the use of cotton sutures is decreasing constantly because of their low strength and occasional tissue reactivity due to contaminants. Monofilaments are important forms of nonabsorbable sutures and are made primarily of polypropylene, nylon, and stainless steel. An interesting application of monofilament sutures is illustrated in the use of polypropylene loops (or haptics) for intraocular lenses. The polypropylene sutures exhibit not only the desirable properties of monofilaments but also the biologic inertness reflected in the minimal tissue reactions associated with their use in almost all surgical sites. With the exception of its natural tendency to undergo hydrolytic degradation and, hence, continued loss of mechanical strength postoperatively, nylon monofilament has similar attributes to those of polypropylene. Because of their exceptionally high modulus, stainless steel sutures are not used in soft-tissue repair because they can tear these tissues. All sutures can be sterilized by gamma radiation except those made of synthetic absorbable polymers, polypropylene, or cotton, which are sterilized by ethylene oxide.

Related to the suture is the tissue suture anchor, used to attach soft tissue to bone. The anchor is embedded into bone and the suture can be used to reattach the soft tissue. The most common anchor is polylactide-based and is used in shoulder repair.

Nonsuture Fibrous and Microporous Implants

Woven PET and polypropylene fabrics are commonly used as surgical meshes for abdominal wall repair and similar surgical procedures where surgical "patching" is required. Braid forms and similar construction made of multifilament PET yarns have been used for repairing tendons and ligaments. Microporous foams of polytetrafluoroethylene (PTFE) are used as pledgets (to aid in anchoring sutures to soft tissues) and in repair of tendons and ligaments. Microporous collagen-based foams are used in wound repair to accelerate healing.

Clips, Staples, and Pins

Ligating clips are most commonly used for temporary or long-term management of the flow in tubular tissues. Titanium clips are among the oldest and still-versatile types of clips. Thermoplastic polymers such as nylon can be injection-molded into different forms of ligating clips. These are normally designed to have a latch and living hinge. Absorbable polymers made of lactide/glycolide copolymers and polydioxanone have been successfully converted to ligating clips with different design features for a broad range of applications.

Metallic staples were introduced about three decades ago as strong competitors to sutures for wound augmentation; their use has grown considerably over the past 10 years for everything from skin closure procedures to a multiplicity of internal surgical applications. Major advantages associated with the use of staples are ease of application and minimized tissue trauma. Metallic staples can be made of tantalum, stainless steel, or titanium–nickel alloys. Staples are widely used to facilitate closure of large incisions produced in procedures such as Caesarean sections and intestinal surgery. Many interesting applications of small staples have been discovered for ophthalmic and endoscopic use, a fast-growing area of minimally invasive surgery.

Thermoplastic materials based on lactide/glycolide copolymers have been used to produce absorbable staples for skin and internal wound closures. These staples consist primarily of two interlocking components, a fastener and receiver. They are advantageous in that they provide a quick means of closure with comparable infection resistance. They are limited to locations which do not have large tensile loads and/or thicker or more sensitive tissue.

A new form of ligating device is the subcutaneous pin. This is designed with a unique applicator to introduce the pin parallel to the axis of the wound. During its application, the linear pin acquires a zig-zag-like configuration for stabilized tissue anchoring. The pins are made of lactide/glycolide polymers.

Surgical Tapes

Surgical tapes are intended to minimize necrosis, scar tissue formation, problems of stitch abscesses, and weakened tissues. The problems with surgical tapes are similar to those experienced with traditional skin tapes. These include (1) misaligned wound edges, (2) poor adhesion due to moisture or dirty wounds, and (3) late separation of tapes when hematoma or wound drainage occur.

Wound strength and scar formation in skin may depend on the type of incision made. If the subcutaneous muscles in the fatty tissue are cut and the overlying skin is closed with tape, then the muscles retract. This, in turn, increases the scar area, causing poor cosmetic appearance when compared to a suture closure. Tapes also have been used successfully for assembling scraps of donor skin for skin graft.

Tissue Adhesives

The constant call for tissue adhesives is particularly justified when dealing with the repair of exceptionally soft tissues. Such tissues cannot be easily approximated by sutures, because sutures inflict substantial mechanical damage following the traditional knotting scheme and associated shear stresses. However, the variable biological environments of soft tissues and their regenerative capacity make the development of an ideal tissue adhesive a difficult task. Experience indicates that an ideal tissue adhesive should (1) be able to wet and bond to tissues; (2) be capable of onsite formation by the rapid polymerization of a liquid monomer without producing excessive heat or toxic byproducts; (3) be absorbable; (4) not interfere with the normal healing process; and (5) be easily applied during surgery. The two common types of tissue adhesives currently used are based on alkyl-*o*-cyanoacrylates and fibrin. The latter is a natural adhesive derived from fibrinogen, which is one of the clotting components of blood. Although fibrin is used in Europe, its use in the U.S. has not been approved because of the risk of its contamination with hepatitis and/or immune disease viruses. Due to its limited mechanical strength (tensile strength and elastic modulus of 0.1 and 0.15 MPa, respectively), fibrin is used mostly as a sealant and for adjoining delicate tissues as in nerve anastomoses. Meanwhile, two members of the cyanoacrylate family of adhesives, *n*-butyl- and *iso*-butyl-cyano-acrylates, are used in a number of countries as sealants, adhesives, and blocking agents. They are yet to be approved for use in the U.S. because of the lack of sufficient safety data. Due to a fast rate of polymerization and some limited manageability in localizing the adhesive to the specific surgical site, the *in vivo* performance of cyanoacrylates can be unpredictable. Because of the low strength of the adhesive joints or sealant films produced on *in vivo* polymerization of these cyanoacrylates, their applications generally are limited to use in traumatized fragile tissues (such as spleen, liver, and kidney) and after extensive surgery on soft lung tissues. A major safety concern of these alkyl cyanoacrylates is related to their nonabsorbable nature. Hence, a number of investigators have directed their attention to certain alkoxy-alkyl cyanoacrylates which can be converted to polymeric adhesives with acceptable absorbable profiles and rheological properties. Methoxypropyl cyanoacrylate, for example, has demonstrated both the absorbability and high compliance that are advantageous to soft tissue repair.

Percutaneous and Skin Implants

The need for percutaneous (*trans* or through the skin) implants has been accelerated by the advent of artificial kidneys and hearts and the need for prolonged injection of drugs and nutrients. Artificial skin is urgently needed to maintain the body temperature and prevent infection in severely burned patients. Actual permanent replacement of skin by biomaterials is still a great clinical challenge.

Percutaneous Devices

The problem of obtaining a functional and viable interface between the tissue (skin) and an implant (percutaneous device) is primarily due to the following factors. First, although initial attachment of the tissue into the interstices of the implant surface occurs, attachment cannot be maintained for a sustained time since the dermal tissue cells turn over continuously. Downgrowth of epithelium around the implant or overgrowth on the implant leads to extrusion or invagination, respectively. Second, any opening near the implant that is large enough for bacteria to penetrate may result in infection, even though initially there may be a tight seal between skin and implant. Several factors are involved in the development of percutaneous devices:

1. Type of end use—this may deal with transmission of information (biopotentials, temperature, pressure, blood flow rate), energy (electrical stimulation, power for heart-assist devices), transfer of matter (cannula for blood), and load (attachment of a prosthesis);
2. Engineering factors—these may address materials selection (polymers, ceramics, metals, and composites), design variation (button, tube with and without skirt, porous or smooth surface), and mechanical stresses (soft and hard interface, porous or smooth interface);
3. Biologic factors—these are determined by the implant host (human, dog, hog, rabbit, sheep), and implant location (abdominal, dorsal, forearm);
4. Human factors—these can pertain to postsurgical care, implantation technique, and esthetic look.

No percutaneous devices are completely satisfactory. Nevertheless, some researchers believe that hydroxyapatite may be part of a successful approach. In one experimental trial, a hydroxyapatite-based percutaneous device was associated with less epidermal downgrowth (1 mm after 17 months vs. 4.6 mm after 3 months) when compared with a silicone rubber control specimen in the dorsal skin of canines. Researchers have also investigated coatings such as laminin-5 which has been shown to enhance epithelial attachment.

Artificial Skins

Artificial skin is another example of a percutaneous implant, and the problems are similar to those described above. Important for this application is a material which can adhere to a large (burned) surface and thus prevent the loss of fluids, electrolytes, and other biomolecules until the wound has healed.

In one study on wound-covering materials with controlled physicochemical properties, an artificial skin was designed with a crosslinked collagen-polysaccharide (chondroitin 6-sulfate) composite membrane. This was specifically chosen to have controlled porosity (5–150 μm in diameter), flexibility (by varying crosslink density), and moisture flux rate.

Several polymeric materials and reconstituted collagen have also been examined as burn dressings. Among the synthetic ones are the copolymers of vinyl chloride and vinyl acetate as well as polymethyl cyanoacrylate (applied as a fast-polymerizing monomer). The latter polymer and/or its monomer were found to be too brittle and histotoxic for use as a burn dressing. The ingrowth of tissue into the pores of polyvinyl alcohol sponges and woven fabric (nylon and silicone rubber velour) was also attempted without much success. Nylon mesh bonded to a silicone rubber membrane, another design attempt, prevented water evaporation but has not been found to induce fibrovascular growth.

Rapid epithelial layer growth by culturing cells *in vitro* from the skin of the burn patient for covering the wound area may offer a practical solution for less severely burned patients. Implantation of an allogenic fibroblast/polymer construct has proven useful for providing long-term skin replacement. Related to this, temporary tissue engineered replacements are possible alternatives for burns requiring larger area coverage. These can be similar to the synthetic dressing, a nylon mesh and silicone rubber component, but incorporates allogeneic fibroblasts. This temporary covering hopefully will stimulate or allow fibrovascular growth into the wound bed by providing the appropriate matrix proteins and growth factors.

Maxillofacial Implants

There are two types of maxillofacial implants: extraoral and intraoral. The former deals with the use of artificial substitutes for reconstructing defective regions in the maxilla, mandible, and face. Useful polymeric materials for extraoral implants require: (1) match of color and texture with those of the patient; (2) mechanical and chemical stability (i.e., material should not creep or change color or irritate skin); and (3) ease of fabrication. Copolymers of vinyl chloride and vinyl acetate (with 5 to 20% acetate), polymethyl methacrylate, silicones, and polyurethane rubbers are currently used. Intraoral implants are used for repairing maxilla, mandibular, and facial bone defects. Material requirements for the intraoral implants are similar to those of the extraoral ones. For the latter group of implants, metallic materials such as tantalum, titanium, and Co–Cr alloys are commonly used. For soft tissues, such as gum and chin, polymers such as silicone rubber and polymethylmethacrylate are used for augmentation.

Ear and Eye Implants

Implants can be used to restore conductive hearing loss from otosclerosis (a hereditary defect which involves a change in the bony tissue of the ear) and chronic otitis media (the inflammation of the middle ear which can cause partial or complete impairment of the ossicular chain). A number of prostheses are available for correcting these defects. The porous polyethylene total ossicular implant is used to achieve a firm fixation by tissue ingrowth. The tilt-top implant is designed to retard tissue ingrowth into the section of the shaft which may diminish sound conduction. Materials used in fabricating these implants include polymethyl methacrylate, polytetrafluoroethylene, polyethylene, silicone rubber, stainless steel, and tantalum. More recently, polytetrafluoroethylene-carbon composites, porous polyethylene, and pyrolytic carbon have been described as suitable materials for cochlear (inner ear) implants.

Artificial ear implants capable of processing speech have been developed with electrodes to stimulate cochlear nerve cells. Cochlear implants also have a speech processor that transforms sound waves into electrical impulses that can be conducted through coupled external and internal coils. The electrical impulses can be transmitted directly by means of a percutaneous device.

Eye implants are used to restore the functionality of damaged or diseased corneas and lenses. Usually the cornea is transplanted from a suitable donor. In cataracts, eye lenses become cloudy and can be removed surgically. Intraocular lenses (IOL) are implanted surgically to replace the original eye lens and to restore function. IOL are made from transparent acrylics, particularly polymethyl methacrylate, which has excellent optical properties. Infection and fixation of the lens to the tissues are frequent concerns, and a number of measures are being used to address them. Transplantation of retinal pigmented epithelium can be used in the treatment of adult onset blindness; the challenge is developing readily detachable or absorbable materials on which to culture sheets of these cells.

Space-Filling Implants

Breast implants are common space-filling implants. At one time, the enlargement of breasts was done with various materials such as paraffin wax and silicone fluids, by direct injection or by enclosure in a rubber balloon. Several problems have been associated with directly injected implants, including progressive instability and ultimate loss of original shape and texture as well as infection and pain. One of the early efforts in breast augmentation was to implant a sponge made of polyvinyl alcohol. However, soft tissues grew into the pores and then calcified with time, and the so-called marble breast resulted. Although the enlargement or replacement of breasts for cosmetic reasons alone is not recommended, prostheses have been developed for patients who have undergone radical mastectomy or who have nonsymmetrical deformities. The development of the tissue-engineered breast is ongoing, where fat or normal breast tissue may be derived from the patient and combined with an absorbable scaffold for transplantation. A silicone rubber bag filled with silicone gel and backed with polyester mesh to permit tissue ingrowth for fixation is a widely used prosthesis, primarily for psychological reasons. The artificial penis, testicles, and vagina fall into the same category as breast implants, in that they make use of silicones and are implanted for psychological reasons rather than to improve physical health.

Fluid-Transfer Implants

Fluid transfer implants are required for cases such as hydrocephalus, urinary incontinence, glaucoma-related elevated intraocular pressure, and chronic ear infection. Hydrocephalus, caused by abnormally high pressure of the cerebrospinal fluid in the brain, can be treated by draining the fluid (essentially an ultrafiltrate of blood) through a cannula. Earlier shunts had two one-way valves at either end. However, the more recent Ames shunt has simple slits at the discharging end, which opens when enough fluid pressure is exerted. The Ames shunt empties the fluid in the peritoneum while others drain into the blood stream through the right internal jugular vein or right atrium of the heart. The simpler peritoneal shunt shows less incidence of infection.

The use of implants for correcting the urinary system has not been successful because of the difficulty of adjoining a prosthesis to the living system for achieving fluid tightness. In addition, blockage of the passage by deposits from urine (salt, for example) and constant danger of infection are major concerns. Several materials have been used for producing these implants, with limited long-term success; these include Dacron™, glass, polyvinyl alcohol, polyethylene, rubber, silver, tantalum, Teflon™, and Vitallium™. Tissue engineered devices also have application in urinary repair; for example, an alginate-chondrocyte system has been used clinically to treat vesicoureteral reflux. Preliminary results suggest that by transplanting the hydrogel system as a bulking agent below a refluxing ureter, neocartilage gradually develops to correct the reflux. Uroepithelial cells, combined with porous, absorbable polyester matrices show promise in the replacement of urologic tissues.

Drainage tubes, which are impermanent implants for chronic ear infection, can be made from poly-tetrafluoroethylene (Teflon™). Glaucoma-related elevated intraocular pressure may be relieved by implanting a tube connecting the anterior eye chamber to the external subconjunctival space in order to direct aqueous humor. Complications can arise with occlusion of the tube due to wound healing processes; however, researchers are investigating combining this device with an absorbable drug delivery plug to regulate flow and deliver drugs to regulate the wound healing process.

Technologies of Emerging Interest

A new process for uniaxial solid-state orientation, using a range of compressive forces and temperatures, has been developed to produce stock sheets of polyether-ether ketone (PEEK) for machining dental implants with substantially increased strength and modulus as compared to their unoriented counterparts.

Surface treatment of materials is another emerging interest, a process potentially influencing surface charge, topography, and conductivity. The former has obvious effects on cell adhesion and integration of traditional implants with surrounding tissues, and it has a profound effect on the success or failure of a tissue-engineered device.

Pertinent to the effect of surface chemistry and texture on tissue regeneration/ingrowth, recent studies on surface-phosphonylation to create hydroxyapatite-like substrates show that (1) surface-microtextured polypropylene and polyethylene transcortical implants in goat tibia having phosphonate functionalities (with or without immobilized calcium ions) do induce bone ingrowth, and (2) microtexture and surface phosphonylated (with and without immobilized calcium ions) rods made of PEEK and similarly treated rods of carbon fiber-reinforced PEEK induce bone ingrowth when implanted in the toothless region of the lower jaw of goats. The use of surface-phosphonylated and post-treated (with a bridging agent) UHMW-PE fibers and fabric do produce high strength and modulus composites at exceptionally low filler loading. Among these composites are those based on methyl methacrylate matrices, similar to those used in bone cement.

Conductivity manipulation may be extremely useful in such areas as biosensor design. Surface-conducting phosphonylated, ultra-high-molecular-weight polyethylene may be formed by exposure to aqueous pyrole solution. Preliminary results suggest that this is a stable process, yielding no apparent cytotoxic effects due to the material or leachables. New surface treatments will be instrumental in the development of the two rapidly expanding areas of biosensor design and tissue engineering, both areas which encompass non-blood-interfacing soft tissue implants.

Further Information

Allan, J., 1993. The molecular binding of inherently conducting polymers to thermoplastic substrates. M.S. thesis, Clemson University, Clemson, SC.

Allan, J.M., Wrana, J.S., Dooley, R.L., Budsberg, S., and Shalaby, S.W., 1999. Bone ingrowth into surface-phosphonylated polyethylene and polypropylene. *Trans. Soc. Biomat.* 468.

Allan, J.M., Wrana, J.S., Linden, D.E., Dooley, R.L., Farris, H., Budsberg, S., and Shalaby, S.W., 1999. Osseointegration of morphologically and chemically modified polymeric dental implants. *Trans. Soc. Biomater.* 37.

Allan, J.M., Kline, J.D., Wrana, J.S., Flagle, J.A., Corbett, J.T., and Shalaby, S.W., 1999. Absorbable gel-forming sealant/adhesives as a staple adjuvant in wound repair. *Trans. Soc. Biomater.* 374.

Chvapil, M., 1982. Considerations on manufacturing principles of a synthetic burn dressing: a review. *J. Biomed. Mater. Res.* 16:245.

Deng, M., Allan, J.M., Lake, R.A., Gerdes, G.A. and Shalaby, S.W., 1999. Effect of phosphonylation on UHMW-PE fabric-reinforced composites. *Trans. Soc. Biomater.* 470.

Deng, M., Wrana, J.S., Allan, J.M., and Shalaby, S.W., 1999. Tailoring mechanical properties of polyether-ether ketone for implants using solid-state orientation, *Trans. Soc. Biomater.* 477.

El-Ghannam, A., Starr, L., and Jones, J. 1998. Laminin-5 coating enhances epithelial cell attachment, spreading, and hemidesmosome assembly on Ti-6Al-4V implant material *in vitro*. *J. Biomed. Mater. Res.* 41:30.

Gantz, B.J., 1987. Cochlear implants: an overview. *Acta Otolaryng. Head Neck Surg.* 1:171.

Holder, W.D., Jr., Gruber, H.E., Moore, A.L., Culberson, C.R., Anderson, W., Burg, K.J.L., and Mooney, D.J. 1998. Cellular ingrowth and thickness changes in poly-l-lactide and polyglycolide matrices implanted subcutaneously in the rat. *J. Biomed. Mater. Res.* 41:412-421.

Kablitz, C., Kessler, T., Dew, P.A. et al., 1979. Subcutaneous peritoneal catheter: 1 1/2-years experience. *Artif. Org.* 3:210.

Lanza, R.P., Langer, R., and Chick, W.L., Eds., 1997. *Principles of Tissue Engineering,* Academic Press, San Diego, CA.

Lynch, W., 1982. *Implants: Reconstructing the Human Body.* Van Nostrand-Reinhold, New York.

Park, J.B. and Lakes, R.S., 1992. *Biomaterials Science and Engineering,* 2nd ed., Plenum Press, New York.

Postlethwait, R.W., Schaube, J.F., and Dillan, M.L. et al., 1959. An evaluation of surgical suture material. *Surg. Gyn. Obstet.* 108:555.

Shalaby, S.W., 1985. Fibrous materials for biomedical applications. In Lewin, M. and Preston, J., Eds., *High Technology Fibers: Part A,* Marcel Dekker, New York.

Shalaby, S.W., 1988. Bioabsorbable polymers. In Boylan, J.C. and Swarbrick, J., Eds., *Encyclopedia of Pharmaceutical Technology,* Vol. 1, Marcel Dekker, New York.

Shalaby, S.W., Ed., 1994. *Biomedical Polymers: Designed-To-Degrade Systems,* Hanser, New York.

Shall, L.M. and Cawley, P.W., 1994. Soft tissue reconstruction in the shoulder. Comparison of suture anchors, absorbable staples, and absorbable tacks. *Amer. J. Sports Med.* 22:715.

VonRecum, A.G. and Park, J.B., 1979. Percutaneous devices. *Crit. Rev. Bioeng.* 5:37.

Yannas, I.V. and Burke, I.F., 1980. Design of an artificial skin: l. Basic design principles. *J. Biomed. Mater. Res.* 14:107.

8

Hard Tissue Replacements

Sang-Hyun Park
University of California, Los Angeles

Adolfo Llinás
Pontificia Universidad Javeriana

Vijay K. Goel
University of Toledo

John C. Keller
University of Iowa

8.1 Bone Repair and Joint Implants

Sang-Hyun Park, Adolfo Llinás, and Vijay K. Goel

The use of biomaterials to restore the function of traumatized or degenerated connective tissues and thus improve the quality of life of a patient has become widespread. In the past, implants were designed with insufficient cognizance of biomechanics. Accordingly, the clinical results were not very encouraging. An upsurge of research activities into the mechanics of joints and biomaterials has resulted in better designs with better *in vivo* performance. The improving long-term success of total joint replacements for the lower limb is testimony to this. As a result, researchers and surgeons have developed and used fixation devices for the joints, including artificial spine discs. A large number of devices are also available for the repair of the bone tissue. This chapter provides an overview of the contemporary scientific work related to the use of biomaterials for the repair of bone (e.g., fracture) and joint replacements ranging from a hip joint to a spine.

Long Bone Repair

The principal functions of the skeleton are to provide a frame to support the organ-systems, and to determine the direction and range of body movements. Bone provides an anchoring point (insertion) for most skeletal muscles and ligaments. When the muscles contract, long bones act as levers, with the joints functioning as pivots, to cause body movement.

Bone is the only tissue able to undergo spontaneous regeneration and to remodel its micro- and macro-structure. This is accomplished through a delicate balance between an *osteogenic* (bone forming) and *osteoclastic* (bone removing) process [Brighton, 1984]. Bone can adapt to a new mechanical environment by changing the equilibrium between osteogenesis and osteoclasis. These processes will respond to changes in the static and dynamic stress applied to bone; that is, if more stress than the physiological is applied, the equilibrium tilts toward more osteogenic activity. Conversely, if less stress is applied the equilibrium tilts toward osteoclastic activity (this is known as Wolff's law of bone remodeling) [Wolff, 1986].

Nature provides different types of mechanisms to repair fractures in order to be able to cope with different mechanical environments about a fracture [Hulth, 1989; Schenk,1992]. For example, incomplete fractures (cracks), which only allow micromotion between the fracture fragments, heal with a small amount of fracture-line *callus*, known as *primary healing*. In contrast, complete fractures which are unstable, and therefore generate macromotion, heal with a voluminous callus stemming from the sides of the bone, known as *secondary healing* [Hulth, 1989; Brighton, 1984].

The goals of fracture treatment are obtaining rapid healing, restoring function, and preserving cosmesis without general or local complications. Implicit in the selection of the treatment method is the need to avoid potentially deleterious conditions, for example, the presence of excessive motion between bone fragments which may delay or prevent fracture healing [Brand and Rubin, 1987; Brighton, 1984].

Each fracture pattern and location results in a unique combination of characteristics ("fracture personality") that require specific treatment methods. The treatments can be non-surgical or surgical. Examples of non-surgical treatments are immobilization with casting (plaster or resin) and bracing with a plastic apparatus. The surgical treatments are divided into external fracture fixation, which does not require opening the fracture site, or internal fracture fixation, which requires opening the fracture.

With external fracture fixation, the bone fragments are held in alignment by pins placed through the skin onto the skeleton, structurally supported by external bars. With internal fracture fixation, the bone fragments are held by wires, screws, plates, and/or intramedullary devices. Figures 8.1a and b show radiographs of externally and internally fixed fractures.

All the internal fixation devices should meet the general requirement of biomaterials, that is, biocompatability, sufficient strength within dimensional constraints, and corrosion resistance. In addition, the device should also provide a suitable mechanical environment for fracture healing. From this perspective, stainless steel, cobalt-chrome alloys, and titanium alloys are most suitable for internal fixation. Detailed mechanical properties of the metallic alloys are discussed in the chapter on metallic biomaterials. Most internal fixation devices persist in the body after the fracture has healed, often causing discomfort and requiring removal. Recently, biodegradable polymers, e.g., polylactic acid (PLA) and polyglycolic acid (PGA), have been used to treat minimally loaded fractures, thereby eliminating the need for a second surgery for implant removal. A summary of the basic application of biomaterials in internal fixation is presented in Table 8.1. A description of the principal failure modes of internal fixation devices is presented in Table 8.2.

Wires

Surgical wires are used to reattach large fragments of bone, like the greater trochanter, which is often detached during total hip replacement. They are also used to provide additional stability in long-oblique or spiral fractures of long bones which have already been stabilized by other means (Fig. 8.1b). Similar approaches, based on the use of wires, have been employed to restore stability in the lower cervical spine region and in the lumbar segment as well (Fig. 8.1c).

Twisting and knotting is unavoidable when fastening wires to bone; however, by doing so, the strength of the wire can be reduced by 25% or more due to stress concentration [Tencer et al., 1993]. This can be partially overcome by using a thicker wire, since its strength increases directly proportional to its diameter. The deformed regions of the wire are more prone to corrosion than the un-deformed because of the higher strain energy. To decrease this problem and ease handling, most wires are annealed to increase the ductility.

Braided multistrain (multifilament) wire is an attractive alternative because it has a similar tensile strength than a monofilament wire of equal diameter, but more flexibility and higher fatigue strength [Taitsman and Saha, 1977]. However, bone often grows into the grooves of the braided multistrain wire, making it exceedingly difficult to remove, since it prevents the wire from sliding when pulled. When a wire is used with other metallic implants, the metal alloys should be matched to prevent galvanic corrosion [Park and Lakes, 1992].

FIGURE 8.1 Radiographs of (a) tibial fracture fixed with four pins and an external bar; (b) a total hip joint replacement in a patient who sustained a femoral fracture and was treated with double bone plates, screws, and surgical wire (arrows); (c) application of wires, screws, and plates in the spine.

TABLE 8.1 Biomaterials Applications in Internal Fixation

Material	Properties	Application
Stainless steel	Low cost, easy fabrication	Surgical wire (annealed)
		Pin, plate, screw
		IM nail
Ti alloy	High cost	Surgical wire
	Low density and modulus	Plate, screws, IM nails
	Excellent bony contact	
Co–Cr alloys (wrought)	High cost	Surgical wire
	High density and modulus	IM nails
	Difficult fabrication	
Polylactic acid	Resorbable	Pin, screw
Polyglycolic acid	Weak strength	
Nylon	Non-resorbable plastic	Cerclage band

TABLE 8.2 Failure Modes of Internal Fixation Devices

Failure Mode	Failure Location	Reasons for Failure
Overload	Bone fracture site	Small size implant
	Implant screw hole	Unstable reduction
	Screw thread	Early weight bearing
Fatigue	Bone fracture site	Early weight bearing
	Implant screw hole	Small size implant
	Screw thread	Unstable reduction
		Fracture non-union
Corrosion	Screw head-plate hole	Different alloy implants
	Bent area	Over-tightening screw
		Misalignment of screw
		Over-bent
Loosening	Screw	Motion
		Wrong choice of screw type
		Osteoporotic bone

Pins

Straight wires are called Steinmann pins; however, if the pin diameter is less than 2.38 mm, it is called Kirschner wire. They are widely used primarily to hold fragments of bones together provisionally or permanently and to guide large screws during insertion. To facilitate implantation, the pins have different tip designs which have been optimized for different types of bone (Fig. 8.2). The trochar tip is the most efficient in cutting; hence, it is often used for cortical bone.

The holding power of the pin comes from elastic deformation of surrounding bone. In order to increase the holding power to bone, threaded pins are used. Most pins are made of 316L stainless steel; however, biodegradable pins made of polylactic or polyglycolic acid have been employed for the treatment of minimally loaded fractures.

The pins can be used as part of elaborate frames designed for external fracture fixation (Fig. 8.1a). In this application, several pins are placed above and below the fracture, but away from it. After the fracture fragments are manually approximated (reduced) to resemble the intact bone, the pins are attached to various bars, which upon assembly will provide stability to the fracture.

Screws

Screws are the most widely used devices for fixation of bone fragments. There are two types of bone screws: (1) cortical bone screws, which have small threads, and (2) cancellous screws, which have large threads to get more thread-to-bone contact. They may have either V or buttress threads (Fig. 8.3). The cortical screws are subclassified further according to their ability to penetrate, into self-tapping and

FIGURE 8.2 Types of metallic pin tip: (a) trochar end, and (b) diamond end.

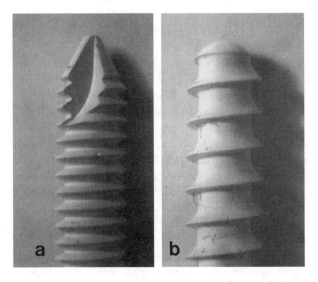

FIGURE 8.3 Bone screws: (a) a self-tapping V-threaded (has a cutting flute), and (b) a non-self-tapping, buttress threaded screw.

non-self-tapping (Fig. 8.3). The self-tapping screws have cutting flutes which thread the pilot drill-hole during insertion. In contrast, the non-self-tapping screws require a tapped pilot drill hole for insertion.

The holding power of screws can be affected by the size of the pilot drill hole, the depth of screw engagement, the outside diameter of the screw, and quality of the bone [Cochran, 1982; DeCoster et al., 1990].

Therefore, the selection of the screw type should be based on the assessment of the quality of the bone at the time of insertion. Under identical conditions, self-tapping screws provide a slightly greater holding power than non-self-tapping screws [Tencer et al., 1993].

Screw pullout strength varies with time after insertion *in vivo*, and it depends on the growth of bone into the screw threads and/or resorption of the surrounding bone [Schatzker et al., 1975]. The bone immediately adjacent to the screw often undergoes *necrosis* initially, but if the screw is firmly fixed, when the bone revascularizes, permanent secure fixation may be achieved. This is particularly true for titanium alloy screws or screws with a roughened thread surface, with which bone ongrowth results in an increase in removal torque [Hutzschenreuter and Brümmer, 1980]. When the screw is subject to micro- or macro-movement, the contacting bone is replaced by a membrane of fibrous tissue, the purchase is diminished, and the screw loosens.

The two principal applications of bone screws are (1) as interfragmentary fixation devices to "lag" or fasten bone fragments together, or (2) to attach a metallic plate to bone. Interfragmentary fixation is used in most fractures involving cancellous bone and in those oblique fractures in cortical bone. In order to lag the fracture fragments, the head of the screw must engage the cortex on the side of insertion without gripping the bone, while the threads engage cancellous bone and/or the cortex on the opposing side. When screws are employed for bone plate fixation, the bone screw threads must engage both cortices. Screws are also used for the fixation of spine fractures (for plate fixation or compression of bone fragment; Fig. 8.1c).

Plates

Plates are available in a wide variety of shapes and are intended to facilitate fixation of bone fragments. They range from the very rigid, intended to produce primary bone healing, to the relatively flexible, intended to facilitate physiological loading of bone.

The rigidity and strength of a plate in bending depend on the cross-sectional shape (mostly thickness) and material of which it is made. Consequently, the weakest region in the plate is the screw hole, especially if the screw hole is left empty, due to a reduction of the cross-sectional area in this region. The effect of the material on the rigidity of the plate is defined by the elastic modulus of the material for bending, and by the shear modulus for twisting [Cochran, 1982]. Thus, given the same dimensions, a titanium alloy plate will be less rigid than a stainless steel plate, since the elastic modulus of each alloy is 110 GPa and 200 GPa, respectively.

Stiff plates often shield the underlying bone from the physiological loads necessary for its healthful existence [O'Slullivan et al., 1989; Perren et al., 1988]. Similarly, flat plates closely applied to the bone prevent blood vessels from nourishing the outer layers of the bone [Perren, 1988]. For these reasons, the current clinical trend is to use more flexible plates (titanium alloy) to allow micromotion, and low-contact plates (only a small surface of the plate contacts the bone, LCP) to allow restoration of vascularity to the bone [Uhthoff and Finnegan, 1984; Claes, 1989]. The underlying goals of this philosophical change are to increase the fracture healing rate, to decrease the loss of bone mass in the region shielded by the plate, and consequently to decrease the incidence of re-fractures which occur following plate removal.

The interaction between bone and plate is extremely important since the two are combined into a composite structure. The stability of the plate-bone composite and the service life of the plate depends upon accurate fracture reduction. The plate is most resistant in tension; therefore, in fractures of long bones, the plate is placed along the side of the bone which is typically loaded in tension. Having excellent apposition of the bone fragments, as well as developing adequate compression between them, is critical in maintaining the stability of the fixation and preventing the plate from repetitive bending and fatigue failure. Interfragmentary compression also creates friction at the fracture surface, increasing resistance to torsional loads [Perren, 1991; Tencer et al., 1993]. On the contrary, too much compression causes micro fractures and necrosis of contacting bone due to the collapse of vesicular canals.

Compression between the fracture fragments can be achieved with a special type of plate called a *dynamic compression plate* (DCP). The dynamic compression plate has elliptic shape screw holes with

FIGURE 8.4   Principle of a dynamic compression plate for fracture fixation. During tightening a screw, the screw head slides down on a ramp in a plate screw hole which results in pushing the plate away from a fracture end and compressing the bone fragments together.

its long axis oriented parallel to that of the plate. The screw hole has a sliding ramp to the long axis of the plate. Figure 8.4 explains the principle of the dynamic compression plate.

Bone plates are often contoured in the operating room in order to conform to an irregular bone shape to achieve maximum contact of the fracture fragments. However, excessive bending decreases the service life of the plate. The most common failure modes of a bone plate-screw fixation are screw loosening and plate failure. The latter typically occurs through a screw hole due to fatigue and/or crevice corrosion [Weinstein et al., 1979].

In the vicinity of the joints, where the diameter of long bones is wider, the cortex thinner, and cancellous bone abundant, plates are often used as a buttress or retaining wall. A buttress plate applies force to the bone perpendicular to the surface of the plate, and prevents shearing or sliding at the fracture site. Buttress plates are designed to fit specific anatomic locations and often incorporate other methods of fixation besides cortical or cancellous screws, for example, a large lag screw or an I-beam. For the fusion of vertebral bodies following diskectomy, spinal plates are used along with bone grafts. These plates are secured to the vertebral bodies using screws (Fig. 8.1c). Similar approaches have been employed to restore stability in the thoracolumbar and cervical spine region as well. Figure 8.5 illustrates a variety of types of bone plates.

Intramedullary Nails

Intramedullary devices (IM nails) are used as internal struts to stabilize long bone fractures. IM nails are also used for fixation of femoral neck or intertrochanteric bone fractures; however, this application requires the addition of long screws. A gamut of designs are available, going from solid to cylindrical, with shapes such as cloverleaf, diamond, and "C" (slotted cylinders). Figure 8.6 shows a variety of intramedullary devices.

Compared to plates, IM nails are better positioned to resist multi-directional bending than a plate or an external fixator, since they are located in the center of the bone. However, their torsional resistance is less than that of the plate [Cochran, 1982]. Therefore, when designing or selecting an IM nail, a high polar moment of inertia is desirable to improve torsional rigidity and strength. The torsional rigidity is proportional to the elastic modulus and the moment of inertia. For nails with a circular cross-section, torsional stiffness is proportional to the fourth power of the nail's radius. The wall thickness of the nail also affects the stiffness. A slotted, open section nail is more flexible in torsion and bending, and it allows easy insertion into a curved medullary canal for example, that of the femur [Tencer, 1993]. However, in bending, a slot is asymmetrical with respect to rigidity and strength. For example, a slotted nail is strongest when bending is applied so that the slot is near the neutral plane; the nail is weakest when oriented so that the slot is under tension.

In addition to the need to resist bending and torsion, it is vital for an IM nail to have a large contact area with the internal cortex of the bone to permit torsional loads to be transmitted and resisted by shear stress. Two different concepts are used to develop shear stress: (1) a three-point, high pressure contact, achieved with the insertion of curved pins; and (2) a positive interlocking between the nail and intra-medullary canal, to produce a unified structure. Positive interlocking can be enhanced by reaming the

FIGURE 8.5 Bone plates: (a) dynamic compression plate, (b) hybrid compression plate (lower part has dynamic compression screw holes), (c) reconstruction bone plate (easy contouring), (d) buttress bone plate, (e) L-shaped buttress plate, (f) nail plate (for condylar fracture), and (g) dynamic compression hip screw.

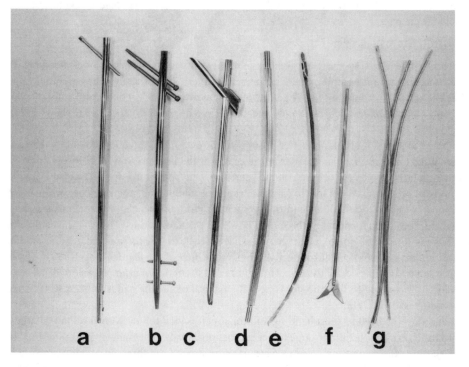

FIGURE 8.6 Intramedullary devices: (a) Gross–Kempf (slotted), (b) Uniflex (Ti alloy, slotted), (c) Kuntscher, (d) Samson, (e) Harris, (f) Brooker–Wills distal locking pin, and (g) Enders pins.

intramedullary canal. Reaming permits a larger, longer, nail-bone contact area and allows the use of a larger nail, with increased rigidity and strength [Kessler et al., 1986].

The addition of screws through the bone and nail, proximal and distal to the fracture, known as *interlocking*, increases torsional stability and prevents shortening of the bone, especially in unstable fractures [Perren, 1989]. The IM nail which has not been interlocked allows interfragmentary compressive force due to its low resistance to axial load. Another advantage of IM nails is that they do not require opening the fracture site, since they can be inserted through a small skin incision, typically located in one extreme of the bone. The insertion of an intramedullary nail, especially those that require reaming of the medullary canal, destroys the intramedullary vessels which supply two thirds of the cortex. However, this is not of clinical significance because revascularization occurs rapidly [Kessler et al., 1986; O'Slullivan et al., 1989].

Joint Replacements

Our ability to replace damaged joints with prosthetic implants has brought relief to millions of patients who would otherwise have been severely limited in their most basic activities and doomed to a life in pain. It is estimated that about 16 million people in the U.S. are affected by osteoarthritis, one of the various conditions that may cause joint degeneration and may lead a patient to a total joint replacement.

Joint degeneration is the end-stage of a process of destruction of the articular cartilage, which results in severe pain, loss of motion, and occasionally, an angular deformity of the extremity [Buckwalter et al., 1993]. Unlike bone, cartilage has a very limited capacity for repair [Salter, 1989]. Therefore, when exposed to a severe mechanical, chemical, or metabolic injury, the damage is permanent and often progressive.

Under normal conditions, the functions of cartilage are to provide a congruent articulation between bones, to transmit load across the joint, and to allow low-friction movements between opposing joint surfaces. The sophisticated way in which these functions are performed becomes evident from some of the mechanical characteristics of normal cartilage. For example, due to the leverage geometry of the muscles and the dynamic nature of human activity, the cartilage of the hip is exposed to about eight times body weight during fast walking [Paul, 1976]. Over a period of 10 years, an active person may subject the cartilage of the hip to more than 17 million weight bearing cycles [Jeffery, 1994]. From the point of view of the optimal lubrication provided by synovial fluid, cartilage's extremely low frictional resistance makes it 15 times easier to move opposing joint surfaces than to move an ice-skate on ice [Mow and Hayes, 1991; Jeffery, 1994].

Cartilage functions as a unit with subchondral bone, which contributes to shock absorption by undergoing viscoelastic deformation of its fine trabecular structure. Although some joints, like the hip, are intrinsically stable by virtue of their shape, the majority require an elaborate combination of ligaments, meniscus, tendons, and muscles for stability. Because of the large multidirectional forces that pass through the joint, its stability is a dynamic process. Receptors within the ligaments fire when stretched during motion, producing an integrated muscular contraction that provides stability for that specific displacement. Therefore, the ligaments are not passive joint restraints as once believed. The extreme complexity and high level of performance of biologic joints determine the standard to be met by artificial implants.

Total joint replacements are permanent implants, unlike those used to treat fractures, and the extensive bone and cartilage removed during implantation make this procedure irreversible. Therefore, when faced with prosthesis failure and the impossibility to reimplant, the patient will face severe shortening of the extremity, instability or total rigidity of the joint, and difficulty in ambulation and often will be confined to a wheel chair.

The design of an implant for joint replacement should be based on the kinematics and dynamic load transfer characteristic of the joint. The material properties, shape, and methods used for fixation of the implant to the patient determine the load transfer characteristics. This is one of the most important elements that determines long-term survival of the implant, since bone responds to changes in load transfer with a remodeling process, mentioned earlier as Wolff's law. Overloading the implant–bone

TABLE 8.3   Biomaterials for Total Joint Replacements

Material	Application	Properties
Co–Cr alloy	Stem, head (ball)	Heavy, hard, stiff
(casted or wrought)	Cup, porous coating	High wear resistance
	Metal backing	
Ti alloy	Stem, porous coating	Low stiffness
	Metal backing	Low wear resistance
Pure titanium	Porous coating	Excellent osseointegration
Tantalum	Porous structure	Excellent osseointegration
		Good mechanical strength
Alumina	Ball, cup	Hard, brittle
		High wear resistance
Zirconia	Ball	Heavy and high toughness
		High wear resistance
UHMWPE	Cup	Low friction, wear debris
		Low creep resistance
PMMA	Bone cement fixation	Brittle, weak in tension
		Low fatigue strength

Note: Stem: femoral hip stem/chondylar knee stem; head: femoral head of the hip stem; cup: acetabular cup of the hip.

TABLE 8.4   Types of Total Joint Replacements

Joint	Type
Hip	Ball and socket
Knee	Hinged, semiconstrained, surface replacement
	Unicompartment or bicompartment
Shoulder	Ball and socket
Ankle	Surface replacement
Elbow	Hinged, semiconstrained, surface replacement
Wrist	Ball and socket, space filler
Finger	Hinged, space filler

interface or shielding it from load transfer may result in *bone resorption* and subsequent loosening of the implant [Sarmiento et al., 1990]. The articulating surfaces of the joint should function with minimum friction and produce the least amount of wear products [Charnley, 1973]. The implant should be securely fixed to the body as early as possible (ideally immediately after implantation); however, removal of the implant should not require destruction of a large amount of surrounding tissues. Loss of tissue, especially of bone, makes re-implantation difficult and often shortens the life span of the second joint replacement [Dupont and Charnley, 1972].

Decades of basic and clinical experimentation have resulted in a vast number of prosthetic designs and material combinations (Tables 8.3 and 8.4) [Griss, 1984]. In the following section, the most relevant achievements in fixation methods and prosthetic design for different joints will be discussed at a conceptual level. Most joints can undergo partial replacement (hemiarthroplasty), that is, reconstruction of only one side of the joint while retaining the other. This is indicated in selected conditions when global joint degeneration has not taken place. This section will focus on total joint replacement, since this allows for a broader discussion of the biomaterials used.

Implant Fixation Method

The development of a permanent fixation mechanism of implants to bone has been one of the most formidable challenges in the evolution of joint replacement. There are three types of methods of fixation: (1) mechanical interlock, which is achieved by press-fitting the implant [Cameron, 1994a], by using polymethylmethacrylate, which is called bone cement, as a grouting agent [Charnley, 1979], or by using threaded components [Albrektsson et al., 1994]; (2) biological fixation, which is achieved by using textured or porous surfaces, which allow bone to grow into the interstices [Cameron, 1994b]; and (3) direct chemical bonding between implant and bone, for example, by coating the implant with calcium hydroxyapatite, which has a mineral composition similar to bone [Morscher, 1992]. Direct bonding with bone was observed with Bioglass, a glass-ceramic, through selective dissolution of the surface film [Hench, 1994]; however, the likelihood of its clinical application is still under investigation.

Each of the fixation mechanisms has an idiosyncratic behavior, and their load transfer characteristics as well as the failure mechanisms are different. Further complexity arises from prostheses which combine two or more of the fixation mechanisms in different regions of the implant. Multiple mechanisms of fixation are used in an effort to customize load transfer to requirements of different regions of bone in an effort to preserve bone mass. Loosening, unlocking, or de-bonding between implant and bone constitute some of the most important mechanisms of prosthetic failure.

Bone Cement Fixation

Fixation of implants with polymethylmethacrylate (PMMA, bone cement) provides immediate stability, allowing patients to bear all of their weight on the extremity at once. In contrast, implants which depend on bone ingrowth require the patient to wait about 12 weeks to bear full weight.

Bone cement functions as a grouting material; consequently, its anchoring power depends on its ability to penetrate between bone trabeculae during the insertion of the prosthesis [Charnley, 1979]. Being a viscoelastic polymer, it has the ability to function as a shock absorber. It allows loads to be transmitted uniformly between the implant and bone, reducing localized high-contact stress.

Fixation with bone cement creates bone–cement and cement–implant interfaces, and loosening may occur at either one. The mechanisms to enhance the stability of the metal–cement interface constitute an area of controversy in joint replacement. Some investigators have focused their efforts on increasing the bond between metal and cement by roughening the implant, or pre-coating it with PMMA to prevent sinking of the prosthesis within the cement mantle, and circulation of debris within the interface [Park et al., 1978; Barb et al., 1982; Harris, 1988]. In contrast, others polish the implant surfaces and favor wedge-shaped designs which encourage sinking of the prosthesis within the cement, to profit from the viscoelastic deformation of the mantle by loading the cement in compression [Ling, 1992].

The problems with bone–cement interface may arise from intrinsic factors, such as the properties of the PMMA and bone, as well as extrinsic factors such as the cementing technique. Refinements in the cementing technique, such as pulsatile lavage of the medullary canal, optimal hemostasis of the cancellous bone, as well as drying of the medullary canal and pressurized insertion of the prosthesis, can result in a cement–bone interface free of gaps, with maximal interdigitation with cancellous bone [Harris and Davies, 1988]. Despite optimal cementing technique, a thin *fibrous membrane* may appear in various regions of the interface, due to various factors such as the toxic effect of free methylmethacrylate monomer, necrosis of the bone resulting from high polymerization temperatures, or devascularization during preparation of the canal [Goldring et al., 1983]. Although a fibrous membrane in the bone cement interface may be present in a well-functioning implant, it may also increase in width over time (most probably as a result of the accumulation of polyethylene wear debris from the bearing couple), and may result in macromotion, bone loss, and eventual loosening [Ebramzadeh et al., 1994]. Finally, the cement strength itself may be improved by removing air bubbles by mixing monomer and polymer under vacuum and/or centrifuging it [Harris, 1988]. During implantation, various devices are used to guarantee uniform thickness of the mantle to minimize risk of fatigue failure of the cement [Oh et al., 1978].

Porous Ingrowth Fixation

Bone ingrowth can occur with inert implants which provide pores larger than 25 μm in diameter, which is the size required to accommodate an osteon. For the best ingrowth in clinical practice, pore size range should be 100 to 350 μm and pores should be interconnected with each other with similar size of opening [Cameron, 1994b]. Implant motion inhibits bony ingrowth and large bone-metal gaps prolong or prevent the *osseointegration* [Curtis et al., 1992]. Therefore, precise surgical implantation and prevention of post-operative weight bearing for about 12 weeks are required for implant fixation.

FIGURE 8.7   Scanning electron micrographs of four different types of porous structures: (a) plasma sprayed coating (7×), (b) sintered wire mesh coating (7×), (c) sintered beads coating (20×), and (d) Hedrocell porous tantalum (50×).

The porous coated implants require active participation of the bone in the fixation of the implant, in contrast to cementation where the bone has a passive role. Therefore, porous coated implants are best indicated in conditions where the bone mass is near normal. The implant design should allow ingrown bone to be subjected to continuous loading within a physiologic range in order to prevent loss of bone mass due to *stress shielding*. Porous ingrowth prostheses are notoriously difficult to remove, and substantial bone damage often results from the removal process. For this reason, they should be optimized to provide predictable ingrowth with a minimal area of surgically accessible porous coated surface.

Commercially pure titanium, titanium alloy, tantalum, and calcium hydroxyapatite (HA) are currently used as porous coating materials. With pure titanium, three different types of porosity can be achieved: (1) plasma spray coating, (2) sintering of wire mesh, or (3) sintering of beads on an implant surface (Fig. 8.7) [Morscher, 1992]. Thermal processing of the porous coating may weaken the underlying metal (implant). Additional problems may result from flaking of the porous coating materials, since loosened metal particles may cause severe wear when they migrate into the articulation (bearing couple) [Agins et al., 1988]. A thin calcium hydroxyapatite coating over the porous titanium surface has been used in an effort to enhance osseointegration; however, it improves only early-stage interfacial strength [Friedman, 1992; Capello and Bauer, 1994]. The long-term degradation and/or resorption of hydroxyapatite is still under investigation.

Recently, a cellular, structural biomaterial comprised of 15 to 25% tantalum (75 to 85% porous) has been developed. The average pore size is about 550 μm, and the pores are fully interconnected. The porous tantalum is a bulk material (i.e., not a coating) and is fabricated via a proprietary chemical vapor infiltration process in which pure tantalum is uniformly precipitated onto a reticulated vitreous carbon skeleton. The porous tantalum possesses sufficient compressive strength for most physiological loads, and tantalum exhibits excellent biocompatibility [Black, 1994]. This porous tantalum can be mechanically attached or diffusion bonded to substrate materials such as Ti alloy. Current commercial applications include polyethylene-porous tantalum acetabular components for total hip joint replacement and repair of defects in the acetabulum.

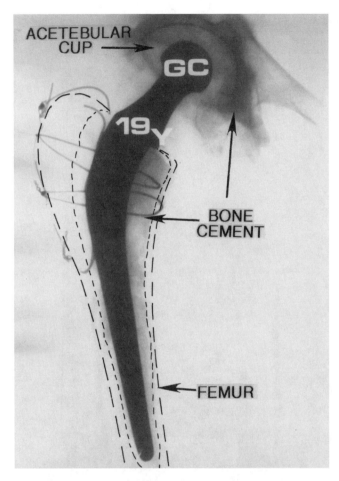

FIGURE 8.8(a)   Radiograph of bone cement fixed Charnley hip joint (monolithic femoral and acetabular component, 15-year follow-up).

Total Joint Replacements

Hip Joint Replacement

The prosthesis for total hip replacement consists of a femoral component and an acetabular component (Fig. 8.8a). The femoral stem is divided into head, neck, and shaft. The femoral stem is made of Ti alloy or Co–Cr alloy (316L stainless steel was used earlier) and is fixed into a reamed medullary canal by cementation or press fitting. The femoral head is made of Co–Cr alloy, alumina, or zirconia. Although Ti alloy heads function well under clean articulating conditions, they have fallen into disuse because of their low wear resistance to third bodies, e.g., bone or cement particles. The acetabular component is generally made of ultra-high-molecular-weight polyethylene (UHMWPE).

The prostheses can be monolithic when they consist of one part, or modular when they consist of two or more parts and require assembly during surgery. Monolithic components are often less expensive, and less prone to corrosion or disassembly. However, modular components allow customizing of the implant intraoperatively and during future revision surgeries, for example, modifying the length of an extremity by using a different femoral neck length after the stem has been cemented in place, or exchanging a worn polyethylene bearing surface for a new one without removing the well-functioning part of the prosthesis from the bone. In modular implants (Fig. 8.8b), the femoral head is fitted to the femoral neck with a Morse taper, which allows changes in head material and size and neck length. Table 8.5 illustrates the most frequently used combinations of material in total hip replacement.

FIGURE 8.8(b)   Modular total hip system: head, femoral stem, porous coated proximal wedge, porous coated metal backing for cup, UHMWPE cup, and fixation screws.

TABLE 8.5   Possible Combination of Total Hip Replacements

Femoral Component			Acetabular Component		
Fixation	**Stem**	**Ball**	**Cup**	**Backing**	**Fixation**

PMMA

Bone Ingrowth

Press fitting

Co–Cr alloy

Ti alloy

Co–Cr alloy

Alumina

Zirconia

Co–Cr alloy

UHMWPE

Alumina

Metal

None

PMMA

Screw, or press fitting

Bone ingrowth

When the acetabular component is monolithic, it is made of UHMWPE; when it is modular, it consists of a metallic shell and a UHMWPE insert. The metallic shell seeks to decrease the microdeformation of the UHMWPE and to provide a porous surface for fixation of the cup [Skinner, 1992]. The metallic shell allows worn polyethylene liners to be exchanged. In cases of repetitive dislocation of the hip after surgery, the metallic shell allows replacing the old liner with a more constrained one, to provide additional stability. Great effort has been placed on developing an effective retaining system for the insert, as well as on maximizing the congruity between insert and metallic shell (Fig. 8.8b). Dislodgment of the insert results in dislocation of the hip and damage of the femoral head, since it contacts the metallic shell directly. Micromotion between insert and shell produces additional polyethylene debris which can eventually contribute to bone loss [Friedman, 1994].

The hip joint is a ball-and-socket joint, which derives its stability from congruity of the implants, pelvic muscles, and capsule. The prosthetic hip components are optimized to provide a wide range of motion without impingement of the neck of the prosthesis on the rim of the acetabular cup to prevent dislocation. The design characteristics must enable implants to support loads that may reach more than eight times body weight [Paul, 1976]. Proper femoral neck length and correct restoration of the center of motion and femoral offset decrease the bending stress on the prosthesis–bone interface. High-stress concentration or stress shielding may result in bone resorption around the implant. For example, if the femoral stem is designed with sharp corners (diamond shaped in a cross-section), the bone in contact with the corners of the implant may necrose and resorb.

Load bearing and motion of the prosthesis produces wear debris from the articulating surface, and from the interfaces where there is micromotion, e.g., stem–cement interface. Bone chip, cement chip, or broken porous coating are often entrapped in the articulating space and cause severe polyethylene wear (third-body wear). The principal source of wear under normal conditions is the UHMWPE bearing surface in the cup. Approximately 150,000 particles are generated with each step and a large proportion of these particles are smaller than 1 μm. Cells from the immune system of the host, for example, *macrophages*, are able to identify the polyethylene particles as foreign and initiate a complex inflammatory response. This response may lead to rapid focal bone loss (*osteolysis*), bone resorption, loosening, and/or fracture of the bone. Recently, low-wear UHMWPE has been developed using a cross-linking of polyethylene molecular chains. There are several effective methods of cross-linking polyethylene, including irradiation of cross-linking, peroxide cross-linking, and silane cross-linking [Shen et al., 1996]. However, none of the cross-linked polyethylene has been clinically tested yet. Numerous efforts are underway to modify the material properties of articulating materials to harden and improve the surface finish of the femoral head [Friedman, 1994]. There is growing interest in metal–metal and ceramic–ceramic hip prostheses as a potential solution to the problem of osteolysis induced by polyethylene wear debris.

Knee Joint Replacements

The prosthesis for total knee joint replacement consists of femoral, tibial, and/or patellar components. Compared to the hip joint, the knee joint has a more complicated geometry and movement biomechanics, and it is not intrinsically stable. In a normal knee, the center of movement is controlled by the geometry of the ligaments. As the knee moves, the ligaments rotate on their bony attachments and the center of movement also moves. The eccentric movement of the knee helps distribute the load throughout the entire joint surface [Burstein and Wright, 1993].

The prostheses for total knee replacement (Fig. 8.9) can be divided according to the extent to which they rely on the ligaments for stability: (1) Constrained: these implants have a hinge articulation, with a fixed axis of rotation, and are indicated when all of the ligaments are absent, for example in reconstructive procedures for tumoral surgery. (2) Semiconstrained: these implants control posterior displacement of the tibia on the femur and medial-lateral angulation of the knee, but rely on the remaining ligaments and joint capsule to provide the rest of the constraint. Semiconstrained prostheses are often used in patients with severe angular deformities of the extremities or in those who require revision surgery, when moderate ligamentous instability has developed. (3) Nonconstrained: these implants provide minimal or no constraint. The prosthesis that provides minimal constraint requires resection of

FIGURE 8.9 Various types of knee joints: (a) metal hinged, (b) hinged with plastic liner, (c) intramedullary fixed semiconstrained, (d) surface replacement, (e) uni-compartmental replacement, and (f) bi-compartmental replacement.

the posterior cruciate ligament during implantation, and the prosthetic constraint reproduces that normally provided by this ligament. The ones that provide no constraint spare the posterior cruciate ligament. These implants are indicated in patients who have joint degeneration with minimal or no ligamentous instability. As the degree of constraint increases with knee replacements, the need for the use of femoral and tibial intramedullary extensions of the prosthesis is greater, since the loads normally shared with the ligaments are then transferred to the prosthesis–bone interface.

Total knee replacements can be implanted with or without cement, the latter relying on porous coating for fixation. The femoral components are typically made of Co–Cr alloy and the monolithic tibial components are made of UHMWPE. In modular components, the tibial polyethylene component assembles onto a titanium alloy tibial tray. The patellar component is made of UHMWPE, and a titanium alloy back is added to components designed for uncemented use. The relatively small size of the patellar component compared to the forces that travel through the extensor mechanism, and the small area of bone available for anchorage of the prosthesis, make the patella vulnerable.

The wear characteristic of the surface of tibial polyethylene is different from that of acetabular components. The point contact stress and sliding motion of the components result in delamination and fatigue wear of the UHMWPE [Walker, 1993]. Presumably because of the relatively larger particle size of polyethylene debris, osteolysis around a total knee joint is less frequent than in a total hip replacement.

Ankle Joint Replacement

Total ankle replacements have not met with as much success as total hip and knee replacements, and typically loosen within a few years of service [Claridge et al., 1991]. This is mainly due to the high load transfer demand over the relatively small ankle surface area, and the need to replace three articulating surfaces (tibial, talar, and fibular). The joint configurations that have been used are cylindrical, reverse cylindrical, and spherical. The materials used to construct ankle joints are usually Co–Cr alloy and UHMWPE. Degeneration of the ankle joint is currently treated with fusion of the joint, since prostheses for total ankle replacement are still considered to be under initial development. Figure 8.10 shows ankle and other total joint replacements.

FIGURE 8.10 Miscellaneous examples of prostheses for total joint replacement: (a) ankle, (b) socket-ball shoulder joint, (c) hinged elbow joint, and (d) encapsulated finger joint.

Shoulder Joint Replacements

The prostheses for total shoulder replacement consist of a humeral and a glenoid component. Like the femoral stem, the humeral component can be divided into head, neck, and shaft. Variations in the length of the neck result in changes in the length of the extremity. Even though the patient's perception of length of the upper extremity is not as accurate as that of the lower extremity, the various lengths of the neck are used to fine-tune the tension of the soft tissues to obtain maximal stability and range of motion.

The shoulder has the largest range of motion in the body, which results from a shallow ball and socket joint, which allows a combination of rotation and sliding motions between the joint surfaces. To compensate for the compromise in congruity, the shoulder has an elaborate capsular and ligamentous structure, which provides the basic stabilization. In addition, the muscle girdle of the shoulder provides additional dynamic stability. A decrease in the radius of curvature of the implant to compensate for soft tissue instability will result in a decrease in the range of motion [Neer, 1990].

Elbow Joint Replacements

The elbow joint is a hinge-type joint allowing mostly flexion and extension, but having a polycentric motion [Goel and Blair, 1985]. The elbow joint implants are either hinged, semiconstrained, or unconstrained. These implants, like those of the ankle, have a high failure rate and are not used commonly. The high loosening rate is the result of high rotational moments, limited bone stock for fixation, and minimal ligamentous support [Morrey, 1993]. In contrast to fusions of the ankle which function well, fusions of the elbow result in a moderate degree of incapacitation.

Finger Joint Replacements

Finger joint replacements are divided into three types: (1) hinge, (2) polycentric, and (c) space-filler. The most widely used are the space-filler type. These are made of high performance silicone rubber (polydimethylsiloxane) and are stabilized with a passive fixation method. This method depends on the development of a thin, fibrous membrane between implant and bone, which allows pistoning of the prosthesis. This fixation can provide only minimal rigidity of the joint [Swanson, 1973]. Implant wear

FIGURE 8.11   Experimental artificial discs used to restore function of the degenerated spine disc.

and cold flow associated with erosive cystic changes of adjacent bone have been reported with silicone implants [Carter et al., 1986; Maistrelli, 1994].

Prosthetic Intervertebral Disk

Because of adjacent-level degeneration and other complications, such as non-fusion, alternatives to fusions have been proposed. One of the most recent developments for non-fusion treatment alternatives is replacement of the intervertebral discs [Hedman et al., 1991]. The goal of this treatment alternative is to restore the original mechanical function of the disc. One of the stipulations of artificial disc replacement is that remaining osseous spinal and paraspinal soft tissue components are not compromised by pathologic changes. Several artificial disk prostheses have been developed to achieve these goals (Fig. 8.11).

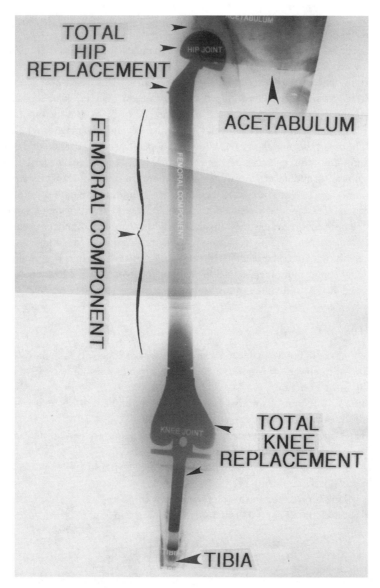

FIGURE 8.12 Radiographic appearance (montage) of a modular endoprosthetic replacement. Entire femur, hip joint, and knee joint of the bone tumor patient were replaced with prostheses for a limb salvage.

Prostheses for Limb Salvage

Prosthetic implant technology has brought new lifestyles to thousands of patients who would lose their limbs due to bone cancer. In the past, the treatment for primary malignant bone cancer of the extremities was amputation. Significant advances in bone tumor treatment have taken place during the last two decades. The major treatment methods for limb reconstruction following bone tumor resection are resection arthrodesis (fusion of two bones), allograft–endoprosthetic composite, and endoprosthetic reconstruction. Endoprosthetic reconstruction is an extension of a total joint replacement(s) component to the resected bone area and is the most popular option due to an advantage of fast postoperative recovery (Fig. 8.12). Therefore, material and fixation methods for limb salvage endoprostheses are exactly the same as for total joint replacements. Femur, tibia, humerus, pelvis, and scapular are often resected and replaced endoprostheses. Similar to total joint replacements, disadvantages of the endoprosthetic reconstruction are prosthesis loosening due to polyethylene wear and cement failure, and mechanical failure of the prostheses.

   Most of the endoprostheses for limb salvage are of the expandable type [Ward et al., 1996]. Expandable endoprostheses are required for children who have a potential for skeletal growth. Several expandable prostheses require an open surgical procedure to be lengthened, whereas others have been developed that can be lengthened by servomechanisims within the endoprosthesis. The modular segmental system is a new option for expandable endoprosthesis. They can be revised easily to elongate modular components to gain length over time. The modular segmental system has several advantages over the mechanically expandable one. The use of the modular system allows intraoperative customization of the endoprosthesis during surgery. It minimizes discrepancies between custom implants and actual skeletal defects due to the radiographic magnification and uncertainty of margin of tumor resection. It allows the surgeon to assemble the prosthesis intraoperatively. The cost of the modular system is less than the cost of an expandable custom endoprosthesis. The modular system allows for simpler and less expensive revision when failures occur, obviating the need for an entirely new prosthesis when only one part needs to be replaced. On the other hand, the modular system has a high chance of corrosion failure at the Morse tapers and dislodgment at the Morse taper fittings. It can be lengthened only in certain increments. The modular component system has additional applications: metastatic bone disease, failure of internal fixation, severe acute fractures with poor bone quality, and failure of total joints with insufficient bone stock.

Defining Terms

Bone resorption: A type of bone loss due to the greater osteoclastic activity than the osteogenic activity.
Callus: Unorganized meshwork of woven bone which is formed following fracture of bone to achieve early stability of the fracture.
Fibrous membrane: Thin layer of soft tissue which covers an implant to isolate it from the body.
Necrosis: Cell death caused by enzymes or heat.
Osseointegration: Direct contact of bone tissues to an implant surface without fibrous membrane.
Osteolysis: Dissolution of bone mineral from the bone matrix.
Primary healing: Bone healing in which union occurs directly without forming callus.
Secondary healing: Bone union with a callus formation.
Stress shielding: Bone is protected from stress by the stiff implant.
Wolff's law: Bone develops or adapts its structure to that most suited to resist the forces acting upon it.

References

Agins HJ, Alcock NW, Bansal M et al. 1988. Metallic wear in failed titanium-alloy total hip replacements. A histological and quantitative analysis. *J Bone Joint Surg* 70-A(3):347.

Albrektsson T, Carlsson LV, Morberg P et al. 1994. Directly bone-anchored implants. In *Bone Implant Interface*, Ed. R Hurley, pp. 97–120, Mosby, St. Louis, MO.

Barb W, Park JB, von Recum AF et al. 1982. Intramedullary fixation of artificial hip joints with bone cement precoated implants: I. Interfacial strengths. *J Biomed Mater Res* 16:447.

Black J. 1994. Biological performance of tantalum. *Clin Mater* 16:167.

Brand RA, Rubin, CT. 1987. Fracture healing, In *Scientific Basics of Orthopaedics*, 2nd ed., Eds. J Albert and R Brand, pp. 325–340, Appleton & Lange, Norwalk, CT.

Brighton CT. 1984. Principle of fracture healing, In *Instructional Course Lectures*, Ed. J. Murray, pp. 60–106, The American Academy of Orthopaedic Surgeons, Northfield, IL.

Buckwalter JA, Woo S et al. 1993. Soft-tissue aging and musculoskeletal function. *J Bone Joint Surg* 75A(10):1533.

Burstein AH, Wright TH. 1993. Biomechanics. In *Surgery of the Knee*, 2nd ed., Vol 7, Eds. J Insall, R Windsor, W Scott et al., pp. 43–62, Churchill Livingstone, New York.

Cameron HU. 1994a. Smooth metal-bone interface. In *Bone Implant Interface*, Ed. R Hurley, pp. 121–144, Mosby, St. Louis, MO.

Cameron HU. 1994b. The implant-bone interface: porous metals. In *Bone Implant Interface*, Ed. R Hurley, pp. 145–168, Mosby, St. Louis, MO.

Capello WN, Bauer TW. 1994. Hydroxyapatite in orthopaedic surgery. In *Bone Implant Interface*, Ed. R Hurley, pp. 191–202, Mosby, St. Louis, MO.

Carter P, Benton L, Dysert P. 1986. Silicone rubber carpal implants: a study of the incidence of late osseous complications, *J Hand Surg* 11A(5):639.

Charnley J. 1979. *Low Friction Arthroplasty of the Hip*, Springer-Verlag, Berlin.

Claes L. 1989. The mechanical and morphological properties of bone beneath internal fixation plates of differing rigidity. *J Orthop Res* 7:170.

Claridge R J, Hart MB, Jones RA et al. 1991. Replacement arthroplasties of the ankle and foot. In *Disorder of the Foot and Ankle*, 2nd ed., Ed. M Jahss, pp. 2647–2664, Saunders, Philadephia, PA.

Cochran GVB. 1982. Biomechanics of orthopaedic structures. In *Primer in Orthopaedic Biomechanics*, pp. 143–215, Churchill Livingstone, New York.

Curtis MJ, Jinnah RH, Wilson VD, Hungerford DS. 1992. The initial stability of uncemented acetabular components. *J Bone Joint Surg* 74B(3):372.

DeCoster TA, Heetderks DB et al. 1990. Optimizing bone screw pullout force. *J Orthop Trauma* 4(2):169.

Dupont JA, Charnley J. 1972. Low-friction arthroplasty of the hip for the failures of previous operations. *J Bone Joint Surg* 54B(1):77.

Ebramzadeh E, Sarmiento A, McKellop HA et al. 1994. The cement mantle in total hip arthroplasty. Analysis of long-term radiographic results. *J Bone Joint Surg* 76A(1):77–87.

Friedman RF, Black J, Galante JO et al. 1994. Current concepts in orthopaedic biomaterials and implant fixation. In *Instructional Course Lectures*, Ed. JM Schafer, pp. 233–255, The American Academy of Orthopaedic Surgeons, Northfield, IL.

Friedman RJ. 1992. Advanced in biomaterials and factors affecting implant fixation. In *Instructional Course Lectures*, Ed. RE Eilert, pp. 127–135, The American Academy of Orthopaedic Surgeons, Northfield, IL.

Goel VK, Blair W. 1985. Biomechanics of the elbow joint. *Automedica* 6:119.

Goldring SR., Schiller AL, Roelke M et al. 1983. The synovial-like membrane at the bone–cement interface in loose total hip replacements and its proposed role in bone lysis. *J Bone Joint Surg* 65A(5):575.

Griss P. 1984. Assessment of clinical status of total joint replacement. In *Functional Behavior of Orthopaedic Biomaterials*, Eds. P Ducheyne and GW Hastings, pp. 21–48, CRC Press, Boca Raton, FL.

Harris WH, Davies JP.1988. Modern use of modern cement for total hip replacement. *Orthop Clin North Am* 19(3):581.

Hedman TP, Kostuik PJ, Fernie GR et al. 1991. Design of an intervertebral disc prosthesis. *Spine* 16:256.

Hench LL. 1994. Bioactive glasses, ceramics and composites. In *Bone Implant Interface*, Ed. R Hurley, pp. 181–190, Mosby, St. Louis, MO.

Hulth A. 1989. Current concepts of fracture healing. *Clin Orthop* 249:265.

Hutzschenreuter P, Brümmer H. 1980. Screw design and stability. In *Current Concepts of Internal Fixation*, Ed. H Uhthoff, pp. 244–250, Springer-Verlag, Berlin.

Jeffery AK. 1994. Articular cartilage and the orthopaedic surgeon. Part 1: Structure and function. *Curr Orthop* 8:38.

Kessler SB, Hallfeldt KK, Perren SM et al. 1986. The effects of reaming and intramedullary nailing on fracture healing. *Clin Orthop* 212:18.

Ling RS. 1992. The use of a collar and precoating on cemented femoral stems is unnecessary and detrimental. *Clin Orthop* 285:73.

Maistrelli GL. 1994. Polymer in orthopaedic surgery, In *Bone Implant Interface*, Ed. R Hurley, pp. 169–190, Mosby, St. Louis, MO.

McKellop HA, Campbell P, Park SH et al. 1995. The origin of submicron polyethylene wear debris in total hip arthroplasty. *Clin Orthop* 311:3.

Morrey BF. 1993. *The Elbow and Its Disorders*, 2nd ed., Saunders, Philadelphia, PA.

Morscher EW. 1992. Current status of acetabular fixation in primary total hip arthroplasty. *Clin. Orthop* 274:172.

Mow VC, Hayes WC. 1991. *Basic Orthopaedic Biomechanics*, Raven Press, New York.

Neer CS. 1990. *Shoulder Reconstruction*, Saunders, Philadelphia, PA.

Oh I, Carlson CE, Tomford WW et al. 1978. Improved fixation of the femoral component after total hip replacement using a methacrylate intramedullary plug. *J Bone Joint Surg* 60A(5):608.

O'Slullivan ME, Chao EYS, Kelly PJ. 1989. Current concepts review: the effects of fixation on fracture healing. *J Bone Joint Surg* 71A(2):306.

Park JB, Lakes RS. 1992. *Biomaterials: An Introduction*, 2nd ed., Plenum Press, London.

Park JB, Malstrom CS, von Recum AF. 1978. Intramedullary fixation of implants precoated with bone cement: a preliminary study. *Biomater Med Dev Artif Org* 6(4):361.

Paul JP. 1976. Loading on normal hip and knee joints and joint replacement. In *Advances in Hip and Knee Joint Technology*, Eds. M Schaldach and D Hohmann, pp. 53–77, Springer-Verlag, Berlin.

Perren SM, 1989. The biomechnics and biology of internal fixation using plates and nails. *Orthopaedics* 12(1):21.

Perren SM. 1991. Basic aspects of internal fixation. In *Manual of Internal Fixation*, 3rd ed., Eds. M Müller, M Allgöwer, R Schneider, and H Willenegger, pp. 1–112, Springer-Verlag, Berlin.

Salter RB. 1988. The biologic concept of continuous passive motion of synovial joints. The first 18 years of basic research and its clinical application. *Clin Orthop* 242:12.

Sarmiento A, Ebramzadeh E, Gogan WJ et al. 1990. Cup containment and orientation in cemented total hip arthroplasties. *J Bone Joint Surg* 72B(6):996.

Schatzker J, Sanderson R, Murnaghan JP. 1975. The holding power of orthopaedic screws *in vivo*. *Clin Orthop* 108:115.

Schenk RK. 1992. Biology of fracture repair. In *Skeletal Trauma*, Eds. B Browner, J Jupitor, A Levine, and P Trafton, pp. 31–75, Saunders, Philadephia, PA.

Shen FW, McKellop H, Salovey R. 1996. Irradiation of chemically crosslinked ultrahigh molecular weight polyethylene. *J Polymer Sci B: Polymer Phys* 34:1063.

Skinner HB. 1992. Current biomaterial problems in implants. In *Instructional Course Lectures*, Ed. RE Eilert, pp. 137–144, The American Academy of Orthopaedic Surgeons, Northfield, IL.

Swanson AB. 1973. Concepts of flexible implant design. In *Flexible Implant Reconstruction Arthroplasty in the Hand and Extremity*, Ed. A Swanson, pp. 47–59, Mosby, St. Louis, MO.

Taitsman JP, Saha S. 1977. Tensile strength of wire-reinforced bone cement and twisted stainless-steel wire. *J Bone Joint Surg*. 59A:419.

Tencer AF, Johnson KD, Kely RF et al. 1993. Biomechanics of fractures and fracture fixation. In *Instructional Course Lectures*, Ed. JD Heckman, pp. 19–55, The American Academy of Orthopaedic Surgeons, Northfield, IL.

Uhthoff HK, Finnegan MA. 1984. The role of rigidity in fracture fixation. *Arch Orthop Trauma Surg* 102:163.

Walker PS. 1993. Design of total knee arthroplasty. In *Surgery of the Knee*, 2nd ed, Vol 7, Eds. J Insall, R Windsor, W Scott et al., pp. 723–738, Churchill Livingstone, New York.

Ward WG, Yang RS., Eckart JJ. 1996. Endoprosthetic bone reconstruction following malignant tumor resection in skeletally immature patients. *Orthop Clin North Am* 27:493.

Weinstein AM, Spires WP Jr, Klawitter et al. 1979. Orthopaedic implant retrieval and analysis study. In *Corrosion and Degradation of Implant Materials*, Eds. BC Syrett, A Acharya, pp. 212–228, American Society for Testing and Materials Tech. Pub. No. 684, Philadelphia, PA.

Wolff J. 1986. *The Law of Bone Remodeling*, R Maquet, R Furlong (trans.), Springer-Verlag, Berlin.

8.2 Dental Implants: The Relationship of Materials Characteristics to Biologic Properties

John C. Keller

As dental implants have become an acceptable treatment modality for partially and fully edentulous patients, it has become increasingly apparent that the interaction of the host tissue with the underlying implant surface is of critical importance for long-term prognosis [Smith, 1993; Young, 1988]. From the anatomical viewpoint, it is generally accepted that dental implants must contact and become integrated with several types of host tissues. Due largely to the work of Branemark and his colleagues [Albrektsson et al., Branemark, 1983], the importance of developing and maintaining a substantial bone–implant interface for mechanical retention and transmission of occlusal forces was realized. Despite documented long-term success of dental implants, longer-term implant failures are noted due to poor integration of connective and epithelial tissues and subsequent failure to develop a permucosal seal akin to that with natural tooth structures. From a biologic point of view, the characteristics of the implant substrate which permit hard and soft tissue integration and prevent adhesion of bacteria and plaque need to be further understood. It is likely that as a more complete understanding of the basic biologic responses of host tissues becomes known, refinements in the currently employed materials as well as new and improved materials will become available for use in the dental implant field.

It is important to realize that the overall biologic response of host tissue to dental implants can be divided into two distinct but interrelated phases (as given in Table 8.6). Phase I consists of the tissue responses which occur during the clinical healing phase immediately following implantation of dental implants. During this healing phase, the initial biologic processes of protein and molecular deposition on the implant surface are followed by cellular attachment, migration, and differentiation [Stanford and Keller, 1991]. It is therefore important to understand the characteristics of the implant material which affect the initial formation of the host tissue–implant interface. The characteristics include materials selection and the physical and chemical properties of the implant surface. These initial tissue responses lead to the cellular expression and maturation of extracellular matrix and ultimately to the development of bony interfaces with the implant material. After the initial healing phase is complete, usually between 3 and 6 months according to the two-stage Branemark implant design, the bone interface remodels under the occlusal forces placed on the implant during the Phase II functional period [Brunski, 1992; Skalak, 1985]. The overall bioresponses including bone remodeling during the functional phase of implant service life are then strongly influenced by the characteristics of loading and distribution of stress at the interface [Brunski, 1992]. The ability of the maturing interface to "remodel" as stresses are placed on the implant thus depend in large part on the original degree of tissue–implant surface interaction.

TABLE 8.6 Correlation between the Clinical Phases of Implant Service Life with Biologic Events and Important Implant Materials Characteristics

Clinical Phase	Biological Events	Influential Materials Characteristics
I (healing)	Protein deposition	Materials selection
	Cell attachment	Metals
	Cell migration	Ceramics
	Development of extracellular matrix	Chemical and physical characteristics
	Bone deposition	Topography
		Micro
		Macro
		Surface chemistry
		Inert
		Dissolution
II (functional)	Matrix and bone remodeling	

This section focuses on the factors concerning dental implants which affect biologic properties of currently available dental implant materials. As pertains to each major topic, the influence of the materials properties on biologic responses will be emphasized.

Effects of Materials Selection

Metals and Alloys

Previously, dental implants have been fabricated from several metallic systems, including stainless steel and cobalt–chrome alloys as well as from the titanium family of metals. Several studies have reported on the ability of host bone tissues to "integrate" with various metal implant surfaces [Albrektsson et al., 1983; Johansson et al., 1989; Katsikeris et al., 1987]. In current paradigms, the term *osseointegration* refers to the ability of host tissues to form a functional interface with implant surfaces without an intervening layer of connective tissue akin to a foreign body tissue capsule observable at the light microscopic level [Albrektsson et al., 1983; Branemark, 1983]. By this definition, it becomes apparent that several biomedical materials including Ti and Ti alloy fulfill this general criterion. Ultrastructural investigations using transmission electron microscopy (TEM) approaches have further refined descriptions of the tissue implant interface, and the early work by Albrektsson and colleagues [1983] has become the descriptive standard by which other materials interfaces are compared. When bone was allowed to grow on Ti, a partially calcified amorphous ground substance was deposited in immediate contact with the implant, followed by a collagenous fibril-based extracellular matrix, osteoblast cell processes, and a more highly calcified matrix generally 200–300 Å from the implant surface.

However, other metallic materials have fallen from favor for use as dental implants due to widely differing mechanical properties compared to bone (Table 8.7), which can result in a phenomenon termed *stress shielding* [Brunski, 1992; Slalak, 1985], and the propensity for formation of potentially toxic corrosion products due to insufficient corrosion resistance properties [Lucas et al., 1987; Van Orden, 1985]. Ultrastructurally, the interface between bone and 316L stainless steel was described as consisting of a multiple-cell layer separating the bone from metal. Inflammatory cells were prominent in this layer, and a thick proteoglycan noncollagenous coating was present. This histologic appearance resembled that of a typical foreign body reaction and typifies a nonosseointegration-type response. The poor biologic response to stainless steel alloys has been reconfirmed by recently conducted *in vitro* studies which related the inability of host tissue to attach to the metal surface to the toxicity associated with metal ion release [Vrouwenvelder et al., 1993].

Due in large measure to the introduction and overall clinical success of the Branemark system, the range of metallic materials utilized for dental implants has become limited largely to commercially pure titanium (cpTi > 99.5%) and its major alloy, Ti-6A1-4V [De Porter et al., 1986; Keller et al., 1987]. Controversy remains, largely due to commercial advertising interests, as to which material provides a more suitable surface for tissue integration. Early work by Johansson and coworkers [1989] reported that sputtercoated Ti alloy surfaces resulted in wide (5000 Å) *amorphous zones* devoid of collagen

TABLE 8.7   Approximate Room Temperature Mechanical Properties of Selected Implant Materials Compared to Bone

	Elastic Modulus (MPa × 10³)	Proportional Limit (MPa)	Ultimate Tensile Strength (MPa)	Percent Elongation
316L SS				
Annealed	200	240	550	50
Cold worked	200	790	965	20
CoCrMo(ASTM-F75)	240	500	700	10
Ti(ASTM-F67)	100	520	620	18
Ti-6A1-4V(ASTM-F136)	110	840	900	12
Cortical bone	18	130	140	1

Source: Keller and Lautenshlager [1986].

TABLE 8.8 Surface Characterizations of cpTi and Ti Alloy (means ± standard deviations)

	cpTi	Ti-6A1-4V
Surface roughness (Ra) (µm)		
Sandblasted	0.9 ± 0.2	0.7 ± 0.03
600 grit polish	0.2 ± 0.02	0.1 ± 0.02
Smooth, 1 µm polish	0.04 ± 0.01	0.03 ± 0.01
Atomic ratios to Ti		
C	1.5 ± 0.2	1.2 ± 0.1
O	2.8 ± 0.1	3.1 ± 0.2
N	0.08 ± 0.01	0.05 ± 0.01
Al	—	0.2 ± 0.04
V[a]	—	(0.02)[a]
Oxide thickness (Å)	32 ± 8	83 ± 12
Wetting angles (°)	52 ± 2	56 ± 4

[a] One specimen.

filaments, compared to the thinner 200- to 400-Å collagen-free amorphous zone surrounding cpTi surfaces. Subsequent studies revealed differences in the oxide characteristics between these sputtercoated cpTi and Ti alloy surfaces used for histologic and ultrastructural interfacial analyses. Significant surface contamination and the presence of V was observed in the Ti alloy surface, which led to an overall woven bone interface compared to the cpTi surface which had a more compact bone interface. Orr and colleagues [1992] demonstrated a similar ultrastructural morphology for interfaces of bone to Ti and Ti alloy, respectively. In each case an afibrillar matrix with calcified globular accretions, similar in appearance to cement lines in Haversian systems, were observed in intimate contact with the oxide surface. Any slight differences in morphology were attributed to minor differences in surface topography or microtexture rather than chemical differences between the two surface oxides.

This is an area that is still under investigation, although recent research indicates that the stable oxide of cpTi and Ti alloy provide suitable surfaces for biologic integration [Keller et al., 1994]. Studies involving comprehensive surface analyses of prepared bulk cpTi and Ti alloy indicated that although the oxide on Ti alloy is somewhat thicker following standard surface preparations (polishing, cleaning, and acid passivation), the overall topography, the chemical characteristics, including presence and concentration of contaminants, and surface energetics were virtually identical for both materials as given in Table 8.8. *In vitro* experiments confirmed that the inherently clean condition of these oxides supports significant osteoblast cell attachment and migration and provides a hospitable surface to allow in vitro mineralization processes to occur [Orr et al., 1992].

In vitro experiments designed to study the ultrastructural details of bone–implant interfaces made from cpTi and Ti alloy may provide additional clues as to the histologic and ultrastructural differences which have been observed with these materials. Since clinical implants made from both materials appear to be successful [Branemark, 1983; De Porter et al., 1986], it is possible that because of the difference in mechanical properties between unalloyed and Ti alloy material, the longer-term tissue interface results from differences in bone remodeling due to the local biomechanical environment surrounding these materials [Brunski, 1992]. This hypothesis requires continued investigation for more definitive answers.

Ceramics and Ceramic Coatings

The use of single crystal sapphire or Al_2O_3 ceramic implants has remained an important component in the dental implant field [Driskell et al., 1973]. Although this material demonstrates excellent biologic compatibility, implants fabricated from Al_2O_3 have not reached a high degree of popularity in the United States. Morphologic analyses of the soft tissue interface with Al_2O_3 revealed a hemidesmosomal external lamina attachment adjacent to the *junctional epithelium*–implant interface [Steflik et al., 1984]. This ultrastructural description is often used for comparison purposes when determining the extent of soft-tissue interaction with dental implants. Similarly, *in vivo* studies of the bone–Al_2O_3 implant interface reveal high levels of bone-to-implant contact, with areas of intervening fibrous connective tissue. Although fibrous tissue was present at the interface, the implant remained immobile, and the interface was consistent with a dynamic support system. More recent ultrastructural studies have demonstrated a mineralized matrix in immediate apposition to the Al_2O_3 implants similar to that described for Ti implants [Steflik et al., 1993].

An approach to enhancing tissue responses at dental implant interfaces has been the introduction of ceramics like *calcium-phosphate-containing (CP) materials* as implant devices. The use of calcium-phosphate materials, in bulk or particulate form or as coatings on metal substrates has taken a predominant position in the biomedical implant area and has been the focus of several recent reviews [Kay, 1992; Koeneman et al., 1990]. One of the most important uses of CP materials has been as a coating on metallic (cpTi and Ti alloy) substrates. This approach has taken advantage of thin-film-coating technology to apply thin coatings of hydroxyapatite (HA) and tricalcium phosphate (TCP) materials to the substrate in order to enhance bone responses at implant sites. The most popular method of coating has been the *plasma spray* process [Herman, 1988]; although this process has some advantages, there are reports of nonuniform coatings, interfacial porosity, and vaporization of elements in the powder [Cook et al., 1991; Kay, 1992].

The use of this class of materials is based on the premise that a more natural hydroxyapatite (HA-like) could act as a scaffold for enhanced bone response—osseointegration—and thereby minimize the long-term healing periods currently required for uncoated metal implants.

Numerous *in vivo* investigations have clearly demonstrated that HA-like coatings can enhance bone responses at implant interfaces [Cook et al., 1991; Jarcho et al., 1997], although the mechanisms responsible for the development of the interface between hard tissue and these ceramic coatings are not well understood [Jansen et al., 1993]. Histologically, the overall bone-coating interface is similar in appearance and chronologic development to that reported for uncoated implant surfaces. Initially, an immature, trabecular, woven bone interface is formed followed by more dense, compact lamellar supporting bone structure. Ultrastructurally, the interface is reported to consist of a globular, afibrillar matrix directly on the HA surface, an electron-dense, proteoglycan rich layer (20–60 nm thick) and the presence of a mineralized collagenous matrix [De Bruijn et al., 1993]. Although the morphologic descriptions of the HA and Ti interfaces are similar, numerous studies have shown that the bone response to HA coatings is more rapid than with uncoated Ti surfaces, requiring approximately one-third to one-half the time to establish a firm osseous bed as uncoated Ti. Likewise, the extent of the bone response to HA coatings is superior and, according to some studies, leads to a several-fold increase in interfacial strength compared to uncoated Ti [Cook et al., 1991].

The cellular events which take place and lead to the interfacial ultrastructure with bone tissue and ceramic surfaces are under current investigation. Based upon preliminary findings, the advantageous biologic properties of HA coatings do not appear to be related to recruitment of additional cells during the early attachment phase of healing. Although recent work indicated that bone cells and tissue form normal cellular focal contacts during attachment to HA coatings, the level of initial *in vitro* attachment generally only approximates that observed with Ti [Keller et al., 1992; Puleo et al., 1991]. Rather, the mechanisms for the enhanced *in vitro* cell responses appear to be related, to a certain degree, to the degradation properties and release of Ca^{+2} and PO_4^{-3} ions into the biologic milieu. This surface corrosion is associated with highly degradable amorphous components of the coating and leads to surface irregularities which may enhance the quality of cell adhesion to these roughened materials [Bowers et al., 1992; Chehroudi et al., 1992]. Cellular events which occur following attachment may be influenced by the nature of the ceramic surface. Emerging evidence from a number of laboratories suggests that cellular-mediated events, including proliferation, matrix expression, and bone formation are enhanced following attachment to HA coatings and appear to be related to the gene expression of osteoblasts when cultured on different ceramic materials. These early cellular events lead to histologic and ultrastructural descriptions of bone healing which take place on these surfaces and are very similar to those reported from *in vivo* studies [Orr et al., 1992; Steflik et al., 1993].

As determined from *in vitro* dissolution studies, there is general agreement that the biodegradation properties of the pertinent CP materials can be summarized as α-TCP > β-TCP >>> HA, whereas amorphous HA is more prone to biodegradation than crystalline HA [Koeneman et al., 1990]. Considerable attempts to investigate the effects of coating composition (relative percentages of HA, TCP) on bone integration have been undertaken. Using an orthopedic canine total hip model, Jasty and coworkers (1992) reported that by 3 weeks, a TCP/HA mixed coating resulted in significantly more woven bone apposition to the implants than uncoated implants. As determined by x-ray diffraction, the mixed coating consisted of 60% TCP, 20% crystalline HA, and 20% unknown Ca-PO$_4$ materials. Jansen and colleagues [1993] reported that, using HA-coated implants (90% HA, 10% amorphous CP), bony apposition was extensive in a rabbit tibia model by 12 weeks. However, significant loss of the coating occurred as early as 6 weeks after implantation. Maxian and coworkers [1993] reported that poorly crystallized HA (60% crystalline) coatings demonstrated significant degradation and poor bone apposition *in vivo* compared to amorphous coatings. Both these reports suggest that although considerable bioresorption of the coating occurred in the cortical bone, there was significant bone apposition (81 ± 2% for amorphous HA at 12 weeks, 77% for crystalline HA, respectively) which was not significantly affected by bioresorption.

From these *in vivo* reports, it is clear that HA coatings with relatively low levels of crystallinity are capable of significant bone apposition. However, as reported in a 1990 workshop report, the FDA is strongly urging commercial implant manufacturers to use techniques to increase the postdeposition crystallinity and to provide adequate adhesion of the coating to the implant substrate [Filiaggi et al., 1993]. Although the biologic responses to HA coatings are encouraging, other factors regarding HA coatings continue to lead to clinical questions regarding their efficacy. Although the overall bone response to HA-coated implants occurs more rapidly than with uncoated devices, with time an equivalent bone contact area is formed for both materials [Jasty et al., 1992]. These results have questioned the true need for HA-coated implants, especially when there are a number of disadvantages associated with the coating concept. Clinical difficulties have arisen due to failures within the coating itself and with continued dissolution of the coating, and to catastrophic failure at the coating–substrate interface [Koeneman et al., 1988].

Recent progress is reported in terms of the improvements in coating technology. Postdeposition heat treatments are often utilized to control the crystallinity (and therefore the dissolution characteristics) of the coatings, although there is still debate as to the relationship between compositional variations associated with differing crystallinity and optimization of biologic responses. Additional coating-related properties are also under investigation in regard to their effects on bone. These include coating thickness, level of acceptable porosity in the coating, and adherence of the coating to the underlying substrate. However, until answers concerning these variables have been more firmly established, HA coatings used for dental implants will remain an area of controversy and interest.

Effects of Surface Properties

Surface Topography

The effects of surface topography are different than the overall three-dimensional design or geometry of the implant, which is related to the interaction of the host tissues with the implant on a macroscopic scale as shown in Fig. 8.13. This important consideration in overall biologic response to implants is discussed later in this chapter. In this discussion the concept of *surface topography* refers to the surface texture on a microlevel. It is on this microscopic level that the intimate cell and tissue interactions leading to osseointegration are based as shown in Fig. 8.14.

The effects of surface topography on *in vitro* and *in vivo* cell and tissue responses have been a field of intense study in recent years. The overall goal of these studies is to identify surface topographies which mimic the natural substrata in order to permit tissue integration and improve clinical performance of the implant. In terms of cell attachment, the *in vitro* work by Bowers and colleagues [1992] established

FIGURE 8.13   Examples of current dental implant designs, illustrating the variety of macroscopic topographies which are used to encourage tissue ingrowth. Left to right: Microvent, Corevent, Screw-vent, Swede-vent, Branemark, IMZ implant.

that levels of short-term osteoblast cell attachment were higher on rough compared to smooth surfaces and cell morphology was directly related to the nature of the underlying substrate. After initial attachment, in many cases, cells of various origin often take on the morphology of the substrate as shown in Fig. 8.15. Increased surface roughness, produced by such techniques as sand or grit blasting or by rough polishing, provided the rugosity necessary for optimum cell behavior.

Work in progress in several laboratories is attempting to relate the nature of the implant surface to cell morphology, intracellular cytoskeletal organization, and extracellular matrix development. Pioneering work by Chehroudi and coworkers [1992] suggests that microtextured surfaces (via micromachining or other techniques) could help orchestrate cellular activity and osteoblast mineralization by several mechanisms including proper orientation of collagen bundles and cell shape and polarity. This concept is related to the theory of *contact guidance* and the belief that cell shape will dictate cell differentiation through gene expression. In Chehroudi's work, both tapered pitted and grooved surfaces (with specific orientation and sequence patterns) supported mineralization with ultrastructural morphology similar in appearance to that observed by Davies and colleagues [1990]. However, mineralization was not observed on smooth surfaces in which osteoblastlike cells did not have a preferred growth orientation. Thus the control of surface microtopography by such procedures as micromachining may prove to be a valuable technology for the control and perhaps optimization of bone formation on implant surfaces.

It is apparent that macroscopic as well as microscopic topography may affect osteoblast differentiation and mineralization. In a recent study by Groessner-Schrieber and Tuan [1992], osteoblast growth, differentiation, and synthesis of matrix and mineralized nodules were observed on rough, textured, or porous coated titanium surfaces. It may be possible therefore, not only to optimize the interactions of host tissues with implant surfaces during the Phase I tissue responses but also to influence the overall bone responses to biomechanical forces during the remodeling phase (Phase II) of tissue responses.

Based on these concepts, current implant designs employ microtopographically roughened surfaces with macroscopic grooves, threads, or porous surfaces to provide sufficient bone ingrowth for mechanical stabilization and the prevention of detrimental micromotion as shown in Figs. 8.16 and 8.17 [Brunski, 1992; De Porter et al., 1986; Keller et al., 1987; Pilliar et al., 1991].

FIGURE 8.14 Laboratory-prepared cpTi surfaces with (a–c, top to bottom) smooth (1-μm polish), grooved (600-grit polish), and rough (sandblasted) surfaces.

FIGURE 8.15 Osteoblastlike cell morphology after 2 h attachment on (a–c, top to bottom) smooth, grooved, and rough cpTi surfaces.

Surface Chemistry

Considerable attention has focused on the properties of the oxide found on titanium implant surfaces following surface preparation. Sterilization procedures are especially important and are known to affect not only the oxide condition but also the subsequent *in vitro* [Stanford et al., 1994; Swart et al., 1992] and *in vivo* [Hartman et al., 1989] biologic responses. Interfacial surface analyses and determinations of surface energetics strongly suggest that steam autoclaving is especially damaging to titanium oxide surfaces. Depending upon the purity of the autoclave water, contaminants have been observed on the metal oxide and are correlated with poor tissue responses on a cellular [Keller et al., 1990, 1994] and tissue [Baier et al., 1984; Hartman et al., 1989; Meenaghan et al., 1979] level.

The role of multiple sterilization regimens on the practice of implant utilization is also under scrutiny. Many implants and especially bone plate systems are designed for repackaging if the kit is not exhausted. However, early evidence indicates that this practice is faulty and, depending on the method of sterilization, may affect the integrity of the metal oxide surface chemistry [Vezeau et al., 1991]. *In vitro* experiments have verified that multiple-steam-autoclaved and ethylene-oxide-treated implant surfaces adversely affected cellular and morphologic integration. However, the effects of these treatments on long-term biological responses including *in vivo* situations remain to be clarified.

Other more recently introduced techniques such as radiofrequency argon plasma cleaning treatments have succeeded in altering metal oxide chemistry and structure [Baier et al., 1984; Swart et al., 1992]. Numerous studies have demonstrated that PC treatments produce a relatively contaminant-free surface with improved surface energy (wettability), but conflicting biologic results have been reported with these surfaces. Recent *in vitro* studies have demonstrated that these highly energetic surfaces do not necessarily improve cellular responses such as attachment and cell expression. This has been confirmed by *in vivo* studies which indicate that the overall histologic and ultrastructural morphology of the bone–implant interface is similar for plasma-cleaned and dry-heat-sterilized implant surfaces [Albrektsson et al., 1983]. Another promising technique for the sterilization of implant materials is the exposure of the implant surface to ultraviolet light [Singh and Schaff, 1989] or gamma irradiation [Keller et al., 1994]. Both these methods of sterilization produce a relatively contaminant-free thin oxide layer which fosters high levels of cell attachment [Keller et al., 1994] and inflammatory-free long-term *in vivo*

FIGURE 8.16 Light microscopic photomicrograph of a bone–smooth cpTi interface with intervening layer of soft connective tissue. This implant was mobile in the surgical site due to lack of tissue ingrowth. (Original magnification, 50×.)

responses [Hartman et al., 1989]. Currently, gamma irradiation procedures are widely used for the sterilization of metallic dental implant devices.

Metallic Corrosion

Throughout the history of the use of metals for biomedical implant applications, electrochemical corrosion with subsequent metal release has been problematic [Galante et al., 1991]. Of the biomedical metal systems available today, Ti and its major medical alloy, Ti-6A1-4V, are thought to be the most corrosion resistant; however, Ti metals are not totally inert *in vivo* [Woodman et al., 1984]. Release of Ti ions from Ti oxides can occur under relatively passive conditions [Ducheyne, 1988]. Whereas other factors such as positioning of the implant and subsequent biomechanical forces may play important roles in the overall tissue response to implants, it is not unreasonable to predict that electrochemical interactions between the implant surface and host tissue may affect the overall response of host bone [Blumenthal and Cosma, 1989]. For example, it has been shown by several groups [De Porter et al., 1986; Keller et al., 1987] that the percentages of intimate bony contact with the implant is inconsistent, at best, and generally averages approximately 50% over a 5-year period. Continued studies involving the effects of

FIGURE 8.17 Light microscopic photomicrograph of a bone–porous Ti alloy implant interface. Note significant bone ingrowth in open porosity at the apical end of the implant. (Original magnification, 10×.)

dissolution products on both local and systemic host responses are required in order to more fully understand the consequences of biologic interaction with metal implants.

Future Considerations for Implant Surfaces

It is clear that future efforts to improve the host tissue responses to implant materials will focus, in large part, on controlling cell and tissue responses at implant interfaces. This goal will require continued acquisition of fundamental knowledge of cell behavior and cell response to specific materials' characteristics. It is likely that a better understanding of the cellular-derived extracellular matrix–implant interface will offer a mechanism by which biologic response modifiers such as growth and attachment factors or hormones may be incorporated. Advancements of this type will likely shift the focus of future research from implant surfaces which as osseoconductive (permissive) to those which are osseoinductive (bioactive).

Defining Terms

Amorphous zone: A region of the tissue-implant interface immediately adjacent to the implant substrate. This zone is of variable thickness (usually <1000 Å), is free of collagen, and is comprised of proteoglycans of unknown composition.

Calcium phosphate: A family of calcium- and phosphate-containing materials of synthetic or natural origin which are utilized for implants and bone augmentation purposes. The most prominent materials are the tricalcium-phosphate- and hydroxyapatite-based materials, although most synthetic implants are a mixture of the various compositions.

Contact guidance: The theory by which cells attach to and migrate on substrates of specific microstructure and topographic orientation. The ability of the cell to attach and migrate on a substrate is related to the cytoskeletal and attachment molecules present on the cell membrane.

Junctional epithelium: The epithelial attachment mechanism which occurs with teeth and has been observed infrequently with implants by some researchers. Less than 10 cell layers thick, the hemidesmosomal attachments of the basal cells to the implant surface provide a mechanical attachment for epithelium and prevent bacterial penetration into the sulcular area.

Osseointegration: A term developed by P.I. Branemark and his colleagues indicating the ability of host bone tissues to form a functional, mechanically immobile interface with the implant. Originally described for titanium only, several other materials are capable of forming this interface, which presumes a lack of connective tissue (foreign body) layer.

Plasma spray: A high-temperature process by which calcium-phosphate-containing materials are coated onto a suitable implant substrate. Although the target material may be of high purity, the high-temperature softening process can dramatically affect and alter the resultant composition of the coating.

References

Albrektsson T, Branemark PI, Hansson HA et al. 1983. The interface zone of inorganic implants *in vivo:* titanium implants in bone. *Ann Biomed Eng* 11:1.

Albrektsson T, Hansson HA, Ivarsson B. 1985. Interface analysis of titanium and zirconium bone implants. *Biomaterials* 6:97.

Baier RE, Meyer AE, Natiella JR et al. 1984. Surface properties determine bioadhesive outcomes. *J Biomed Mater Res* 18:337.

Blumenthal NC, Cosma V. 1989. Inhibition of appetite formation by titanium and vanadium ions. *J Biomed Mater Res* 23(A1):13.

Bowers KT, Keller JC, Michaels CM et al. 1992. Optimization of surface micromorphology for enhanced osteoblast responses *in vitro*. *Int J Oral Maxillofac Implants* 7:302.

Branemark PI. 1983. Osseointegration and its experimental background. *J Pros Dent* 59(3):399.

Brunski JB. 1992. Biomechanical factors affecting the bone-dental implant interface. *Clin Mater* 10:153.

Chehroudi B, Ratkay J, Brunette DM. 1992. The role of implant surface geometry on mineralization *in vivo* and *in vitro*: a transmission and scanning electron microscopic study. *Cells Mater* 2(2):89–104.

Cook SD, Kay JF, Thomas KA et al. 1987. Interface mechanics and histology of titanium and hydroxyl-apatite coated titanium for dental implant applications. *Int J Oral Maxillofac Implants* 2(1):15.

Cook SD, Thomas KA, Kay JF. 1991. Experimental coating defects in hydroxylapatite coated implants. *Clin Orthop Rel Res* 265:280.

Davies JE, Lowenberg B, Shiga A. 1990. The bone-titanium interface *in vitro*. *J Biomed Mater Res* 24:1289–1306.

De Bruijn JD, Flach JS, deGroot K et al. 1993. Analysis of the bony interface with various types of hydroxyapatite *in vitro*. *Cells Mater* 3(2):115.

De Porter DA, Watson PA, Pilliar RM et al. 1986. A histological assessment of the initial healing response adjacent to porous-surfaced, titanium alloy dental implants in dogs. *J Dent Res* 65(8):1064.

Driskell TD, Spungenberg HD, Tennery VJ et al. 1973. Current status of high density alumina ceramic tooth roof structures. *J Dent Res* 52:123.

Ducheyne P. 1988. Titanium and calcium phosphate ceramic dental implants, surfaces, coatings and interfaces. *J Oral Implantol* 19(3):325.

Filiaggi MJ, Pilliar RM, Coombs NA. 1993. Post-plasma spraying heat treatment of the HA coating/Ti-6A1-4V implant system. *J Biomed Mater Res* 27:191.

Galante JO, Lemons J, Spector M et al. 1991. The biologic effects of implant materials. *J Orthop Res* 9:760.

Groessner-Schreiber B, Tuan RS. 1992. Enhanced extracellular matrix production and mineralization by osteoblasts cultured on titanium surfaces *in vitro*. *J Cell Sci* 101:209.

Hartman LC, Meenaghan MA, Schaaf NG et al. 1989. Effects of pretreatment sterilization and cleaning methods on materials properties and osseoinductivity of a threaded implant. *Int J Oral Maxillofac Implants* 4:11.

Herman H. 1988. Plasma spray deposition processes. *Mater Res Soc Bull* 13:60.

Jansen JA, van der Waerden JPCM, Wolke JGC. 1993. Histological and histomorphometrical evaluation of the bone reaction to three different titanium alloy and hydroxyapatite coated implants. *J Appl Biomater* 4:213.

Jarcho M, Kay JF, Gumaer KI et al. 1977. Tissue, cellular and subcellular events at a bone-ceramic hydroxylapatite interface. *J Bioeng* 1:79.

Jasty M, Rubash HE, Paiemont GD et al. 1992. Porous coated uncemented components in experimental total hip arthroplasty in dogs. *Clin Orthop Rel Res* 280:300.

Johansson CB, Lausman J, Ask M et al. 1989. Ultrastructural differences of the interface zone between bone and Ti-6Al-4V or commercially pure titanium. *J Biomed Eng* 11:3.

Katsikeris N, Listrom RD, Symington JM. 1987. Interface between titanium 6-A1-4V alloy implants and bone. *Int J Oral Maxillofac Surg* 16:473.

Kay JF. 1992. Calcium phosphate coatings for dental implants. *Dent Clinic N Amer* 36(1):1.

Keller JC, Lautenschlager EP. 1986. Metals and alloys. In A Von Recon (Ed.), *Handbook of Biomaterials Evaluation*, pp. 3–23, Macmillan, New York.

Keller JC, Young FA, Natiella JR. 1987. Quantitative bone remodeling resulting from the use of porous dental implants. *J Biomed Mater Res* 21:305.

Keller JC, Draughn RA, Wightman JP et al. 1990. Characterization of sterilized cp titanium implant surfaces. *Int J Oral Maxillofac Implants* 5:360.

Keller JC, Niederauer GG, Lacefield WR et al. 1992. Interaction of osteoblast-like cells with calcium phosphate ceramic materials. *Trans Acad Dent Mater* 5(3):107.

Keller JC, Stanford CM, Wightman JP et al. 1994. Characterization of titanium implant surfaces. III. *J Biomed Mater Res* 28(8):939.

Koeneman J, Lemons JE, Ducheyne P et al. 1990. Workshop of characterization of calcium phosphate materials. *J Appl Biomater* 1:79.

Lucas LC, Lemons JE, Lee J et al. 1987. *In vivo* corrosion characteristics of Co–Cr–Mu/Ti-6A1-4V-Ti alloys. In JE Lemons (Ed.), *Quantitative Characterization and Performance of Porous Alloys for Hard Tissue Applications*, pp. 124–136, ASTM, Philadelphia.

Maxian SH, Zawadsky JP, Durin MG. 1993. Mechanical and histological evaluation of amorphous calcium phosphate and poorly crystallized hydroxylapatite coatings on titanium implants. *J Biomed Mater Res* 27:717.

Meenaghan MA, Natiella JR, Moresi JC, et al. 1979. Tissue response to surface treated tantalum implants: preliminary observations in primates. *J Biomed Mater Res* 13:631.

Orr RD, de Bruijn JD, Davies JE. 1992. Scanning electron microscopy of the bone interface with titanium, titanium alloy and hydroxyapatite. *Cells Mater* 2(3):241.

Pilliar RM, DePorter DA, Watson PA et al. 1991. Dental implant design—effect on bone remodeling. *J Biomed Mater Res* 25:647.

Puleo DA, Holleran LA, Doremus RH et al. 1991. Osteoblast responses to orthopedic implant materials *in vitro*. *J Biomed Mater Res* 25:711.

Singh S, Schaaf NG. 1989. Dynamic sterilization of titanium implants with ultraviolet light. *Int J Oral Maxillofac Implants* 4:139.

Skalak R. 1985. Aspects of biomechanical considerations. In PI Branemark, G Zarb, T Albrektsson (Eds.), *Tissue Integrated Prostheses*, pp. 117–128, Quintessence, Chicago.

Smith DC. 1993. Dental implants: materials and design considerations. *Int J Prosth* 6(2):106.

Stanford CM, Keller JC. 1991. Osseointegration and matrix production at the implant surface. *CRC Crit Rev Oral Biol Med* 2:83.

Stanford CM, Keller JC, Solursh M. 1994. Bone cell expression on titanium surfaces is altered by sterilization treatments. *J Dent Res* 73(5):1061.

Steflik DE, McKinney RV, Koth DL et al. 1984. Biomaterial-tissue interface: a morphological study utilizing conventional and alternative ultrastructural modalities. *Scanning Electron Microscopy* 2:547.

Steflik DE, Sisk AL, Parr GR et al. 1993. Osteogenesis at the dental implant interface: high voltage electron microscopic and conventional transmission electric microscopic observations. *J Biomed Mater Res* 27:791.

Swart KM, Keller JC, Wightman JP et al. 1992. Short-term plasma cleaning treatments enhance *in vitro* osteoblast attachment to titanium. *J Oral Implant* 18(2):130.

Van Orden A. 1985. Corrosive response of the interface tissue to 316L stainless steel, Ti-based alloy and cobalt-based alloys. In R McKinney, JE Lemons (Eds.), *The Dental Implant*, pp. 1–25, PSG, Littleton.

Vezeau PJ, Keller JC, Koorbusch GF. 1991. Effects of multiple sterilization regimens on fibroblast attachment to titanium. *J Dent Res* 70:530.

Vrouwenvelder WCA, Groot CG, Groot K. 1993. Histological and biochemical evaluation of osteoblasts cultured on bioactive glass, hydroxylapatite, titanium alloy and stainless steel. *J Biomed Mater Res* 27:465–475.

Woodman JL, Jacobs JJ, Galante JO et al. 1984. Metal ion release from titanium-based prosthetic segmental replacements of long bones in baboons: a long-term study. *J Orthop Res* 1:421–430.

Young FA. 1988. Future directions in dental implant materials research. *J Dent Ed* 52(12):770.

9
Preservation Techniques for Biomaterials

Robin Coger

Massachusetts General Hospital,
Harvard University Medical
School, and the Shriners
Burn Institutes

Mehmet Toner

Massachusetts General Hospital,
Harvard University Medical
School, and the Shriners
Burn Institutes

Biomaterials—i.e., proteins, cells, tissues, and organs—are used daily to preserve life. Uses such as blood transfusions, artificial insemination, burn repair, transplantation, and pharmaceuticals rely on their availability. Natural materials, however, are labile and often deteriorate over time. To counter this effect, preservation procedures for retarding deterioration rates have been developed. Furthermore, since each biomaterial is characterized by unique compositional and physical complexities, a variety of storage techniques exists.

Table 9.1 lists examples of biomaterials that have been preserved successfully using various procedures. The list, although abbreviated, illustrates the wide range of cells, tissues, organs, and macromolecule structures that have been stored successfully and demonstrates how, in some cases (e.g., red blood cells), multiple preservation techniques may be appropriate. In the discussion that follows, four biomaterial storage procedures—nonfreezing, freeze–thaw, freeze-drying (lyophilization), and vitrification—are summarized. Nonfreezing techniques enable biomaterial storage by retarding metabolic processes and chemical reactions during cooling from physiologic to nonfreezing temperatures. With freeze-thaw techniques, the biomaterial is stored at low temperatures (usually less than –70°C) in crystalline form and then thawed for actual use. Lyophilized biomaterials are first frozen, then dehydrated by sublimation for storage at ambient temperature, and finally reconstituted for use. With vitrification, the biomaterials is cooled to subzero temperature in such a way that it is transformed to an amorphous solid for storage and then rewarmed for use. Each procedure—i.e., its applications and risks—will be described in more detail below. This discussion is not a comprehensive review but a general overview of the principles governing each of these four common biomaterial storage techniques.

9.1 Phase Behavior

As mentioned previously, biomaterials in their naturally occurring forms tend to deteriorate over time. Hence to achieve safe long-term storage, it is generally necessary to alter the physicochemical state of the biomaterial. One approach is to promote the transformation of the original substance to a form that can be stored safely and then, when needed, restored to its original state. These types of transformations can best be represented using phase diagrams.

0-8493-1491-7/03/$0.00+$.50
© 2003 by CRC Press LLC

TABLE 9.1 Some Examples of Biomaterials Stored
Using Various Storage Techniques

Nonfreezing	Liver
	Kidney
	Heart valves
	Protein solutions
Freeze–thaw	Red blood cells
	Cartilage
	Bone marrow
	Skin
Lyophilization (freeze-dry)	Red blood cells
	Platelets
	Penicillin
	Collagen
	Liposomes
Vitrification	Embryos
	Islets of Langerhans
	Corneal tissue
	Drosophila melanogaster

FIGURE 9.1 Phase diagram for a hypothetical solute additive. (Adapted from [Fahy et al., 1984].)

Figure 9.1 illustrates a temperature vs. concentration phase diagram, where concentration corresponds to the quantity of a hypothetical solute additive present in the solution. The diagram is particularly useful for describing phase transformations in which a thermodynamic phase of reduced energy nucleates within a parent phase. Crystallization is one example of this type of phase transformation and is a two-step process of nucleation of the new phase and its subsequent growth. If the formation of the new phase is catalyzed from the surface of foreign particles or a substrate, the growth process is triggered by heterogeneous nucleation (T_{HET}). If, however, the new phase develops from the clustering of individual water molecules, growth of the new phase occurs from homogeneous nucleation (T_{HOM}) [Hobbs, 1974]. The latter type of nucleation requires higher activation energies than heterogeneous nucleation and thus occurs at lower temperatures. Figure 9.1 also illustrates the relative positions of the melting (T_M) and the glass-transition (T_G) temperature curves. The melting-temperature curve shows the melting-point depression of a crystalline sample relative to solute concentration. The glass-transition curves signifies the temperatures for which a supercooled solution becomes glassy during cooling. The final curve in

Fig. 9.1 (T_D) demonstrates the devitrification temperature profile and illustrates the conditions for which a substance may experience crystallization damage during warming. For glasslike solids, damage is incurred as the glass transforms to a crystalline form at T_D, while for previously crystalline or partially vitrified solids, recrystallization (the coalescence of small crystals during warming) produces damage. The described elements of the phase diagram are relevant because all the biomaterial storage techniques described in this chapter involve either a phase transformation or its avoidance. Furthermore, if a phase transformation is improperly controlled, the effects can be detrimental to the biomaterial. Four techniques relevant to biomaterial storage are now described.

9.2 Nonfreezing Storage: Hypothermic

Given the high cost of organ transplantation, longer preservation times are urgently needed to make the procedure cost-effective [Evans, 1993] and expand the geographic area over which organs can be harvested and transplanted. Presently, hypothermic storage is the clinically employed organ preservation technique.

There are essentially two techniques for hypothermic preservation of organs for subsequent transplantation. The first is static cold storage by ice immersion at ~4°C—to reduce metabolism as much as possible without the formation of deleterious ice crystals [Belzer and Southard, 1988]. The second procedure is continuous cold machine perfusion at ~10°C to provide diminished metabolism and to remove deleterious end products [Southard and Belzer, 1988]. The perfusate used for static cold storage mimics the intracellular ionic composition of the organ and has impermeant solutes added to prevent cell swelling. However, for perfusion preservation techniques in general, modified plasma or solutions of plasma-like composition usually have been preferred. This is presumably due to the slightly higher temperatures used in perfusion techniques that permit some degree of metabolism to occur during storage.

In most practical instances, simple cold storage is the preservation mode of choice, since the storage time is only slightly increased by using continuous perfusion. Furthermore, the development of the University of Wisconsin (UW) solution has dramatically extended the preservation times. In the case of human liver, for example, the storage time increased from less than 10 to about 30 hours, thus alleviating the need for continuous-perfusion storage. As a result of extensive studies, it seems that lactobionate is an essential component of the UW solution, which is believed to act as an effective osmotic agent while suppressing cell swelling in metabolically depressed cells and tissues [Southard and Belzer, 1993].

Another nonfreezing technique that can be used to retard the chemical reaction rates of a biomaterial is undercooled storage. During undercooled storage, the biomaterial is exposed to subzero temperatures in the absence of deleterious ice crystal formation. Such a method may be particularly applicable to the medium-term (months) storage of proteins. Small droplets of aqueous-based solutions are dispersed in an inert oil phase, and the final preparation is then put into test tubes for freezer storage at $T \geq -20°C$. By keeping the quantity of aqueous droplets much greater than the number of heterogeneous nucleation sites in the bulk solution, one can effectively deter heterogeneous nucleation during storage. When needed, the dispersions are removed from the freezer and warmed to room temperature and reconstituted [Franks, 1988].

Unfortunately, a chief problem in using the undercooled storage technique in biochemical application lies in the scale-up of the procedure to the larger volumes needed for clinical and commercial applications. Furthermore, methods for "efficiently" separating the innocuous oil from the biomaterial are a problem that must be solved if the previously stored protein solutions are to be used in therapeutic applications. Apparently, it is also difficult to conduct all steps of the undercool procedure under sterile conditions [Franks, 1988].

9.3 Freeze–Thaw Technology

Freeze–thaw technology is the most commonly used method for storing cells and tissues; hence, it is an important cryopreservation methodology. When a transplantation emergency arises, the preserved biomaterial can be thawed and used to save lives. In addition, the development of cell and tissue transplantation procedures also benefits the growing field of tissue engineering—where frozen biomaterials are utilized in organ replacement devices (e.g., bioartificial liver) [Borel-Rinkes et al., 1992; Karlsson et al., 1993]. Even the simple cell, however, is thermophysically complex. Consequently, the design of feasible cryopreservation protocols must incorporate knowledge from biology, engineering, and medicine to be successful.

In 1949, Polge and coworkers made an important contribution to biomaterial preservation research. In work with sperm, they were the first to report the protective effects of additives or cryoprotectant agents (CPAs), i.e., glycerol, on biomaterials at low temperatures. The mechanisms by which CPAs protect cells from freeze injury are of fundamental importance but are, unfortunately poorly understood. There are four major protective actions of these compounds. First, CPAs act to stabilize the proteins of biomaterials under low-temperature conditions. Experimental evidence indicates that for cells, this effect results from the interaction of sugars with the polar head groups of phospholipids [McGann, 1978]. Recent thermodynamic analyses demonstrate that the preferential exclusion of CPAs from the protein hydration shell, at low temperatures, results in stabilization [Arakawa et al., 1990]. Second, CPAs lower the electrolyte concentration of the suspending medium of the cell at a given temperature by altering the phase relationship during cooling. Third, CPAs reduce the temperature at which cells undergo lethal intracellular ice formation. Fourth, CPAs promote the formation of the vitreous, rather than crystalline, phases inside the cell during cooling and help prevent intracellular ice formation (see Fig. 9.1) [Karlsson et al., 1994].

Unfortunately, the addition and removal of CPAs from the biomaterial introduce a separate set of problems. In the case of penetrating additives (i.e., dimethyl sulfoxide and glycerol), the permeability of the cell membrane is typically several orders of magnitude less than the permeability of the membrane to water [McGrath, 1988]. During the prefreeze addition of these compounds, the biomaterial recognizes the CPA as another extracellular solute. Hence the cell responds by initiating the rapid transport of water across the cell membrane and into the extracellular medium. Meanwhile, if the CPA is permeable, it gradually diffuses into the cell, thus contributing to the state of chemical nonequilibrium experienced by the cell. These transport processes continue (usually for minutes) until equilibrium is regained, at which time the volume of the biomaterial returns to normal. If the initial concentration of CPA is too large, the cell volume variations may be so severe that the biomaterial experiences osmotic stress damage. The reverse process, of cell swelling and the subsequent return to normal volume, is observed during the removal of CPAs. Osmotic injury from the addition or removal of penetrating compounds can be minimized by incrementally increasing or decreasing, respectively, their concentration.

Unfortunately, the benefits of using stepwise CPA addition and removal in reducing osmotic damage is counterbalanced by the increased risk of toxic damage to the biomaterial from longer exposure times [Fahy, 1986]. Also, in some cases, a single-step CPA removal process has been shown to be effective [Friedler et al., 1988]. The balance between these considerations can be optimized if both the permeability of the biomaterial to CPAs and the effects of the CPA on the biomaterial are known. Methodologies for measuring these critical parameters are discussed in McGrath [1988].

In the case of impermeable CPAs (i.e., polyvinylpyrrolidone, hydroxyethyl starch), the potentially injurious effects of exosmosis are also experienced. However, because impermeable CPAs remain in the extracellular medium, they are relatively easier to remove from the biomaterial than permeable additives. Their major disadvantage is believed to be their inability to afford direct protection to intracellular structures during freezing.

Figure 9.2 illustrates extrema observed when cooling biologic substances to subzero temperatures. To minimize cryoinjury, a suitable CPA is added to the biomaterial before the actual freeze-thaw protocol is begun. Cooling then proceeds at a controlled rate. As the material is cooled along the freezing path (Fig. 9.2), ice formation initiates first in the extracellular medium. This phase transformation is initiated either by external seeding or by heterogeneous nucleation from the walls of the container and is crucial because it corresponds to the initial temperature at which physicochemical changes occur within the biomaterial during cooling. The formation of extracellular ice results in a chemical potential gradient across the cell membrane that can be balanced by exosmosis of the intracellular water. If the freezing process occurs at slow cooling rates, the intracellular fluid has sufficient time to leave the cell. However,

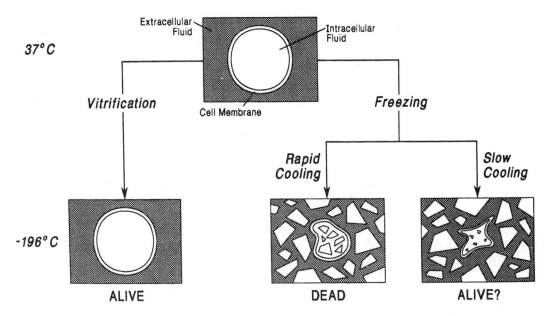

FIGURE 9.2 Schematic of the physicochemical processes experienced by cells during cryopreservation.

if excessive exosmosis occurs, the result is excessive cell dehydration and shrinkage and subsequent cell death from the high concentration of solutes remaining within the cell after water diffusion. If the freezing rate is rapid, however, water entrapped in the cell becomes supercooled. Then, at some subzero temperature, thermodynamic equilibrium is achieved through intracellular ice formation. Unfortunately, intracellular ice formation is usually associated with irreversible cell damage. Although the exact damage mechanism is not known, mechanical effects and high electrolyte concentrations caused by the crystal formation are believed to be major modes of cell damage [Mazur, 1984].

Figure 9.3 schematically illustrates the relationship between cell survival and cooling rate during a freeze-thaw protocol. As shown, cell damage at suboptimal cooling rates is predominantly caused by "solution" effects (e.g., exposure to high electrolyte concentrations, decreased unfrozen fractions, excessive dehydration), until a range of peak survival is obtained at the optimal cooling rate. Experimental evidence suggests that the optimal cooling rate for maximum cellular survival is the fastest rate that will not result in intracellular ice formation. Beyond this peak, cells are exposed to supraoptimal cooling conditions, in which damage from intracellular ice formation dominates.

Theoretical models have been developed to describe both the kinetics of water loss and the probability of intracellular ice formation [Mazur, 1984; Pitt, 1992; Muldrew and McGann, 1993]. The value of these models in designing effective freezing protocols for biomaterial preservation also has been demonstrated [e.g., Karlsson et al., 1993].

Once a cell or tissue sample has been frozen successfully, it can then be stored in liquid nitrogen in a −70°C freezer until needed. This step is usually not very crucial, since, as long as the freezer temperature is kept stable, storage does not cause cell damage.

The next challenge in freeze–thaw technology is to thaw the biomaterial using a warming protocol that minimizes the risk of recrystallization, or devitrification if applicable, and promotes high survival. The optimal thawing rate correlates directly with the rate at which the sample was cooled before storage. If the material was frozen slowly at a suboptimal rate (Fig. 9.3), a wide range of thawing rates usually can be utilized with negligible effects on survival. If the biomaterial experienced slightly supraoptimal cooling rates (Fig. 9.3), rapid thawing is almost exclusively required to avoid recrystallization of small intracellular ice crystals formed during the initial cooling step. The rapid thawing of volumes of appreciable size is particularly difficult because the thermal mass of the specimen dictates the warming rate that can be achieved.

FIGURE 9.3 A diagram illustrating the relationship between cell survival and cooling rate during a freeze–thaw protocol.

9.4 Freeze-Drying

Freeze-drying, or lyophilization, is a dehydration storage technique that is advantageous because it produces a final product that can be stored at suprazero temperatures and reconstituted with the addition of an appropriate solvent. The procedure is commonly applied to protein products (e.g., collagen, penicillin) and less frequently applied to cells (e.g., platelets, red blood cells) [Doebbler et al., 1966; Goodrich and Sowemimo-Coker, 1993]. Freeze-drying techniques also have been applied to liposomes—vesicles utilized in drug delivery systems that can trap water-soluble substances within their lumina. Lyophilization is a dual stage process that consists of rapidly cooling the liquid material to its solid form and subsequent drying (or removing) of the solidified solvent. The intricacies of the procedures employed directly influence the shelf life of the final dehydrated product. The drying stage of the process utilizes vacuum sublimation (transformation of a solid phase directly to the vapor phase) and may itself consist of multiple steps. The complexities of the drying procedure are determined by the continuity of the ice phase throughout the frozen specimen [MacKenzie, 1976]. Franks [1982] explains that the quality of the final lyophilized product partially depends on the freezing protocol experienced by the original sample, the size and distribution of the resultant ice crystals, the degree of heterogeneity, the presence or absence of amorphous regions, and the conditions imposed on the sample during drying. As one might expect, these factors can produce differentiations between the desired goals of the freeze-drying process and the actual final product.

The effects of the freezing protocol and the size and distribution of the resultant crystals are important for the reasons discussed previously. It should be mentioned that in the case of protein lyophilization, carbohydrates are often added for protection, while for cells, glycerol is a common lyoprotectant. The next two factors—the degree of heterogeneity and presence of amorphous regions—directly relate to the drying procedure. For simple cases in which large areas of ice (e.g., continuous channels) have formed in the sample, ice is removed by direct sublimation. However, for the more complex configurations commonly encountered with biomaterials, sublimation alone is inadequate because the ice crystal formation is discontinuous and amorphous regions are present. The amorphous regions correspond to pockets of water bound by freeze-concentrated solutes and biomaterial components (e.g., cell membranes). Water bound in this way serves to satisfy the hydration shell requirements of the specimen [Steinbrecht and Müller, 1987], hence contributing to the stabilization of the biomaterial. It is now recognized that the formation of amorphous regions is necessary for the successful lyophilization of biomaterials [Crowe et al., 1993a; Levine and Slade, 1992]. Since material destabilization is one source of damage during freeze-drying, this is an important area of lyophilization research.

Regardless of the complexity of the frozen matrix, biomaterial injury can occur during drying. Factors such as the effective drying temperature and the rate of drying are important in determining the degree of damage incurred. The drying step entails the removal of first the free water and then the bound water. However, the complete removal of this bound water during freeze-drying can be injurious to biomaterials and can promote protein denaturation and possibly aggregation into insoluble precipitates. Denaturation is the disruption of the folded structure of a protein and is affected by variables such as pH, surface interactions, and thermal and chemical changes [Darby and Creighton, 1993]. It is unfavorable because the final lyophilized product may no longer resemble the original biomaterial once denaturation occurs. Hence the avoidance of protein denaturation is crucial to effective biomaterial lyophilization. Investigations with liposomes and proteins reveal that the survival of biomaterials in the dry state is linked to the stabilizing influence of disaccharides (such as sucrose and trehalose) present in the system [Crowe et al., 1993b]. However, to minimize denaturation during freeze-drying protocols, lyoprotectants and CPAs should be used [Cleland et al., 1993]. It should be mentioned that the removal of these additives can be problematic in the large-scale industrial use of freeze-drying techniques.

Once a biomaterial has been lyophilized successfully, it is stored for future use. For the special case of protein storage—an area that is of particular interest to the pharmaceutical industry—the stability of the drug or protein must be guaranteed throughout a reasonable shelf life (the time period, measured in years, for which the drug maintains its original physical and functional properties). Two means of biomaterial destabilization during storage are the occurrence of oxidative and chemical reactions after lyophilization. Oxidation effects can be reduced by the exclusion of oxygen from containers of the dried materials and the use of antioxidants. The chemical reactions can be inhibited through the maintenance of low residual moisture levels [Cleland et al., 1993].

The final step, in the use of freeze-drying techniques for biomaterial storage, is the reconstitution of the lyophilized product. If pure water is used as the rehydration solvent, concentration gradients and osmotic imbalances can result in severe injury. To counter these effects, biomaterials are commonly rehydrated using isotonic solutions or media. The effects of using additives in the reconstituting solvent of biomaterials has recently been addressed. Apparently sugars are also effective in reducing damage during this rehydration step [Crowe et al., 1993b].

9.5 Vitrification

The hazards of ice crystal formation are significantly reduced by rapidly cooling the biomaterial to low temperatures at sufficient rates to produce an amorphous solid. This alternative, depicted in Fig. 9.2, was originally proposed in the 1930s and is called *vitrification* [Luyet, 1937; Goetz and Goetz, 1938]. Vitrification is the kinetic process by which a liquid solidifies into a glass. It requires the rapid cooling of the liquid to the glass-transition temperature T_G and is most easily achieved in high-viscosity liquids [Doremus, 1973]. The molecular configuration of the supercooled liquid ($T \geq T_G$) is the same as that of the glass ($T \leq T_G$). Hence, rapid cooling is necessary to prevent the supercooled liquid molecules from reorganizing into a regular (e.g., lattice) configuration. Vitrification is a second-order phase transition. Hence, by definition, the specific volumes of both phases (near T_G) are identical, although the thermodynamic property values (i.e., heat capacity, coefficient of thermal expansion) are not [Kauzmann, 1948].

The difficulty in successfully vitrifying a material lies in reaching its glass transition temperature T_G prior to crystal formation. Hence, reducing the distance between T_M and T_G by increasing the solute concentration (Fig. 9.1) increases the probability that a given liquid will form a glass. Two alternative ways to achieve glassy state are (1) to cool biomaterials at ultrarapid rates such that T_G is reached before nucleation can proceed and (2) to increase the pressure of the system such that the intersection of T_{HOM} and T_G (Fig. 9.1) occurs at lower CPA concentrations [Fahy et al., 1984; Kanno and Angell, 1977]. Since glass formation circumvents the deleterious effects of freeze injury during cooling, it is becoming an increasingly important biomaterial storage technique.

We have already mentioned the roles of viscosity and rapid cooling in vitrification. The more viscous a liquid, the slower it can be cooled to achieve its vitrified form. Fairly large cryoprotectant concentrations are necessary to obtain the vitrified form of aqueous solutions by slow cooling, and the requirement increases with specimen volume. This is undesirable, since high concentrations of CPAs are toxic to biomaterials. Hence, in practical applications of vitrification technology, a balance between the thermodynamic conditions necessary to achieve vitrification and the physicochemical conditions suitable for survival is crucial.

The most common difficulty encountered in attempts to vitrify biologic materials is their susceptibility to ice crystal formation. As mentioned previously, the larger the sample volume, the higher the CPA concentration necessary to reduce the probability of crystallization [Coger et al., 1990]. *Drosophila melanogaster* cells, corneal tissue, and pancreatic islets of Langerhans are three examples of biomaterials that have been vitrified successfully [Steponkus et al., 1990; Bourne, 1986; Jutte et al., 1987]. Of these, only *D. melanogaster* has not been preserved previously by the freeze–thaw technique. In fact, the freeze–thaw technique remains the chief method of cells storage. For many cell and tissue types, the appropriate combination of effective temperature, cryoprotectant concentration, and cooling and warming rate conditions necessary for their vitrification have yet to be determined. For long-term organ storage, the freeze–thaw technique is not an alternative, because the mechanical stress and toxic damage that the organ would incur during freezing would be lethal [Bernard et al., 1988; Fahy et al., 1984]. Organ vitrification attempts, although unsuccessful, have demonstrated that the CPA toxicity limitation is especially evident in organ preservation such that toxic death prevention is an unavoidable challenge in organ vitrification [Fahy, 1986]. With respect to cooling rate, the relatively large volumes of organs require the use of slow cooling protocols to ensure a uniform thermal history throughout the total volume. Organs therefore require high-pressure, high-cryoprotectant concentrations and slow cooling conditions to achieve the vitreous state.

Once a biomaterial has been vitrified successfully, it must be stored at temperatures below T_G (Fig. 9.1) to encourage stability. When restoring the sample to physiologic conditions, special care must be taken to avoid crystallization during the warming protocol. Crystallization under these circumstances, termed *devitrification*, is possible (or even probable) since at temperatures greater than T_G the crystalline phase is more stable than the amorphous solid. If such a transformation occurs, cryoinjury is unavoidable. The probability of devitrification is significantly reduced by warming the biomaterial at rates equivalent to those imposed during the original cooling [Fahy, 1988; MacFarlane et al., 1992]. The use of vitrification as a biomaterial storage technique is an ongoing and important area of cryopreservation research. Presently, it is the only apparent solution for the long-term storage of organs.

9.6 Summary

Biomaterial storage is an exciting research area whose advances are of value to a variety of fields, including medicine, biologic research, and drug design. However, the compositional and physical complexities of the various biosubstances (e.g., proteins, cells, tissues, and organs) require the development of specialized preservation procedures. In the present discussion, four stage techniques—nonfreezing, freeze–thaw, lyophilization, and vitrification—and their relevance to specific biomaterial examples have been reviewed. Although there have been definite advances, important challenges still remain for future investigations.

Defining Terms

Cryopreservation: Techniques utilized to store cells, tissues, and organs under subzero conditions for future use in clinical applications.

Cryoprotectant: Chemical additive used to protect biomaterials during cooling to low temperatures by reducing freezing injury.

Devitrification: Crystallization of an amorphous substance during warming.

Freeze-drying: Dehydration of a sample by vacuum sublimation.

Lyoprotectant: Expedients added to lyophilization formulations to protect the biomaterial from the damaging effects of the process.

Recrystallization: The coalescence of small ice crystals during warming.

Shelf life: Length of time in which the stability of the components of a biomaterial (e.g., pharmaceutical drugs) is guaranteed during storage.

Vitrification: Solidification process in which an amorphous (glasslike) solid, devoid of crystals, is formed.

References

Arakawa T, Carpenter JF, Kita YA, Crowe JH. 1990. The basis for toxicity of certain cryoprotectants: a hypothesis. *Cryobiology* 27:401.

Belzer FO, Southard JH. 1988. Principles of solid-organ preservation by cold storage. *Transplantation* 45:673.

Bernard A, McGrath JJ, Fuller BJ et al. 1988. Osmotic response to oocytes using a microscope diffusion chamber: a preliminary study comparing murine and human ova. *Cryobiology* 25:945.

Borel-Rinkes IHM, Toner M, Tompkins RG, Yarmush ML. 1993. Long-term functional recovery of hepatocytes after cryopreservation in a three-dimensional culture configuration. *Cell Transplant* 1:281.

Bourne WM. 1986. Clinical and experimental aspects of corneal cryopreservation. *Cryobiology* 23:88.

Cleland JL, Powell MF, Shire SJ. 1993. The development of stable protein formulations: a close look at protein aggregation, deamidation, and oxidation. In S Bruck (Ed), *Crit Rev Ther Drug Carrier Syst* 10:307.

Coger R, Rubinsky B, Pegg DE. 1990. Dependence of probability of vitrification on time and volume. *Cryo-Letters* 11:359.

Crowe JH, Crowe LM, Carpenter JF. 1993a. Preserving dry biomaterials: the water replacement hypothesis, part 1. *Biopharm* 6:28.

Crowe JH, Crowe LM, Carpenter JF. 1993b. Preserving dry biomaterials: the water replacement hypothesis, part 2. *Biopharm* 6:40.

Darby NJ, Creighton TE. 1993. *Protein Structure*. Oxford University Press, Oxford.

Doebbler FG, Rowe AW, Rinfret AP. 1966. Freezing of mammalian blood and its constituents. In HT Meryman (Ed), *Cryobiology*, pp. 407–450. Academic Press, London.

Doremus RH. 1973. *Glass Science*. Wiley, New York.

Evans RW. 1993. A cost-outcome analysis of retransplantation the need for accountability. *Transplant Rev* 7:163.

Fahy GM. 1988. Vitrification. In JJ McGrath, KR Diller (Eds), *Low Temperature Biotechnology*, Vols. 10 and 98, pp. 113–146. ASME, New York.

Fahy GM. 1986. The relevance of cryoprotectant "toxicity" to cryobiology. *Cryobiology* 23:1.

Fahy GM, MacFarlane DR, Angell CA, Meryman HT. 1984. Vitrification as an approach to cryopreservation. *Cryobiology* 21:407.

Franks F. 1988. Storage in the undercooled state. In JJ McGrath, KR Diller (Eds), *Low Temperature Biotechnology*, Vols. 10 and 98, pp. 107–112. ASME, New York.

Franks F. 1982. The properties of aqueous solutions at subzero temperatures. In F Franks (Ed), *Water: A Comprehensive Treatise*, Vol. 7, pp. 215–338. Plenum Press, New York.

Friedler S, Giudice L, Lamb E. 1988. Cryopreservation of embryos and ova. *Fertil Steril* 49:473.

Goetz A, Goetz SS. 1938. Vitrification and crystallization of organic cells at low temperatures. *J Appl Physiol* 9:718.

Goodrich RP, Sowemimo-Coker SO. 1993. Freeze drying of red blood cells. In PL Steponkus (Ed), *Advances in Low-Temperature Biology*, Vol. 2, pp. 53–99. JAI Press, London.

Hobbs PV. 1974. *Ice Physics*. Oxford, Oxford University Press.

Jutte NHPM, Heyse P, Jansen HG et al. 1987. Vitrification of human islets of Langerhans. *Cryobiology* 24:403.

Kanno H, Angell CA. 1977. Homogenous nucleation and glass formation in aqueous alkali halide solutions at high pressure. *J Phys Chem* 81(26):2639.

Karlsson JOM, Cravalho EG, Borel-Rinkes IHM et al. 1993. Nucleation and growth of ice crystals inside cultured hepatocytes during freezing in the presence of dimethyl sulfoxide. *Biophys J* 65:2524.

Karlsson JOM, Cravalho EG, Toner M. 1994. A model of diffusion-limited ice growth inside biological cells during freezing. *J Appl Physiol* 75:4442.

Kauzmann W. 1948. The nature of the glassy state and the behavior of liquids at low temperatures. *Chem Rev.* 43:219.

Levine H, Slade L. 1992. Another view of trehalose for drying and stabilizing biological materials. *Biopharm* 5:36.

Luyet B. 1937. The vitrification of organic colloids and of protoplasm. *Biodynamica* 1:1.

MacFarlane DR, Forsyth M, Barton CA. 1992. Vitrification and devitrification in cryopreservation. In PL Steponkus (Ed), *Advances in Low Temperature Biology*, Vol. 1, pp. 221–278. London, JAI Press.

MacKenzie AP. 1976. Principles of freeze-drying. *Transplant Proc* 8(suppl 1):181.

Mazur P. 1984. Freezing of living cells: mechanisms and implications. *Am J Physiol* 143:C125.

McGann LE. 1978. Differing actions of penetrating and nonpenetrating cryoprotective agents. *Cryobiology* 15:382.

McGrath JJ. 1988. Membrane transport properties. In JJ McGrath, KR Diller (Eds), *Low Temperature Biotechnology*, Vols. 10 and 98, pp. 273–330. New York, ASME.

Muldrew K, McGann LE. 1994. The osmotic rupture hypothesis of intracellular freezing injury. *Biophys J* 66:532.

Pitt RE. 1992. Thermodynamics and intracellular ice formation. In PL Steponkus (Ed), *Advances in Low-Temperature Biology*, Vol. 1, pp. 63–99. JAI Press, London.

Polge C, Smith AU, Parkes AS. 1949. Revival of spermatozoa after vitrification and dehydration at low temperatures. *Nature* 164:666.

Rall WP, Mazur P, McGrath JJ. 1983. Depression of the ice-nucleation temperature of rapidly cooled mouse embryos by glycerol and dimethyl sulfoxide. *Biophys J* 41:1.

Southard JH, Belzer FO. 1993. The University of Wisconsin organ preservation solution: components, comparisons, and modifications. *Transplant Rev* 7:176.

Southard JH, Belzer FO. 1988. Kidney preservation by perfusion. In GJ Cerilli (Ed), *Organ Transplantation and Replacement*, pp. 296–311. Lippincott, Philadelphia.

Steponkus PL, Myers SP, Lynch DV et al. 1990. Cryopreservation of *Drosophila melanogaster* embryos. *Nature* 345:170.

Steinbrecht RA, Muller M. 1987. Freeze substitution and freeze-drying. In RA Steinbrecht, K Zierold (Eds), *Cryotechniques in Biological Electron Microscopy*, pp. 149–172. Springer-Verlag, Berlin.

Further Information

In addition to the review works cited throughout the text, the following publications also may be of interest.

For more detailed information concerning lyophilization, as applied specifically to proteins, see "The development of stable protein formulations: a close look at protein aggregation, deamidation, and oxidation," by Cleland et al., an especially helpful article (*Crit. Rev. Ther. Drug Carrier Syst.* 10:307, 1993).

A good introduction to the fields of cryobiology and cryopreservation is presented in *The Clinical Applications of Cryobiology*, by B. J. Fuller and B. W. W. Grout (CRC Press, Boca Raton, FL, 1991). For review work relevant to vitrification and organ preservation, *The Biophysics of Organ Cryopreservation*, edited by D. E. Pegg and A. M. Karow, Jr. (Plenum Press, New York, 1987) should be consulted.

For additional information on the physicochemical processes encountered during cooling of biomaterials, refer to Korber's 1988 review (*Q. Rev. Biophys.* 21:229). For an overview of bioheat transfer processes, refer to Diller's review in *Bioengineering Heat Transfer* 22:157, 1992. For additional information on the fundamental principles of intracellular ice formation, consult the 1993 review by Toner (pp. 1–51 in *Advances in Low Temperature Biology*, Vol. 2, edited by P. L. Steponkus, JAI Press, London).

10

Hip Joint Prosthesis Fixation: Problems and Possible Solutions

Joon B. Park

The University of Iowa

Total hip joint replacement (THR) has been very successful mainly due to the introduction of bone cement for the fixation by Dr. John Charnley on the advice of Dr. Dennis Smith in the late 1950s [Charnley, 1970; Charnley, 1972; Charnley and Cupic, 1973; Eftekhar, 1978; Wroblewski, 1986]. One of the inherent problems of orthopedic joint prosthesis implantation is the fixation and maintenance of a stable interface between the device and the host tissue at the cellular and organ levels [Crowninshield, 1988; Ducheyne, 1988; Park, 1992; Park, 1995]. The fixation can be classified into several categories as given in Table 10.1. Basically, the hip joint can be considered as three parts: (1) *acetabular cup*, (2) *cup–femoral head–articulating surface*, and (3) *femoral stem* (Fig. 10.1). The problems and possible solutions related to each of the three parts will be examined.

Most frequent fixation problems are related to (1) *infection*, (2) *wear and wear particulate*, (3) *migration and failure* of implants, and (4) *loosening* of which the "long-term loosening" of the implant is especially important [Ducheyne, 1988; Park, 1992]. These problems manifest into *osteolysis* in the bone bed which is the major cause of long-term loosening mostly for the femoral stem [Anthony et al., 1990; Harris, 1995; Maloney et al., 1990; Maloney and Smith, 1995]. Some major factors related to (late) loosening are (1) mismatch of the physical properties between tissues and implant, (2) biocompatibility of the implant, (3) deterioration of physical properties of implant materials, (4) surgical techniques, (5) design of the implant, (6) selection of patients, and (7) post surgical care, etc. [Amstutz et al., 1976; Carlsson et al., 1983; Crowninshield, 1988; Dowd et al., 1995; Gruen et al., 1979; Harris and McGann, 1984; Havelin et al., 1995; Lu et al., 1993; Mohler et al., 1995; Mulroy and Harris, 1990; Nilsen and Wiig, 1996; Riegels-Nielsen et al., 1995; Stromberg et al., 1996]. In this review, recently reported clinical cases based on the large studies will be examined, especially the Norwegian Arthroplasty Register, which will shed some light on the *cemented vs. uncemented fixation* of the total hip arthroplasty. This is mainly due to the fact that the individuals reporting and their clinical results could be widely varied and biased.

Variables related to the total (hip) joint replacement are (1) materials (Table 10.2), (2) design, and (3) fixation method (Table 10.3). One should keep in mind that any particular type of prosthesis is made to have a particular fixation method, e.g., the Charnley prosthesis is designed to be used with bone

TABLE 10.1 Summary of Various Methods of Prosthesis Fixation

Methods of Fixation	Examples
1. Mechanical fixation	
a. Active—use of screws, bolts, nuts, wires, etc.	Pre-Charnley implants [Williams and Roaf, 1973]
b. Passive—interference fit and noninterference fit	[Moore, 1952; Mittlemeier, 1975, 1976]
2. Bone cement fixation	
a. Pure cement	[Charnley, 1970; 1972]
b. Modified cement—composite cement	[Dai et al., 1991; Henrich et al., 1993]; resorbable particle impregnated cement [Liu et al., 1987; Park et al., 1986]
3. Biological fixation	
a. Porous ingrowth	[Klawitter and Hulbert, 1972; Sauer et al., 1974; Hirshhorn et al., 1972; Homsy et al., 1972; Smith, 1963]
b. Modified porous ingrowth—electrical and pulsed electromagnetic field (PEMF) stimulation	[Park, 1983; Park and Kenner, 1975; Weinstein et al., 1976]
4. Direct (chemical) bonding fixation	
a. Osteogenic/inductive-glass-ceramics	[Blencke et al., 1978; Hench and Paschall, 1973]
b. Osteoconductive hydroxyapatite	[de Groot, 1983; Kay, 1988]

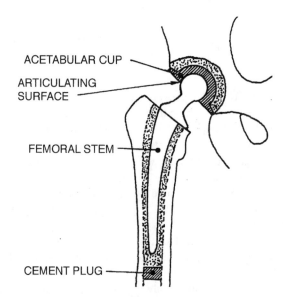

ACETABULAR CUP

ARTICULATING
SURFACE

FEMORAL STEM

CEMENT PLUG

FIGURE 10.1 Schematic diagram showing the three important areas of THR.

cement at both the cup and femoral prosthesis sites while some were designed to be used as uncemented such as the BIAS® femoral stem prosthesis [Onsten et al., 1995]. Also, sometimes the outcome of the THR may depend on the type of bone cement used: (1) low vs. high viscosity, (2) plain vs. antibiotics-impregnated, and (3) low vs. high heat of polymerization cement, etc. A more mitigating problem is that the outcome of the THR could not be clearly attributed to any one specific factor; e.g., the *osteolysis* may be due to the particulates which are due to wear and corrosion products which in turn could be initiated between the articulating surfaces or between the metal backing and polyethylene. However, the critical stage may be reached due to the *accelerated rate* of particulate production due to the *loosening* of the implant, which causes a larger and unnatural motion of the articulation. Once the lysis starts, the cycle becomes more vicious—further aggravating the situation.

The design and fixation related variables are summarized in Table 10.3. It is not that uncommon to find that a prosthesis designed for uncemented fixation is used with cement, making the outcome study more complicated.

TABLE 10.2 Physical Properties of Materials Used for Joint Prosthesis and Bone

Materials	Young's Modulus (GPa)	UTS[a] (MPa)	Elongation (%)	Density (g/cm³)
Metals				
316L S.S. (wrought)	200	1000	9	7.9
CoCrMo (cast)	230	660	8	8.3
CoNiCrMo (wrought)	230	1800	8	9.2
Ti6Al4V	110	900	10	4.5
Ceramics				
Alumina (Al_2O_3, polycrystalline)	400	260	<0.1[b]	3.9
Glass-ceramic (Bioglass®)	200	200	~0.1[b]	2.5[b]
Calcium Phosphate (Dense Hydroxyapatite)	120	200	~0.1[b]	3.2
Polymers				
PMMA[c](Solid)	3	65	5	1.18
PMMA Bone Cement	2	30	3	1.1
UHMW[d] Polyethylene	1	30	200	0.94
Polysulfone	2.5	70	50	1.24
Silicone Rubber	<0.01	6	>350	1.12
Fibers and wires				
Aramid (Kevlar)	130	2700	2	1.45
Carbon	400	2500	1	2
Nylon	5	500	10	1.07
Steel (piano wire)	200	2450	1.2	7.8
Bone				
Femur (compact), long axis	17	130	3	2.0
Femur (compact), tangential	12	60	1	2.0
Spongy bone	0.1	2	2.5	1.0

[a] UTS: ultimate tensile strength, for ceramics the Young's modulus and UTS are for the flexural modulus and bending strength, respectively.

[b] Estimated values.

[c] PMMA: poly(methylmethacrylate)

[d] UHMW: ultra high molecular weight (>2×10^6 g/mole)

Source: Park and Lakes [1992].

TABLE 10.3 List of Design and Fixation Related Variables in THR

Part	Materials Used	Fixation Methods
Cup	All PE	Cemented
	Metal-backed	Uncemented (mechanical)
	Porous-coated	Uncemented (mechanical)
	Screw-holed	Uncemented (mechanical)
	All ceramic	Cemented/uncemented
Articulating surfaces	PE/metal	
	PE/ceramic	
	Ceramic/ceramic	
	Metal/metal	
Femoral stem	Metal	Cemented/uncemented
	Composite	Uncemented
	Smooth	Threaded(rare)
	Textured	Uncemented
	Porous-coated	Uncemented
	PMMA-coated	Cemented
	HA-coated	Uncemented
Head	Metal	Fixed
	Ceramic	Rotated (trunnion/modular)

PE: Polyethylene (ultra high molecular weight).

10.1   Acetabular Cup

The advent of the uncemented acetabular cup necessitated the metal backing of the polyethylene liner although some use all polyethylene without cement [Ritter, 1995]. Due to the relatively new advocacy of the so-called "hybrid" THR, where the femoral prosthesis is cemented and the cup is uncemented, there are fewer cases of comparing the outcome of the cemented vs. uncemented acetabular cup performance. Havelin et al. compared 11 of the most widely used *uncemented* cups (4352 cases) [Havelin et al., 1995]. After 5 years, the overall cumulative revision rate was 3.2% but increased drastically to 7.1% after 6 years with large differences among the designs. Hydroxyapatite and porous (metal) coated cups had a failure rate of less than 0.1%. It is interesting that all polyethylene cups had a cumulative revision rate of 14% while threaded uncoated metal-backed cups varied from 0% (PM® cups) to 21% (Ti-Fit®) after 6 years. They concluded that the coating of the surface is the most important factor for the uncemented cups for the first 6 years of implantation. As is the case with all tissue ingrowth fixation, the most important factor for short-term results with uncemented cups is the immediate stability and possibility for the tissue ingrowth. They also concluded:

> It remains to be seen if the results with some uncemented cups, in some groups of patients, are better than for the best-cemented. Until more is known about their long-term results, uncemented acetabular components should be used as part of randomized trials.

Of course, the performance of the acetabular cup may be closely interrelated to the femoral stem. However, Havelin's study could not detect any outstanding difference with different combinations of the cup and femoral stem.

Espehaug et al. studied 12,179 hip prostheses comparing 10 different brands reported to the Norwegian Arthroplasty Register during 1987–1993 [Espehaug et al., 1995]. The overall revision rate after 5 years was 2.5% while the Charnley prosthesis was 2.9%. Elite cup and Charnley stem combination resulted in much poorer performance (9.84% after 5 years). However, other combinations gave better results. The main cause of revision was aseptic loosening after 5 years (1.8%) followed by infection (0.5% after 5 years). In conclusion, they

> ...observed good overall results of cemented hip prostheses. However, clinically important differences in revision rates were demonstrated among the various cemented total hip prosthesis brands.

Some studied the aseptic loosening of the *cemented* cups and concluded that the mechanism of late loosening is biological (osteolysis) not mechanical, which is the opposite of the femoral stem [Harris, 1995; Schmalzried et al., 1992]. Therefore, the *metal-backed* cup which is designed to reduce the stresses in the bone-bone cement interface would be ineffective. Some clinical studies showed that the all polyethylene cup performed better than the metal-backed cemented cups [Dall et al., 1993; Harris and Penenberg, 1987; Ritter, 1995; Ritter et al., 1990].

Malchau and Herberts reported revision and re-revision rates in THR in Sweden. The reasons for revision were similar to the Norwegian study (Table 10.4), and are as follows: (1) aseptic loosening, which was the major factor (72.3%); (2) infection (7.2%); (3) fracture (4.7%); and (4) dislocation (4.2%), etc. [Malchau and Herberts, 1998]. The loosening of metal-backed and

TABLE 10.4   Reason for Revision of THR in Sweden

Reason	Number	Percent (%)
Aseptic loosening	6965	72.3
Primary deep infection	690	7.2
Fracture only	4.7	—
Dislocation	403	4.2
Two-stage procedure	386	4.0
Technical error	372	3.9
Implant fracture	161	1.7
Secondary infection	94	1.0
Pain	37	0.4
Polyethylene wear	26	0.3
Miscellaneous	33	0.3
Missing	13	0.1
Total	9634	100.0

Source: Malchau and Herberts [1998].

all-polyethylene acetabular cups were compared. Mixed results were obtained, where in one design the all-poly was clearly better, while in others both performed equally well. One would be tempted to advocate the use of all-poly since it is a lot less costly (1/2 to 1/3) and equal or better in clinical performance compared to the metal-backed acetabular cup.

Basically, the Charnley type all polyethylene cup has been the "gold standard" for long-term clinical results. The metal-backed, either cemented or uncemented polyethylene lined acetabular cup is still considered as experimental until long-term follow-up studies (more than 10 years) become available [Malchau and Herberts, 1998]. Also, the benefits of biological fixation due to the lack of long-term follow-up studies are inconclusive at this time, although some designs gave promising results. Other variations such as flanged vs. unflanged, elevated vs. conventional cups, etc., should be proven clinically through long-term trials although the flanged cup performed better in one analysis [Wroblewski, 1993].

In our laboratory we have been developing polymethylmethacrylate pre-coated acetabular cups and tibial plateau of the total knee replacement (TKR) for cemented fixation [Dowd et al., 1995; Gruen et al., 1979; Harris and McGann, 1984; Havelin et al.] It is very difficult to adhere bone cement to the surface of ultra-high-molecular-weight polyethylene (UHMWPE) with PMMA bone cement. Therefore, the acetabular cup is deeply grooved to make a mechanical bonding and thus causes a weak implant. The UHMWPE surface is treated with xylene, polymethylmethacrylate, and a methylmethacrylate monomer for chemical bonding between the two polymers. Preliminary results show that the interface tensile strength between the UHMWPE and bone cement resulted in about 10 MPa which is about one third of the tensile strength of bone cement and UHMWPE [Kang, 1998; Kang and Park, 1998; Park and Lakes, 1992]. Recent studies on the UHMWPE powders treated with the methylmethacrylate (MMA) monomers without the use of xylene showed a high degree of adhesion after sintering at a high temperature (165°C) and pressure (77.4 MPa) [Park and Park, 1998]. Increased interfacial tensile strength by further treating the MMA treated powders with "PMMA + MMA" and "PMMA + MMA + BPO" is evidenced as shown in Table 10.5. The sintering of UHMWPE with a mold is one way of making an acetabular cup and tibial plateau; therefore, the latest results open the possibility of making a graded composite structure of the UHMWPE implants from pure PE articulating surface to the pure PMMA surface to which the acrylic bone cement can be attached directly via chemical bonding as shown in Fig. 10.2 [Park, 1998]. It is also possible to sinter UHMWPE powers which were cross-linked, which also showed improved wear properties [Gul et al.; Marrs et al., 1998; McKellop et al., 1998; Oonishi et al., 1998]. Glow discharge technique could be used for the high and low density polyethylene if one chooses to use this material for the cup as was the case for the early (before the mid-1980s, HDPE) Charnley prostheses [Foerch et al., 1994; Khang et al., 1996]. However, the interfacial strength is not as high as the present values with the UHMWPE.

TABLE 10.5 The Tensile Strength for Molded and Original Specimens (Park, 1998)

Sintered Layers	Sintering Temperature (°C)	PE Powder Treatments	Group	Interfacial Strength (MPa)
PMMA rod/PMMA	165	MMA only	165M	2.1 ± 1.6
Powder/treated PE		MMA+MMA/PMMA	165PM	10.6 ± 3.6
Powder/PMMA		MMA+MMA/PMMA+BPO	165PMB	17.7 ± 2.53
Powder/PMMA rod				
PE rod/PE powder/treated PE	145	MMA+MMA/PMMA+BPO	145PMB	12.4 ± 1.67
Powder/PE powder/PE rod	165	MMA+MMA/PMMA+BPO	165PMB	14.95 ± 0.85
	185	MMA+MMA/PMMA+BPO	185PMB	22.6 ± 1.26
PE rod/pure PE powder/PE rod	205	MMA+MMA/PMMA+BPO	205PMB	22.8 ± 2.5
PMMA rod	205	—	205PE	32.5 ± 1.20
PE rod	—	—	PMMA	75.9 ± 1.00
	—	—	UHMWPE	36.9 ± 1.90

FIGURE 10.2 Schematic diagram showing the graded UHMWPE and PMMA for better fixation and wear [Park, 1998].

10.2 Femoral Stem

Cemented and Uncemented Fixation

The design of the femoral stem also involves the articulating surface with the acetabular cup which could be a more important factor for the longevity of the stem function. The fixation of the stem is largely divided into two categories, i.e., *cemented* and *uncemented*. The uncemented can be classified into interference fit and porous-coated for tissue ingrowth fixation. The porous-coated type can be further coated with a hydroxyapatite layer to aid tissue ingrowth.

A large study involving 14,009 cases of cemented and 1326 uncemented total hip arthroplasties were reported [Havelin et al., 1994]. It was found that the cumulative revision rate for the cemented hip was 2.7% after 4.5 years and 6.5% for the uncemented. For the cup, it was 0.6% for the cemented and 1.7% for the uncemented, and for the femoral components 1.7% and 3.9% after 4.5 years. The results for the uncemented prostheses were less favorable in young patients. In men and women under 60 the revision rates were 6 and 3% for the uncemented and cemented respectively. There were large variations in performance among the individual designs of the uncemented prostheses. However, the early results warrant further clinical trials for the uncemented implants. Malchau and Herberts reported revision and re-revision rates in THR in a large Swedish population consisting of 148,359 people. The reasons for revision were similar to the Norwegian study (Table 10.4): (1) aseptic loosening was the major factor (72.3%), (2) infection (7.2%), (3) fracture (4.7%), and (4) dislocation (4.2%), etc. [Malchau and Herberts, 1998]. The survival at 17 years (1979–1986) was 81.8% and at 9 years (1987–1996) was 95.5% for the cemented implants. The survival at 13 years (1979–1986) was 68.9% and at 9 years (1987–1996) was 87.2% for the uncemented implants [Malchau and Herberts, 1998]. Again the results show a definitively better surgical outcome where cements were used regardless of the various factors involved, such as types of implants, materials, patients, etc.

Using less stiff materials and filling the bone cavity with a custom-designed prosthesis has not met researchers' expectations [Lombardi et al., 1995; Morscher, 1995]. It is believed that the bone reacts to the presence of implants as if they are part of the supporting member of the body weight. Thus, the filling of the femoral cavity would cause a greatly different behavior of the bone since the prosthesis alters the stress pattern completely. Incorporation of the bony tissue into the interstices of pores would also alter the stress pattern of the femur. This also complicates the situation. Any stiff material contacting the surface of the bone will cause *bone density change* due to the altered stress pattern and bone lysis due largely to the particulate generated at the articulating surface between the acetabular cup and femoral head [Maloney et al., 1990; Maloney and Smith, 1995]. Most of the osteolysis is located in the distal and proximal end of the prosthesis. The osteolysis can be accelerated by the aseptic loosening of the implants, which in turn causes the accelerated wear of the UHMWPE cup. The initial mode of failure of the femoral prosthesis is the debonding of the stem/bone cement interface followed by osteolysis at the distal end of the stem where the particulate may accumulate by gravity [Jasty et al., 1991].

It is interesting to note that the firm fixation of the porous and hydroxyapatite coated implants cause a great deal of difficulties during revision surgery, sometimes necessitating cutting of the femora [Bhamra et al., 1996]. This result creates the Catch-22 dilemma for the fixation of implants—to have a stable implant, it should be firmly embedded into the intramedullary cavity, but when it fails one should be able to remove it easily.

Possible Solutions for Cemented Fixation

There are many studies concerning the loosening of the femoral stem of the hip joint replacement but very few facts have been elucidated with respect to the loosening [Amstutz et al., 1976; Carlsson et al., 1983; Crowninshield et al., 1980; Fowler et al., 1988; Harris, 1992; Hedley et al., 1979; Jasty et al., 1991]. For instance, some believe that the strengthening of bone cement may not be beneficial to the enhancement of fixation due to the unfavorable stress distribution [Crowninshield et al., 1980; Crugnola et al., 1979]. On the other hand, the bone cement is the weakest link between bone and prosthesis. Failure of the bone cement itself and interface loosening between cement and stem may be large contributing factors toward the failure of the fixation of the prosthesis [Amstutz et al., 1976; Carlsson et al., 1983; Harris, 1992; Lu et al., 1993; Wykman et al., 1991]. Recent reports on the failure rate of the Boneloc® bone cement implanted prostheses alarmed the European orthopedic community and it was abandoned [Riegels-Nielsen et al., 1995]. The Boneloc® bone cement was designed to give less exothermic heat of polymerization but its mechanical properties were compromised [Thanner et al., 1995; Wykman et al., 1991].

Cement–Prosthesis Interface

Bone cement fixation creates two interfaces: (1) cement–bone and (2) cement–implant. According to an earlier report [Amstutz et al., 1976] the incidence of loosening for the femoral prostheses were evenly divided at about 10 and 11% for cement–bone and cement–implant interfaces, respectively. Jasty et al. reported that the initiation of loosening of the cemented femoral components originates from the prosthesis–cement interface, especially the pores trapped between them [Jasty et al., 1991]. The cement–implant interface loosening can be minimized by "pre-coating" with bone cement or poly-methylmethacrylate polymer [Ahmed et al., 1984; Barb et al., 1982; Park, 1983; Park et al., 1982; Park et al., 1978; Raab et al., 1982]. Pre-coating can achieve a good bonding between the "cement" and prosthesis during the manufacturing process. During surgery, the fresh cement adheres well to the pre-coated cement [Park et al., 1978; Park et al., 1979].

Mohler et al. reported early loosening of the femoral component at the cement–prosthesis interface after 1941 THRs performed between 1980 and 1990 [Mohler et al., 1995]. They analyzed 29 failed hips (27 patients). The femoral stems were matte finished; 20 were PMMA-precoated and 9 were not pre-coated. Initiation of debonding took place in zone 1 of Gruen between cement and prosthesis followed by progressive loosening with maintenance of the bone-cement interface. Extensive osteolysis took place after debonding in many hips (20/29). The average time for revision between the onset of the symptoms after surgery was 9 months. The authors attributed the progressive loosening to the stem geometry (a cylindrical shape, distal to the proximal cobra shape) and matted surface finish. The cylindrical shape allowed the rotation of the prosthesis, permitting the matte-finished surface to grind the bone cement. This results in loosening and osteolysis. It is also not likely that the PMMA-coating would help to avoid rotation of the prosthesis since it is only applied in the proximal region and the resistance to rotation is greatly compromised by the cylindrical shaped stem. Shear strength of the PMMA bone cement is about 1/3 of the tensile strength. Therefore, if the bone cement is subjected to shear, such as rotation of the stem, the cement will not be able to resist the load. It has been suggested that the stem should be more square with a smooth surface finish.

Malchau and Herberts reported inconclusive results on the question of the matte or polished finish on the survival of the implants [Malchau and Herberts, 1998]. It would be reasonable to assume that the matte finish may hold the implants better initially due to the larger surface area but may act to grind the bone cement when the implant becomes loose.

The high strains or stresses on the cement at the tip of the prosthesis are strong indications that this location is a likely site for the initial event of failure [O'Connor et al., 1991]. Others reported that high strains at the proximal and distal tip of the prosthesis appeared to cause debonding between the stem and cement and was associated with radial crack initiation at the debonded surface of the pores in the cement surrounding the areas of debonding [Harrigan et al., 1992]. These radial cracks seemed to be due to stress changes secondary to debonding.

There has been some discussion on the merits of smooth vs. rough finish on the femoral stem surface with regard to the finish's effect on the longevity of the implant [Harris, 1992; Ling, 1992]. Recent studies show that the effect of the surface roughness may depend on the effectiveness of the load transfer from cement to the stem as shown in Fig. 10.3. The smooth surface will generate local stress peaks in the cement

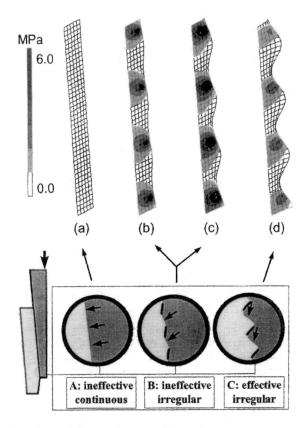

FIGURE 10.3   Illustration of the von Mises stress patterns in the cement mantle from smooth to the rough surface finish (right) and corresponding axial load transfer effectiveness [Verdonschot and Huiskes, 1998].

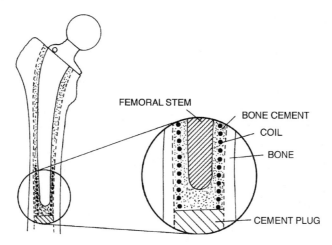

FIGURE 10.4   Illustration of the reinforcement of the bone cement around the prosthesis to resist radial and hoop stress on the cement mantle by incorporating a wire coil conforming to the contours of the femoral stem which can be placed during surgery or prefabricated during manufacturing of the implant [Kim et al., 1994].

mantle as well as ineffective load transfer. The ineffective (rough) irregular surface which has shallow profiles will be ineffective in axial load transfer and will act as a stress inducer. The effective load transfer profile will have deeper surface irregularity as shown in Fig. 10.3c [Verdonschot and Huiskes, 1998].

The cement–prosthesis interface strength could be enhanced by placing reinforcing material around the stem to resist the radial and hoop stress caused by body loading [Park, 1993]. It is also critical that the cement is reinforced to counteract the hoop stress and to some extent the radial stress created by the prosthesis when it is loaded [Ahmed et al., 1984; Mann et al., 1991]. Therefore, a coil or mesh of wire conforming to the contours of the prosthesis could be placed prior to bone cement injection during surgery as shown in Fig. 10.4. It could also be pre-fabricated around the prosthesis. Also, some advocate the use of a mesh reinforcement around the prosthesis which can be fixed with fresh bone cement at the time of surgery. This mesh reinforcement is similar to the coil but is more difficult to incorporate [Davidson, 1988; Willert et al., 1991]. The simple wire coil would resist the hoop stress developed by the prosthesis, which in turn will decrease the stress on the bone cement beyond the wire coil toward the bone.

Changes to the mechanical property of the bone cement by reinforcing the cement with a wire coil in a simulated stem loading condition has been tried [Kim and Park, 1994] instead of the traditional reinforcement of adding wires, fibers, etc. to the bone cement [Saha and Pal, 1984]. The coils were made from 20 gage 302/304 stainless steel wire and were very effective counteracting the static radial and hoop stress as given in Table 10.6. The magnitude of the ultimate load of the control specimens (3.70 ± 1.13 kN) is similar to the ones obtained by Mann et al. (~32 kN), whose specimen was 8 times longer [Mann et al., 1991]. If one extrapolates the ultimate load of the wire reinforced specimens to that of Mann's work (which is closer to the *in vivo* condition) the load to fracture would be about 72 kN, well above the normal loading on the prosthesis even in dynamic loading (6~8 times body weight; 4 kN) [Paul, 1976]. The percentage increases of improvements in mechanical properties are similar or higher than

TABLE 10.6   Summary of the Static Mechanical Property Measurements

Specimen Type	Maximum Strain (%)	Maximum Load (kN)	Stiffness (GNm/m)	Toughness (Nm/m)
Control	2.6 ± 0.5	3.70 ± 1.13	1.73 ± 0.39	49.33 ± 18.63
Wire reinforced	3.2 ± 0.9	7.68 ± 2.33	4.17 ± 1.16	129.48 ± 65.3
Change (%)	+22.7	+107.6	+141.0	+162.5

Source: Kim and Park [1994].

other studies although the increases are not as high as predicted by the composite theory [Taitsman and Saha, 1977; Topoleski et al., 1990].

The fatigue test showed a substantial increase in its cyclic load to failure by the wire coil specimens [Kim and Park, 1996]. It is believed that the beneficial effects of the wire (fiber) layer lie in its ability to inhibit the propagation of fatigue cracks [Manley and Stern, 1985; Manley et al., 1987]. At high stress levels in the cement mantle, fatigue cracks could initiate from defects such as air bubbles and surface discontinuities, and propagate gradually over a large number of load cycles. The presence of the fiber or wire coil increases the energy necessary for crack propagation by crack tip blunting, crack deflection, and the bridging of cracks by intact fibers [Taylor, 1987; Taylor et al., 1989].

Another observation gained from fatigue testing was a subsidence of the stem. The subsidence is due to the creep of the viscoelastic materials such as bone and bone cement [Park and Lakes, 1992]. The net effect from the creep would be a continued subsidence of the implant shortening the leg [Kim and Park, 1996; Manley et al., 1987].

All measured mechanical properties show that the wire coil reinforcement significantly enhanced the strength, fracture strain, stiffness, and toughness over the control [Kim and Park, 1996]. The most significant increases were in the toughness, indicating that the coil reinforced cement mantle will resist the load much more than the non-reinforced control. This may result in a prolonged fixation life of the prosthesis, which is the ultimate goal of all arthroplasties.

Cement–Bone Interface

The problems at the bone–cement interface cannot be easily overcome since these problems arise from the intrinsic properties of the bone cement as well as extrinsic factors such as cementing technique, condition of the bone surface, etc. The toxicity of the monomer, inherent weakness of the cement as a material due to the unavoidable inclusion of the pores (Table 10.7), and blood and tissue debris mixed during surgery can contribute to the problem of loosening at the bone–cement interface [Park, 1983].

The bone–cement interface strength may be enhanced by growing bone into the cement after fixation. Bone cement can be used for immediate fixation yet provides tissue ingrowth space later by incorporating resorbable particles (such as inorganic bone particles) as shown conceptually in Fig. 10.5. Some studies [Dai et al., 1991; Henrich et al., 1993; Liu et al., 1987; Park et al., 1986] indicate that the concept can be used effectively, at least in rabbit and canine models [Kwon et al., 1997]. In one study the bone-particle impregnated bone cement was used to fix femoral stem prostheses in the femora of dogs (one side was experimental, the other was control) and after a pre-determined time period, the femora were harvested and sectioned into disks for the push-out test to measure the interfacial strength between the bone and cement interface [Dai et al., 1991]. The results as shown in Fig. 10.6 indicate that the experimental side increased in strength for up to five months while the control side decreased slightly. The histology also showed the integration of tissues into the spaces of the dissolved particles. Of course, care should be taken to control the amount of particles to balance out the increased viscosity and decreased strength. Table 10.7 illustrates the relationship between the amount of resorbable particle (inorganic bone particles,

TABLE 10.7   Effect of Inorganic Bone Particle Mixed with Acrylic Bone Cement on the Pore Size, Porosity, and Tensile Strength

Particle Amount (%)	Pore Size (μm)	Porosity (%)	Tensile Strength (MPa)
0	154.7 ± 72	7.2 ± 2.5	23.2 ± 2.3
10	160.6 ± 68	5.0 ± 1.7[a]	22.6 ± 2.0[a]
20	172.9 ± 52[a]	4.9 ± 1.5[a]	20.1 ± 1.1[a]
30	218.0 ± 92[a]	2.4 ± 0.7[a]	19.7 ± 1.1[a]

Note: 15 specimens for each group.
[a] Statistically significant vs. control ($p < 0.05$).
Source: Kim et al. [1994].

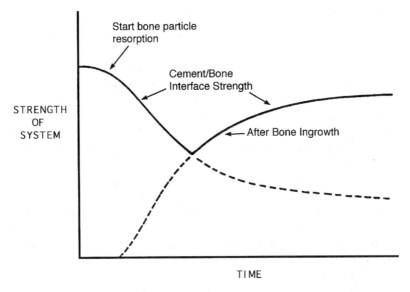

FIGURE 10.5 Basic concept of the bone cement with resorbable particle fixation. Immediate fixation is achieved as in the ordinary bone cement with the enhanced biological fixation to be achieved later for a prolonged stabilization of the implant [Park, 1992 and 1995].

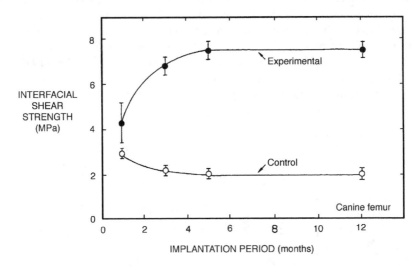

FIGURE 10.6 Maximum interfacial shear strength between bone and bone cement vs. implant period when the femoral stems were implanted with ordinary bone cement and cement with bone particles. In both cases the interfacial strength was stabilized after 5 months for this canine model [Dai et al., 1991].

100–300 μm) and the porosity and pore size [Kim et al., 1994]. As more particles are incorporated onto the bone cement, a lesser amount of porosity resulted, however, the average pore size increased. The tensile strength decreased with an increased amount of bone particles. Fatigue properties improved with higher particle inclusion; however, it was found that about 30% (by weight) of bone particles can provide sufficient interconnected porosity for bony ingrowth and yet give reasonable compromises to other parameters [Liu et al., 1987]. The bone-particle impregnated bone cement has been used clinically but its long-term success remains to be proven since it has been only 5 years without any failures [Dai, 1991 and 1996].

Uncemented Fixation

Efforts to develop a viable interface between the tissue and implants have been made ever since Moore designed a femoral prosthesis which had a fenestrated large hole in the proximal region [Moore, 1952]. Ironically, the fixation itself is by the passive mechanical fixation technique as discussed earlier. Smith [1963] tried to develop a bone substitute with porous aluminate ceramic impregnated with an epoxy resin called Cerocium®. Although the material demonstrated a good adherence to the tissues, the pore size (average 18 μm in diameter) was too small to allow any bony tissue ingrowth. Later, ceramics [Klawitter and Hulbert, 1972; Oonishi et al., 1989; Predecki et al., 1972], metals [Hirshhorn et al., 1972; Niles and Lapitsky, 1975], and polymers [Sauer et al., 1974] were used to test the ingrowth idea. Basically, any biocompatible material will allow bony tissues to grow into any space large enough to accommodate osteons. However, to be continuously *viable* the space must be large enough (more than 75 μm in diameter for the bony tissues) and contiguous to the surface of bone matrix [Heimke, 1990]. In addition, Wolff's law dictates that the ingrown tissues should be subjected to bodily loading in order to prevent resorption, even after the initial ingrowth has taken place. The same principle also makes it difficult to have a uniform tissue ingrowth throughout the implant surface. This is the reason why the tissue ingrowth takes place where the stress transfer occurs, e.g., in the distal lateral region of the femoral stem of the artificial hip joint.

Figure 10.7 shows the general trends of the fixation (interfacial) strength variation with implantation period in animals to be up to six months for metallic implants (Co–Cr alloys, Ti and its alloys, and stainless steel). A few observations can be made from this data. First, the maximum interfacial shear strength between bone and porous implant peaked at about 12 to 13 MPa in about 6 to 8 weeks regardless of the implant material, animal type, or location of the implants (i.e., cortical or cancellous bone and transcortical or intramedullary canal). Second, the data are widely scattered. (The original data showed wide variations, therefore, they are not distinguished among the variables). The *decrease* in interfacial strength with time after the peak for the metallic implants is somewhat distressing since this may also be true with human patients. This may be caused by two factors. The first is that of bone resorption from the initially ingrown area due to the stress shielding. The second is the release of a large number of metal ions due to the increased surface area by making the implant porous. Porous polymers did not

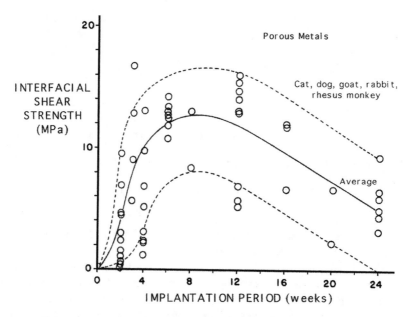

FIGURE 10.7   Maximum interfacial shear strength between bone and porous metal implants vs. implant of various metals and animals, data from [Spector, 1982].

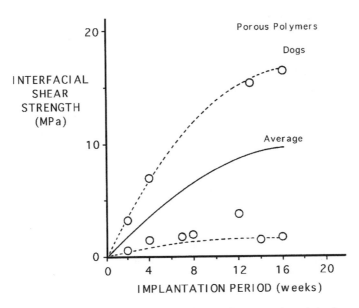

FIGURE 10.8 Maximum interfacial shear strength between bone and porous polymeric implants vs. implant. [Data from Spector, 1982].

have the decreasing trends as shown in Fig. 10.8 [Spector, 1982]. This may be interpreted as the lack of stress shielding (after bone is ingrown into the pores) due to the low modulus of the polymers. However, there are not enough data available to come to a definitive conclusion [Keet and Runne, 1989; Sadr and Arden, 1987; Spector, 1982; Tullos et al., 1984].

Further problems with biological fixation are: (1) the unforgiving nature of the surgery, (2) the long immobilization time for tissue ingrowth, (3) the unpredictable time to ambulate, (4) the difficulty in eradicating infection, and (5) once the interface is destroyed by an accidental overloading, it cannot be regrown with certainty. Moreover, the porous coating may weaken the underlying prosthesis itself and, in case of metals, there is an increased danger of corrosion fatigue due to the increased surface area [Brand, 1987; Morscher, 1984]. Due to these problems and clinical results of porous fixation some investigators have insisted that the bone cement fixation technique is still the gold standard at this time [Johnston, 1987; Wroblewski, 1993].

In order to alleviate these problems several modifications have been attempted.

Pre-Coating the Metallic Porous Surface with Ceramics or Carbons

This method has been tried with limited success [Cranin et al., 1972; Thomas et al., 1985]. The problems of coating deep in the pores and the thermal expansion difference between the metal and ceramic materials both make a uniform and good adherent coating very difficult. An attractive material for coating is hydroxyapatite $[Ca_{10}(PO_4)_6(OH)_2]$ ceramic which is similar to bone mineral. It is not yet conclusive that this material is more beneficial than other ceramics. Some preliminary studies in our laboratory indicate that during the early period of fixation the bioactive hydroxyapatite coating may be more beneficial, but the effect may diminish after 3 weeks, as shown in Fig. 10.9. The result is for the simple cortical bone plug experiment performed on canine femora [Park, 1988]. Others have shown promising results with the same material system used on rabbits instead of canines as in our study [Oonishi et al., 1989].

Pre-Coating with Porous Polymeric Materials on Metal Stem

Theoretically, this method has two distinct advantages over the ceramics or carbon coating methods discussed above [Keet and Runne, 1989; Sadr and Arden, 1987; Spector, 1982; Tullos et al., 1984; Homsy et al., 1972]. First, the low modulus polymeric material could transfer the load from the implant to the

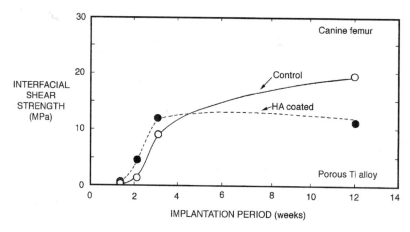

FIGURE 10.9   Maximum interfacial shear strength between bone and bioactive ceramic coated porous plug implants vs. implant period when the plugs with and without (control) coating were implanted in the cortices of canine femora [Park, 1988].

bone more gradually and evenly and thus prevent stress-shielding effects on the ingrown tissues. Second, this method would prevent the metallic-surface ion release, i.e., less corrosion of the metal. One major problem with this technique is the weak interfacial strength between the polymer and metallic stem, especially in dynamic loading conditions *in vivo*.

Enhancement of Porous Ingrowth with Electrical or Electromagnetic Stimulation

This technique combines the porous ingrowth with the stimulating effects of electrical and/or electro-magnetic stimulation [Park and Kenner, 1975; Weinstein et al., 1976]. Direct current stimulation can indeed accelerate tissue ingrowth in the early stages of healing but its effect diminishes over time [Weinstein et al., 1976]. Direct current stimulation has one distinct problem: the invasive nature of the power source. The pulsed electromagnetic field stimulation is a better method since the stimulation can be carried out extracorporeally.

Porous Ingrowth with the Use of Filling Materials

There has been some effort to use filling materials around the porous implant since it is very difficult to prepare the tissue bed with the exact shape of the prosthesis to eliminate the micro-motion of the prosthesis after implantation. Bone matrix proteins (BMP) or demineralized bone and hydroxyapatite crystals can be used for this purpose [Parsons et al., 1987]. The success of this technique has not been fully documented.

Some glass-ceramics tend to achieve *direct bonding* with the bone through a selective dissolution of the surface film [Blencke et al., 1978; Hench and Paschall, 1973; Yamamuro et al., 1990]. Some researchers have reported a direct bonding of tissues to hydroxyapatites [Geesink et al., 1987; Kay, 1988]. It has been difficult to coat a metallic surface with these materials due to the large difference in the thermal expansion coefficient between the coating and base materials although dip-coating can be utilized [West et al., 1990]. The glass-ceramics have not been used to make load bearing implants due to their brittleness.

10.3   Articulating Surface of the Acetabular Cup and Femoral Head

Any articulating joint will involve the friction and wear of the two opposing members. Ever since the total joint replacement has been practiced this subject gave the orthopedic community pause and posed a considerable problem to the biomedical engineers due to the fact that any material or design can avoid this subject. The lowest friction coefficient material such as polytetrafluoroethylene (PTFE), best known as Teflon®, is not sufficient as a member of a joint as it was proved to be disastrous by Dr. J. Charnley. Earlier than Charnley, the all metal-metal combinations were used but abandoned. Some researchers advocate it again [Bohler, 1995; Muller, 1995] claiming that smaller head design resulted in drastically reduced wear after 10 years of implantation (60, 1330, and 2100 μm for CoCrMo/CoCrMo, Al_2O_3/UHM-WPE, and CoCrNo/UHMWPE, respectively). Saikko reported wear of the UHMWPE cup and five different Al_2O_3 ceramic head combinations and found a vastly different wear volume with a different femoral head design and stem fit [Saikko, 1995]. The head on these implants was attached to the Ti-alloy stem by taper-fit. The wear particles from the ceramic and head resulted in severe third-body abrasive wear (3170 mg) compared to minimal wear of others (5.3 to 124 mg) after 26 million cycles. Obviously there was a loosening between the head and the stem collar of the femoral implant for the worst case (Protek®) since others had similar taper-fit. In this respect, the trunnion design of the head and stem should be avoided at all possible costs to eliminate the possibility of third-body wear. Modularity of the head of the femoral stem is sound in principle since it could reduce inventory while providing the surgeons with versatility. The full benefits of such flexibility have not been realized in actual usage. Third body wear of the acetabular cup, increased chance of corrosion, and less than optimal design (although the optimal design remains elusive) contribute to the problem of the modularity [Chmell et al., 1995; Jacobs et al., 1995; Salvati et al., 1995].

Similar problems of third-body wear exist for the cemented polyethylene acetabular cup and metal-baked (porous coated) cup. PMMA bone cement particles were found in autopsies for the cemented cups. Ritter [1995] analyzed uncemented metal-backed vs. a cemented polyethylene cups and found statistically significant better clinical performance of the cemented cup in terms of the linear wear (0.05 vs. 0.11 mm/yr). There were also differences in the wear between *machined* and *molded* cups, indicating that the molding resulted in better polyethylene powder consolidation than the raw material used in the machine from rod stocks.

It is also now widely recognized that gamma radiation causes the polyethylene to lose its original chemical and mechanical properties due to the oxidation about 1 mm below the surface after about three years of implantation [Li et al., 1995; Sutula et al., 1995]. This increases the density by crystallization but causes brittleness of the material. Increased localized wear could result. Inert or vacuum sterilization may minimize the problem unless the sterilization method is changed.

Conclusions

In summary, the wear of the articulating surface in a complex phenomenon like THR could be minimized by having the most consolidated polyethylene (molded) as a cup material with a small femoral head (either ceramic or metal) cemented with bone cement. Although some advocate the use of "hybrid" fixation techniques, i.e., cemented stem and uncemented cup, the final verdict is not yet in. A metal-backed polyethylene lined cup would cause more problems, either cemented or uncemented, due to the increased complexity and decreased shock absorbing capacity of the cup during walking. The same is true with modularity of the femoral stem and head.

It is strongly recommended that all nations follow the example of the Norwegian Arthroplasty Register in obtaining meaningful outcome data of all implantations. Thus, the clinical performance of a particular implant could be determined and disasters like the Boneloc® bone cement and Christianson prosthesis could be avoided more quickly [Linder, 1995].

Orthopedic surgeons often suggest that the fixation of implants should not be too strong since it would be difficult to remove, should it become necessary to have a revision arthroplasty to restore its function. The two requirements could be mutually exclusive since the interface must be strong enough to hold the prosthesis *in vivo* but not so strong that it may impair any remedial measures.

The assessment of success or failure of the prosthesis fixation could be quite difficult clinically as demonstrated by some researchers. For example, some [Ling, 1992] contend that the relative motion between the implant and bone cement and subsidence of the prosthesis are not a direct cause of failure of arthroplasties while others consider it a failure [Harris, 1992].

Another problem is related to the more frequent use of the implants for younger patients, which requires firmer fixation and longer implant life [Park et al., 1995]. The original expectation of uncemented porous ingrowth fixation for the young is tempered somewhat and we need to explore a longer lasting method of fixation.

Acknowledgments

This work was partially funded by the Biomaterials Research Fund and the University of Iowa Research Foundation. A major part of this chapter was presented originally as a paper at the International Symposium on Biomaterials and Drug Delivery Systems held at the Korea Research Institute of Chemical Technology in Taejon, Korea, July 4–5, 1996.

References

Ahmed, A. M., Raab, S., and Miller, J. E. (1984). Metal/cement interface strength in cemented stem fixation. *J. Orthop. Res.* 2, 105–118.

Amstutz, H. C., Markolf, K. L., McNeices, G. M., and Gruen, T. A. W. (1987). Loosening of total hip components: cause and prevention. In: *The Hip*, R. A. Brand, Ed. (St. Louis: Mosby), 102–116.

Anthony, P. P., Gie, G. A., Howie, C. R., and Ling, R. S. M. (1990). Localised endosteal bone lysis in relation to the femoral components of cemented total hip arthroplasties. *J. Bone Joint Surg.* 72B, 971–979.

Barb, W., Park, J. B., von Recum, A. F., and Kenner, G. H. (1982). Intramedullary fixation of artificial hip joints with bone cement precoated implants: I. Interfacial strengths. *J. Biomed. Mater. Res.* 16, 447–458.

Bhamra, M., Rao, G. S., and Robson, M. (1996). Hydroxyapatite-coated hip prostheses: difficulties with revision in four cases. *Acta Orthop. Scand.* 67, 49–52.

Blencke, B. A., Bromer, H., and Deutscher, K. K. (1978). Compatibility and long-term stability of glass ceramic implants. *J. Biomed. Mater. Res.* 12, 307–316.

Bohler, N. (1995). Metal/metal articulating interfaces. *Orthoped.* 18, 879–880.

Brand, R. A. (1987). *The Hip: Non-Cemented Hip Implants* (St. Louis: Mosby).

Carlsson, A. S., Gentz, C. F., and Lindberg, H. O. (1983). Thirty-two noninfected total hip arthroplasties revised due to stem loosening. *Clin. Orthop. Rel. Res.* 181, 196–203.

Charnley, J. (1970). *Acrylic Cement in Orthopaedic Surgery* (Edinburgh: Churchill Livingstone).

Charnley, J. (1972). The long-term results of low-friction arthroplasty of the hip, performed as a primary intervention. *J. Bone Joint Surg.* 54B, 61–76.

Charnley, J. and Cupic, Z. (1973). The nine and ten year results of the low-friction arthroplasty of the hip. *Clin. Orthop. Rel. Res.* 95, 9–25.

Chmell, M. J., Rispler, D., and Poss, R. (1995). The impact of modularity in total hip arthroplasty. *Clin. Orthop. Rel. Res.* 319, 77–84.

Cranin, A. N., Schnitman, P. A., Rabkin, M., Dennison, T., and Onesto, E. J. (1972). Alumina and zirconia coated Vitallium oral endosteal implants. *J. Biomed. Mater. Res. Symp. No. 6*, 257–262.

Crowninshield, R. (1988). An overview of prosthetic materials for fixation. *Clin. Orthop. Rel. Res.* 235, 166–172.

Crowninshield, R. D., Brand, R. A., Johnston, R. C., and Milroy, J. C. (1980). An analysis of femoral component stem design in total hip arthroplasty. *J. Bone Joint Surg.* 62A, 68–78.

Crugnola, A., Ellis, E. J., Radin, E. L., and Rose, R. M. (1979). A second generation of acrylic cements. *Trans. Soc. Biomater.* 3, 91.

Dai, K. R. (1991 and 1996). Personal communications.

Dai, K. R., Liu, Y. K., Park, J. B., and Zhang, Z. K. (1991). Bone particle impregnated bone cement: an *in vivo* weight-bearing study. *J. Biomed. Mater. Res.* 25, 141–156.

Dall, D. M., Learmonth, I. D., Solomon, M., and Davenport, M. (1993). 811 Charnley hips followed for 3–17 years. *Acta Orthop. Scand.* 64, 252–256.

Davidson, J. A. (1988). Bone cement reinforcement and method. U.S. Patent No. 4,735,625.

de Groot, K. (1983). *Bioceramics of Calcium Phosphate* (Boca Raton, FL: CRC Press).

Dowd, J. E., Schwendeman, L., Macaulay, W., Doyle, J. S., Shanbhag, A. S., Wilson, S., Herndon, J. H., and Rubash, H. E. (1995). Aseptic loosening in uncemented total hip arthroplasty in a canine model. *Clin. Orthop. Rel. Res.* 319, 106–121.

Ducheyne, P. (1988). Prosthesis fixation for orthopedics. In: *Encyclopedia of Medical Devices and Instrumentation,* J. G. Webster, Ed. (New York: Wiley-Interscience), 2146–2154.

Eftekhar, N. S. (1978). *Principles of Total Hip Arthroplasty* (St. Louis: Mosby).

Espehaug, B., Havelin, L. I., Engesaeter, L. B., Vollset, S. E., and Langeland, N. (1995). Early revision among 12,179 prostheses: a comparison of ten different brands reported to the Norwegian arthroplasty register, 1987–1993. *Acta Orthop. Scand.* 66, 487–493.

Foerch, R., Kill, G., and Walzak, M. (1994). Plasma surface modification of polymers. In: *Plasma Surface Modification of Polyethylene: Short-Term vs. Long-Term Plasma Treatment,* M. Strobel, C. Lyons, and K. L. Mittal, Eds. (Utrecht, the Netherlands: VSP Press), 99–111.

Fowler, J. L., Gie, G. A., Lee, A. J. C., and Ling, R. S. M. (1988). Experience with Exeter total hip replacement since 1970. *Orthop. Clin. N. Am.* 19, 477–489.

Geesink, R. G., de Groot, K., and Klein, C. (1987). Chemical implant fixation using hydroxyaptite coatings. *Clinic. Orthop. Rel. Res.* 226, 147–170.

Gruen, T. S., McNeice, G. M., and Amstutz, H. A. (1979). "Modes of failure" of cemented stem-type femoral components. *Clin. Orthop. Rel. Res.* 141, 17–27.

Gul, R. M., Muratoglu, O. K., McGarry, F. J., Bragdon, C. R., Jasty, M., and Harris, W. H. (1998). The effect of the peroxide content on the cross-link density, mechanical properties, and wear behavior of UHMWPE. In: *Orthop Res. Soc.* (New Orleans, LA), 99.

Harrigan, T. P., Kareh, J. A., O'Connor, D. O., Burke, D. W., and Harris, W. H. (1992). A finite element study of the initiation of failure of fixation in cemented femoral total hip components. *J. Orthop. Res.* 10, 134–144.

Harris, W. H. (1992). Is it advantageous to strengthen the cement-metal interface and use a collar for cemented femoral components of total hip replacements? *Clin. Orthop. Rel. Res.* 285, 67–72.

Harris, W. H. (1995). The problem is osteolysis. *Clin. Orthop. Rel. Res.* 311, 46–53.

Harris, W. H. and McGann, W. A. (1984). Loosening of the femoral component after use of the medullary-plug cementing technique. *J. Bone Joint Surg.* 67B, 222–224.

Harris, W. H. and Penenberg, B. L. (1987). Further follow-up on socket fixation using a metal-backed acetabular component for total hip replacement. A minimum ten year follow-up study. *J. Bone Joint Surg.* 69A, 1140–1143.

Havelin, L. I., Espehaug, B., Vollset, S. E., and Engesaeter, L. B. (1994). Early failures among 14,009 cemented and 1,326 uncemented prostheses for primary coarthrosis: The Norwegian Arthroplasty Register, 1987–1992. *Acta Orthop. Scand.* 65, 1–6.

Havelin, L. I., Vollset, S. E., and Engesaeter, L. B. (1995). Revision for aseptic loosening of uncemented cups in 4,352 primary total hip prostheses: a report from the Norwegian arthroplasty register, 1987–1993. *Acta Orthop. Scand.* 66, 494–500.

Hedley, A. K., Moreland, J., Bloebaum, R. D., Coster, I., Gruen, T., and Clarke, I. (1979). Press-fit, cemented, and bone ingrowth surface replacement-canine fixation model. *Trans. Orthop. Res. Soc.* 4, 163.

Heimke, G. E. (1990). *Osseo-Integrated Implants,* Vols. I and II (Boca Raton, FL: CRC Press).

Hench, L. L. and Paschall, H. A. (1973). Direct chemical bond of bioactive glass-ceramic materials to bone and muscle. *J. Biomed. Mater. Res. Symposium No. 4,* 25–43.

Henrich, D. E., Cram, A. E., Park, J. B., Liu, Y. K., and Reddi, H. (1993). Inorganic bone and bone morphogenetic protein impregnated bone cement: a preliminary *in vivo* study. *J. Biomed. Mater. Res.* 27, 277–280.

Hirshhorn, J. S., McBeath, A. A., and Dustoor, M. R. (1972). Porous titanium surgical implant materials. *J. Biomed. Mater. Res. Symp. No. 2,* 49–69.

Homsy, C. A., Cain, T. E., Kessler, F. B., Anderson, M. S., and King, J. W. (1972). Porous implant systems for prosthetic stabilization. *Clinic. Orthop. Rel. Res.* 89, 220–231.

Jacobs, J. J., Urban, R. M., Gilbert, J. L., Skipor, A. K., Jasty, M., Black, J., and Galante, J. O. (1995). Local and distant products from modularity. *Clin. Orthop. Rel. Res.* 319, 94–105.

Jasty, M., Maloney, W. J., Bragdon, C. R., O'Connor, D. O., Haire, T., and Harris, W. H. (1991). The initiation of failure in cemented femoral components of hip arthroplasties. *J. Bone Joint Surg.* 73B, 551–558.

Johnston, R. C. (1987). The case for cemented hips. In *The Hip*, R. A. Brand, Ed. (St. Louis: Mosby), 351–358.

Kang, Y. H. (1998). Pre-coating of ultra-high molecular weight polyethylene (UHMWPE) with poly-methylmethacrylate (PMMA). In: *Biomedical Engineering* (Iowa City: The University of Iowa), 1–160.

Kang, Y. H. and Park, J. B. (1998). Interfacial tensile strength of PMMA pre-coated UHMWPE and bone cement. *J. Biomed. Mat. Res. (Appl. Biomat.)* 43, 261–269.

Kay, J. F. (1988). Bioactive surface coatings: cause for encouragement and caution. *J. Oral Implant.* 16, 43–54.

Keet, G. G. M. and Runne, W. C. (1989). The anaform endoprosthesis: a proplast-coated femoral endoprosthesis. *Orthopaedics* 12, 1185–1190.

Khang, G., Kang, Y., Lee, H., and Park, J. (1996). Improved bonding strength of polyethylene/polyme-thylmethacrylate bone cement: A preliminary study. *Biomed. Mater. Eng.* 6, 335–344.

Kim, J. K. and Park, J. B. (1994). Reinforcement of bone cement around prostheses by precoated wire coil: A preliminary study. *Biomed. Mater. Eng.* 4, 369–380.

Kim, J. K. and Park, J. B. (1996a). Fatigue properties and stem subsidence of wire coil reinforced PMMA bone cement: An *in vitro* study. *Biomed. Mater. Eng.* 6, 453–462.

Kim, J. K. and Park, J. B. (1996b). Reinforcement of bone cement around the femoral prosthesis tip by pre-coated wire coil: a human cadaver bone study. *Biomed. Mater. Eng.* 6, 159–164.

Kim, Y. S., Kang, Y. H., Kim, J. K., and Park, J. B. (1994). Effect of bone mineral particles on the porosity of bone cement. *Biomed. Mater. Eng.* 4, 1–10.

Klawitter, J. J., and Hulbert, S. F. (1972). Application of porous ceramics for the attachment of load bearing internal orthopedic applications. *J. Biomed. Mater. Res. Symp. No. 2*, 161–229.

Kwon, S. Y., Kim, Y. S., Woo, Y. K., Kim, S. S., and Park, J. B. (1997). Hydroxyapatite impregnated bone cement: *In vitro* and *in vivo* studies. *Biomed. Mar. Eng.* 7, 129–140.

Li, S., Chang, J. D., Barrena, E. G., Furman, B. D., Wright, T. M., and Salvati, E. (1995). Nonconsolidated polyethylene particles and oxidation in Charnley acetabular cups. *Clin. Orthop. Rel. Res.* 319, 54–63.

Linder, L. (1995). Boneloc®—the Christiansen experience revisited, editorial. *Acta Orthop. Scand.* 66, 205–206.

Ling, R. S. M. (1992). The use of a collar and precoating on cemented femoral stems is unnecessary and detrimental. *Clin. Orthop. Rel. Res.* 285, 73–83.

Liu, Y. K., Njus, G. O., Park, J. B., and Stienstra, D. (1987). Bone particle impregnated bone cement. I. *In vitro* study. *J. Biomed. Mater. Res.* 21, 247–261.

Lombardi, A. V., Mallory, T. H., Eberle, R. W., Mitchell, M. B., Lefkowitt, M. S., and Williams, J. R. (1995). Failure of intraoperatively customized non-porous femoral components inserted without cement in total hip arthroplasty. *J. Bone Joint Surg.* 77A, 1836–1844.

Lu, Z., Ebramzadeh, E., and Sarmiento, A. (1993). The effect of failure of the cement interfaces on gross loosening of cemented total hip femoral components. *Trans. Orthop. Res. Soc.* 18, 519.

Malchau, H. and Herberts, P. (1998). Prognosis of total hip replacement: revision and re-revision rate in IHR: a revision-risk study of 148,359 primary operations. In *65th Annual Amer. Acad. Orthop. Surg.* (New Orleans, LA).

Maloney, W. J. and Smith, R. L. (1995). Periprosthetic osteolysis in total hip arthroplasty: the role of particulate wear debris. *J. Bone Joint Surg.* 77A, 1448–1460.

Maloney, W. J., Jasty, M., Rosenberg, A., and Harris, W. H. (1990). Bone lysis in well-fixed cemented femoral components. *J. Bone Joint Surg.* 72B, 966–970.

Manley, M. T. and Stern, L. S. (1985). The load carrying and fatigue properties of the stem-cement interface with smooth and porous coated femoral components. *J. Biomed. Mater. Res.* 19, 563–575.

Manley, M. T., Stern, L. S., Kotzar, G., and Stulberg, B. N. (1987). Femoral component loosening in hip arthroplasty. *Acta Orthop. Scand.* 58, 485–490.

Mann, K. A., Bartel, D. L., Wright, T. M., and Ingraffea, A. R. (1991). Mechanical characteristics of stem–cement interface. *J. Orthop. Res.*, 798–808.

Marrs, H., Barton, D. C., Ward, I. M., Doyle, C., Fisher, J., and Jones, R. A. (1998). Comparative wear under three different tribological conditions of acetylene crosslinked ultra high molecular weight polyethylene, *Orthop. Res. Soc.*, 100.

McKellop, H. A., Shen, F. W., and Salovey, R. (1998). Extremely low wear of gamma crosslinked/remelted UHMW polyethylene acetabular cups. *Orthop. Res. Soc.* 98.

Mittlemeier, H. (1975). New development of wear-resistant ceramic and metal composite prostheses with ribbed support shafts for cement-free implantation. *Hefte zur Unfallheilkunde: Beiheft zu Monatsschrift für Unfallheilkunde. Versicherungs, Versorgungs und Verkehrsmedizin* 126, 333–336.

Mittlemeier, H. (1976). Anchoring hip endoprosthesis without bone cement. In: *Advances in Artificial Hip and Knee Joint Technology*, M. Schaldach and D. Hohmann, Eds. (Berlin: Springer-Verlag), 387–402.

Mohler, C. G., Callaghan, J. J., Collis, D. K., and Johnston, R. C. (1995). Early loosening of the femoral component at cement-prosthesis interface after total hip replacement. *J. Bone Joint Surg.* 77A, 1315–1322.

Moore, A. T. (1952). Metal hip joint: a new self-locking Vitallium prosthesis. *South. Med. J.* 45, 10–15.

Morscher, E. (1984). *The Cementless Fixation of Hip Endoprosthesis* (Heidelberg: Springer-Verlag).

Morscher, E. W. (1995). The clinical significance of implant stiffness. *Orthopedics* 18, 795–800.

Muller, M. E. (1995). The benefits of metal-on-metal total hip replacements. *Clin. Orthop. Rel. Res.* 311, 54–59.

Mulroy, R. D. and Harris, W. H. (1990). The effect of improved cementing techniques on component loosening in total hip replacement: an eleven year radiographic review. *J. Bone Joint Surg.* 72B, 757–760.

Niles, J. L. and Lapitsky, M. (1975). Biomechanical investigations of bone-porous carbon and metal interfaces. *Biomed. Mater. Res. Symp.* 4, 63–84.

Nilsen, A. R. and Wiig, M. (1996). Total hip arthroplasty with Boneloc®: loosening in 102/157 cases after 0.5–3 years. *Acta Orthop. Scand.* 67, 57–59.

O'Connor, D. O., Burke, D. W., Sedlacek, R. C., and Harris, W. H. (1991). Peak cement strains in cemented femoral total hip. *Trans. Orthop. Res. Soc.* 16, 220.

Onsten, I., Sanzen, L., Carlsson, A., and Besjakov, J. (1995). Migration of uncemented, long-term femoral components in revision hip arthroplasty: a 2–8 year clinical follow-up of 45 cases and radiostereometric analysis of 13 cases. *Acta Orthop. Scand.* 66, 220–224.

Oonishi, H., Yamamoto, M., Ishimaru, H., Tsuji, E., Kushitani, S., Aono, M., and Ukon, Y. (1989). Comparisons of bone ingrowth into porous Ti-6Al-4V beads uncoated and coated with hydroxyapatite. In: *Bioceramics*, H. Ooonoishi, H. Aoki, and K. Sawai, Eds. (Tokyo: Ishiyaku EuroAmerica, Inc.), 400–405.

Oonishi, H., Saito, M., and Kadoya, Y. (1998). Wear of high-dose gamma irradiated polyethylene in total joint replacement. Long-term radiological evaluation. *Orthop. Res. Soc.*, 97.

Park, J. B. (1983a). Acrylic bone cement: *in vitro* and *in vivo* property–structure relationship—a selective review. *Annals Biomed. Eng.* 11, 297–312.

Park, J. B. (1983b). Implant fixation by pulsed electromagnetic field stimulation. Unpublished study (Iowa City, IA: The University of Iowa).

Park, J. B. (1988). *In vivo* evaluation of hydroxyapatite coated implant. Unpublished study (Iowa City: The University of Iowa).

Park, J. B. (1992). Orthopedic prosthesis fixation. *Annals Biomed. Eng.* 20, 583–594.

Park, J. B. (1993). Reinforcement of bone cement around prosthesis by pre-coated wire coil/wire mesh. In Patent Disclosure.

Park, J. B. (1995). Orthopedic prosthesis fixation. In: *Biomedical Engineering Handbook,* J. D. Bronzino, Ed. (Boca Raton, FL: CRC Press), 704–723.

Park, J. B. (1998). Sintering of pure and cross-linked UHMWPE, MMA, and PMMA treated powders to create graded total joint implants for better fixation and wear. In Patent Disclosure (USA).

Park, J. B. and Kenner, G. H. (1975). Effect of electrical stimulation on the tensile strength of the porous implant and bone interface. *Biomater. Med. Dev. Artif. Org.* 3, 233–243.

Park, J. B. and Lakes, R. S. (1992). *Biomaterials: An Introduction,* 2nd ed. (New York: Plenum Press).

Park, J. B., Malstrom, C. S., and von Recum, A. F. (1978). Intramedullary fixation of implants pre-coated with bone cement: a preliminary study. *Biomater. Med. Dev. Artif. Org.* 6, 361–373.

Park, J. B., von Recum, A. F., and Gratzick, G. E. (1979). Pre-coated orthopedic implants with bone cement. *Med. Dev. Artif. Org.* 7, 41–53.

Park, J. B., Barb, W., Kenner, G. H., and von Recum, A. F. (1982). Intramedullary fixation of artificial hip joints with bone cement precoated implants. II. Density and histological study. *J. Biomed. Mater. Res.* 16, 459–469.

Park, J. B., Choi, W. W., Liu, Y. K., and Haugen, T. W. (1986). Bone particle impregnated polymethylmethacrylate: *in vitro* and *in vivo* study. In: *Tissue Integration in Oral and Facial Reconstruction,* D. Van Steenberghe, Ed. (Amsterdam: Excerpta Medica), 118–124.

Park, K. D. and Park, J. B. (1998). Pre-coating UHMWPE powers with PMMA and sintering (Iowa City: The University of Iowa).

Park, S.-H., Llinas, A., and Goel, V. K. (1995). Hard tissue replacement. In: *Biomedical Engineering Handbook,* J. D. Bronzino, Ed. (Boca Raton, FL: CRC Press), 672–691.

Parsons, J. R., Ricci, J. L., Liebrecht, P., Salsbury, R. L., Patras, A. S., and Alexander, H. (1987). Enhanced stabilization of orthopedic implants with spherical hydroxylapatite particulate (Dublin, CA: Ortho-Matrix, Inc.).

Paul, J. P. (1976). Loading on normal hip and knee joints and joint replacements. In: *Advances in Hip and Knee Joint Technology,* M. Schaldach and D. Hohmann, Eds. (Berlin: Springer-Verlag), 53–70.

Predecki, P., Stephan, J. E., Auslander, B. E., Mooney, V. L., and Kirkland, K. (1972). Kinetics of bone growth into cylindrical channels in aluminum oxide and titanium. *J. Biomed. Mater. Res.* 6, 375–400.

Raab, S., Ahmed, A. M., and Provan, J. W. (1982). Thin film PMMA precoating for improved implant bone-cement fixation. *J. Biomed. Mater. Res.* 16, 679–704.

Riegels-Nielsen, P., Sorensen, L., Andersen, H. M., and Lindequist, S. (1995). Boneloc® cemented total hip prostheses: loosening in 28/43 cases after 3–38 months. *Acta Orthop. Scand.* 66, 215–217.

Ritter, M. A. (1995). All polyethylene versus metal backing. *Clin. Orthop. Rel. Res.* 311, 69–75.

Ritter, M. A., Keating, E. M., Faris, P. M., and Brugo, G. (1990). Metal-backed acetabular cups in total hip arthroplasty. *J. Bone Joint Surg.* 72A, 672–677.

Sadr, B. and Arden, G. P. (1987). A comparison of the stability of proplast-coated and cemented Thompson prosthesis in the treatment of subcapital femoral fractures. *Injury* 8, 234–237.

Saha, S. and Pal, S. (1984). Mechanical properties of bone cement: a review. *J. Biomed. Mater. Res.* 18, 435–462.

Saikko, V. (1995). Wear of the polyethylene acetabular cup: the effect of head material, head diameter, and cup thickness studied with a hip simulator. *Acta Orthop. Scand.* 66, 501–506.

Salvati, E. A., Lieberman, J. R., Huk, O. L., and Evans, B. G. (1995). Complications of femoral and acetabular modularity. *Clin. Orthop. Rel. Res.* 319, 85–93.

Sauer, B. W., Weinstein, A. M., Klawitter, J. J., Hulbert, S. F., Leonard, R. B., and Bagwell, J. G. (1974). The role of porous polymeric materials in prosthesis attachment. *J. Biomed. Mater. Res. Symp.* 5, 145–156.

Schmalzried, T. P., Kwong, L. M., Sedlacek, R. C., Jasty, M., Haire, T. C., O'Connor, D. O., Bragdon, C. R., Kabo, J. M., Malcolm, A. J., and Harris, W. H. (1992). The mechanism of loosening of cemented acetabular components in total hip arthroplasty: analyis of specimens retrieved at autopsy. *Clin. Orthop. Rel. Res.* 274, 60–78.

Smith, L. (1963). Ceramic-plastic material as a bone substitute. *Arch. Surg.* 87, 653–661.

Spector, M. (1982a). Bone ingrowth into porous metals. In: *Biocompatibility of Orthopedic Implants*, D. F. Williams, Ed. (Boca Raton, FL: CRC Press), 55–88.

Spector, M. (1982b). Bone ingrowth into porous polymers. In: *Biocompatibility of Orthopedic Implants*, D. F. Williams, Ed. (Boca Raton, FL: CRC Press), 89–128.

Stromberg, C. N., Herberts, P., Palmertz, B., and Garellick, G. (1996). Radiographic risk signs for loosening after cemented THA: 61 loose stems and 23 loose sockets compared with 42 controls. *Acta Orthop. Scand.* 67, 43–48.

Sutula, L. C., Collier, J. P., Saum, K. A., Currier, B. H., Currier, J. H., Sanford, W. M., Mayor, M. B., Wooding, R. E., Spering, D. K., Williams, I. R., Kasprzak, D. J., and Sorprenant, V. A. (1995). Impact of gamma sterilization on clinical performance of polyethylene in the hip. *Clin. Orthop. Rel. Res.* 319, 28–40.

Taitsman, J. P. and Saha, S. (1977). Tensile strength of wire-reinforced bone cement and twisted stainless-steel wire. *J. Bone Joint Surg.* 59A, 419–425.

Taylor, D. (1987). Fatigue failure in bone cements for hip joint implants. *Fatigue* 87, 1353.

Taylor, D., Clarke, F., McCormack, B., and Sheehan, J. (1989). Reinforcement of bone cement using metal meshes. *Eng. Med.* 203, 49–53.

Thanner, J., Freij-Larsson, C., Karrholm, J., Malchau, H., and Wesslen, B. (1995). Evaluation of Boneloc®: chemical and mechanical properties, and a randomized clinical study of 30 total hip arthroplasties. *Acta Orthop. Scand.* 66, 207–214.

Thomas, K. A., Cook, S. D., Renz, E. A., Anderson, R. C., Haddad, R. J. J., Haubold, A. D., and Yapp, R. (1985). The effect of surface treatments on the interface mechanics of LTI pyrolytic carbon implants. *J. Biomed. Mater. Res.* 19, 145–160.

Topoleski, L. D. T., Ducheyne, P., and Cuckler, J. M. (1990). The fracture toughness of short-titanium-fiber reinforced bone cement. *Trans. Soc. Biomat.* 13, 107.

Tullos, H. S., McCaskill, B. L., Dickey, R., and Davidson, J. (1984). Total hip arthroplasty with a low-modulus porous-coated femoral component. *J. Bone Joint Surg.* 66A, 888–898.

Verdonschot, N., and Huiskes, E. T. (1998). Effects of prosthesis surface roughness on the failure process of cemented hip implants after stem-cement debonding *J. Biom. Mater. Res.* 42, 554–559.

Weinstein, A. M., Klawitter, J. J., Cleveland, T. W., and Amos ... ulation of bone growth into porous Al₂O₃. *J. Biomed. Mater. Res.* ...

West, J. K., Clark, A. E., Hall, M. B., and Turner, G. F. (1990). ... Bioglass®-coated titanium alloy. In: *CRC Handbook of Bioactive C* ... *and Glass-Ceramics*, T. Yamamuro, L. L. Hench, and J. Wilson, Ed... 161–166.

Willert, H. G., Koch, R., and Burgi, M. (1991). Reinforcemer... Patent No. 5,035,714.

Williams, D. F. and Roaf, R. (1973). *Implants in Surgery* (Lon...

Wroblewski, B. M. (1986). 15–21 year results of the charnley l... *rthop. Rel. Res.* 211, 30–35.

Wroblewski, B. M. (1993). Cementless versus cemented total hip arthroplasty: a scientific controversy? *Orthop. Clin. North Am.* 24, 591–597.

Wykman, A. G. M., Olsson, A. E., Axdorph, G., and Goldie, I. (1991). Total hip arthroplasty. A comparison between cemented and press-fit noncemented fixation. *J. Arthoplasty* 6, 19–29.

Yamamuro, T., Hench, L. L., and Wilson, J. E. (1990). *CRC Handbook of Bioactive Ceramics*, Vol I: *Bioactive Glasses* and *Glass-Ceramics*; Vol. II: *Calcium Phosphate and Hydroxylapatite Ceramics* (Boca Raton, FL: CRC Press).

Index